ESSENTIALS OF THE
U.S. Health Care System

FIFTH EDITION

LEIYU SHI, DrPH, MBA, MPA
Professor, Bloomberg School of Public Health
Director, Johns Hopkins Primary Care Policy Center
Johns Hopkins University
Baltimore, Maryland

DOUGLAS A. SINGH, PhD, MBA
Associate Professor Emeritus of Management
Judd Leighton School of Business and Economics
Indiana University, South Bend
South Bend, Indiana

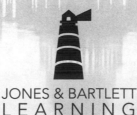

JONES & BARTLETT
LEARNING

World Headquarters
Jones & Bartlett Learning
5 Wall Street
Burlington, MA 01803
978-443-5000
info@jblearning.com
www.jblearning.com

Jones & Bartlett Learning books and products are available through most bookstores and online booksellers. To contact Jones & Bartlett Learning directly, call 800-832-0034, fax 978-443-8000, or visit our website, www.jblearning.com.

29444-6

Production Credits

VP, Product Management: David D. Cella
Director of Product Management: Michael Brown
Product Specialist: Danielle Bessette
Reprints and Special Projects Manager: Tina Chen
Production Editor: Brooke Haley
Associate Production Editor, Navigate: Jamie Reynolds
Senior Marketing Manager: Sophie Fleck Teague
Manufacturing and Inventory Control Supervisor:
  Amy Bacus

Composition: codeMantra U.S. LLC
Cover Design: Kristin E. Parker
Rights & Media Specialist: Merideth Tumasz
Media Development Editor: Shannon Sheehan
Cover Image (Title Page, Chapter Opener):
  © ninjaMonkeyStudio/Getty Images
Printing and Binding: LSC Communications
Cover Printing: LSC Communications

Library of Congress Cataloging-in-Publication Data
Names: Shi, Leiyu, author. | Singh, Douglas A., 1946- author. | Abridgement
  of (work): Shi, Leiyu. Delivering health care in America. Seventh edition.
Title: Essentials of the U.S. health care system / Leiyu Shi, Douglas A. Singh.
Description: Fifth edition. | Burlington, Massachusetts: Jones & Bartlett Learning, [2019] |
  Abridgement of: Delivering health care in America: a systems approach / Leiyu Shi,
  Douglas A. Singh. Seventh edition. 2019.
Identifiers: LCCN 2018014666 | ISBN 9781284156720 (pbk.)
Subjects: | MESH: Delivery of Health Care | Health Policy | United States
Classification: LCC RA395.A3 | NLM W 84 AA1 | DDC 362.10973—dc23
LC record available at https://lccn.loc.gov/2018014666

6048

Printed in the United States of America
22 21 20 19   10 9 8 7 6 5 4 3

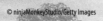

Contents

Chapter 9   Managed Care and Integrated Systems. 205

Chapter 10   Long-Term Care Services 229

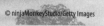

Preface

This text is a condensed and simplified version of our standard text on the U.S. health care system, *Delivering Health Care in America: A Systems Approach, Seventh Edition*. Nevertheless, each new edition of this text is independently revised, with new materials that may not be found in the larger text.

This text retains the systems model to organize the major themes of U.S. health care delivery. The first three chapters lay the foundation that is necessary for understanding the U.S. health care delivery system, which is distinct from any other system in the world. *Major Characteristics of U.S. Health Care Delivery* (Chapter 1) gives an overview of U.S. health care and contrasts the American system with the three most commonly used models of health care delivery in other advanced nations, such as Canada, the United Kingdom, and Germany. *Foundations of U.S. Health Care Delivery* (Chapter 2) explains the different models for understanding health and its determinants. In the context of American beliefs and values, this chapter also discusses the issue of equity using the concepts of market justice and social justice and explains how health services are rationed in both market justice– and social justice–based systems. *Historical Overview of U.S. Health Care Delivery* (Chapter 3) traces the history of U.S. health care from colonial times to the present and includes an added section on health care reform. The key to understanding the nature of the current health care system and its likely future direction is to understand its evolutionary past. This chapter also describes current trends in corporatization, information revolution, and globalization as they pertain to health care delivery.

The next three chapters are about the resources—both human and nonhuman—employed in delivering health care. *Health Care Providers and Professionals* (Chapter 4) addresses the roles played by some of the major types of personnel in health care delivery. It also discusses some key issues pertaining to the number and distribution of physicians and the effect these factors have on the delivery of health care. *Technology and Its Effects* (Chapter 5) focuses on medical technology and the various issues related to its development and dissemination. *Financing and Reimbursement Methods* (Chapter 6) explains the concept of health insurance, the major private and public health insurance programs in the United States, and methods of reimbursing providers.

The next five chapters describe the system processes, beginning with outpatient and primary care services (discussed in Chapter 7) and hospitals (discussed in Chapter 8). *Managed Care and Integrated Systems* (Chapter 9) examines managed care and integrated organizations, such as integrated delivery systems and accountable care organizations, as well as the different types of arrangements found in integrated organizations. *Long-Term Care Services* (Chapter 10) explores the meaning and scope of long-term care and provides an overview of community-based and institution-based long-term care services. *Populations with Special Health Needs* (Chapter 11) highlights vulnerable populations and their special health care needs, including populations with mental health issues.

The next two chapters deal with the main outcomes of the health care system and the ways in which those outcomes are addressed through health policy. The main outcomes associated with health care are presented in the *Cost, Access, and Quality* chapter (Chapter 12). *Health Policy* (Chapter 13) gives an overview of health policy, including the major participants in its development and the process by which it is created, in the United States.

Finally, *The Future of Health Services Delivery* (Chapter 14) explores the future of health care in the United States in the context of forces of future change, health care reform, conflicting issues of cost and access, future models of care delivery, global challenges, and technological innovations.

Leiyu Shi
Douglas A. Singh

▶ New in the *Fifth Edition*

This edition has been updated with the latest health statistics and pertinent information available at the time the manuscript was prepared. Some key additions to the text include the following:

- Chapter 1: Current status of managed care and integrated delivery system under the Affordable Care Act; current status of health care reform; health care systems in selected countries.
- Chapter 2: Implementation of *Healthy People 2020*; assessment of the *Healthy People* initiative; preparation for *Healthy People 2030*; the concept of value-based practice.

- Chapter 3: Coverage of mental health care in its historical context, including a new section "Reform of Mental Health Care." New section: "Health Care Reform in a Flux."
- Chapter 4: Current development of the U.S. physician and health care workforce and challenges; the transition from patient-centered care to population health; the need for chronic disease managers.
- Chapter 5: Introduction to the Drug Supply Chain Security Act of 2013 and the 21st Century Cures Act of 2016. New section: "The FDA in a Global Environment."
- Chapter 6: New sections: "Issues with Medicaid"; "Payment Reform Initiatives."
- Chapter 7: Community health centers' current scope, efficacy and value, and challenges; status of the primary care workforce around the world.
- Chapter 8: Updated section on hospital employment and staffing.
- Chapter 9: Updated sections on integrated delivery systems and accountable care organizations.
- Chapter 10: Updated section on the nursing home industry and expenditures on long-term care.
- Chapter 11: Current disparities described in the literature (racial, socioeconomic status) in terms of access to care, quality of care, and health outcomes; programs (national, regional, local) that address disparities (racial, socioeconomic status) in terms of access to care, quality of care, and health outcomes; the chronically ill; patient safety.
- Chapter 12: Quality initiatives both from the government (e.g., the Agency for Healthcare Research and Quality) and from the private sector; programs to contain health care costs.
- Chapter 13: Updated information on health policy issues and challenges after the ACA.
- Chapter 14: Updated sections on the health care coverage, cost, and access dilemmas; the future of health care reform; movement toward a single-payer system; the cost-control imperative; Medicare's generational impact; and future models of care delivery.

© ninjaMonkeyStudio/Getty Images

Acknowledgments

We gratefully acknowledge Sylvia Shi for creating the cartoons for this text. We are also grateful for the valuable assistance of Hailun Liang. Of course, all errors and omissions remain the responsibility of the authors.

© ninjaMonkeyStudio/Getty Images

List of Exhibits

© ninjaMonkeyStudio/Getty Images

List of Tables

List of Figures

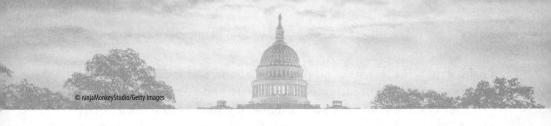

CHAPTER 1
Major Characteristics of U.S. Health Care Delivery

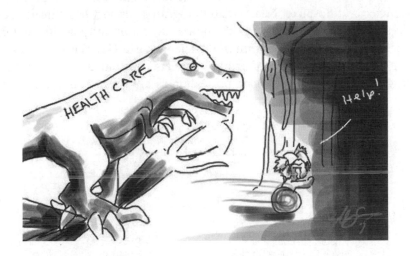

▶ Introduction

The United States has a unique health care delivery system. Nearly all developed countries offer universal health insurance programs, and the government plays a central role in them. Almost all citizens are entitled to routine, basic, and other health care services. In the United States, the Affordable Care Act[1] (ACA) has expanded health insurance but not achieved universal coverage. Furthermore, access to affordable

---

1 The Affordable Care Act, also known as Obamacare, refers to the Patient Protection and Affordable Care Act of 2010 as amended by the Health Care and Education Reconciliation Act of 2010.

health care is inadequate at both individual and national levels—a challenge for academics, health care professionals, and politicians alike.

This chapter provides a general understanding of health care delivery in the United States. The U.S. health care delivery system is complex and massive, with many loosely coordinated components (**FIGURE 1.1**).

Organizations and individuals involved in health care delivery include educational and research institutions, medical suppliers, insurers, payers, and claims processors as well as health care providers. Nearly 12.3 million people work in health care delivery settings, including doctors of medicine (MDs), doctors of osteopathy (DOs), nurses, dentists, pharmacists, and administrators, and about 451,500 physical, occupational, and speech therapists in rehabilitation services. The institutions where health care is delivered include 5,627 hospitals, 15,656 nursing homes, nearly 2,806 inpatient mental health facilities, and 12,400 home health agencies and hospices. Nearly 1,200 programs support basic health services for migrant workers and the homeless, community health centers, black lung clinics, human immunodeficiency virus (HIV) early intervention services, and integrated primary care and substance abuse treatment programs. Various health care professionals are trained in 172 medical

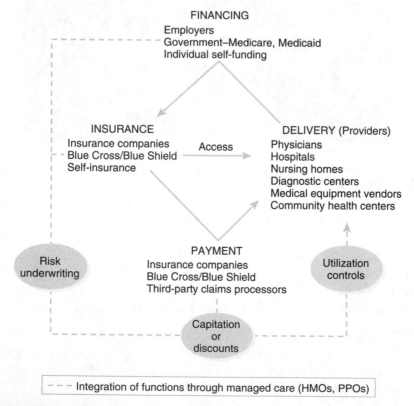

FIGURE 1.1 Managed Care: Integration of Functions

and osteopathic schools, 66 dental schools, 133 schools of pharmacy, and over 1,869 nursing programs throughout the U.S. (Bureau of Labor Statistics, 2016; Bureau of Primary Health Care, 2011; National Center for Health Statistics, 2017).

176.6 million Americans younger than age 65 have private health insurance coverage, with most covered through their employers. Another 110.7 million are covered by two major public health insurance programs, Medicare and Medicaid. Medicare is managed by the U.S. federal government whereas Medicaid is jointly managed by the federal and state governments. Private health insurance can be purchased from roughly 1,000 health insurance companies. The private managed care sector includes approximately 470 licensed health maintenance organizations (HMOs) and 934 preferred provider organizations (PPOs). Multiple government agencies are involved in health care financing, medical and health services research, and regulatory oversight of the health care delivery system (Aventis Pharmaceuticals, 2002; Bureau of Primary Health Care, 2011; Kaiser Family Foundation, 2011, 2016a; National Center for Health Statistics, 2007, 2017; U.S. Bureau of the Census, 1998, 2007).

▶ Subsystems of U.S. Health Care Delivery

In the U.S., multiple subsystems of health care delivery serve to address the health needs of certain populations, through market forces or government action.

Managed Care

As shown in Figure 1.1, *managed care* is the dominant health care delivery system in the United States. Managed care covers most Americans in private and public health insurance programs through contracts with a managed care organization (MCO), such as an HMO or a PPO. The MCO, in turn, contracts with selected health care providers—physicians, hospitals, and others—to deliver health care services to its enrollees. An *enrollee* (member) is an individual covered under a managed care plan. The contract between the MCO and the enrollee—with descriptions of health services for enrollees—is referred to as the *health plan* or simply the *plan*.

Managed care strives for efficiency by integrating basic functions of health care delivery and seeks to control (manage) the utilization and cost of medical services. The MCO pays providers either through a capitation (per head) arrangement, in which providers receive a fixed payment for each enrollee under their care, or through a discounted fee arrangement. Providers are willing to discount services for MCO patients to be included in the MCO network and be guaranteed a patient population. Health plans depend on the expected cost of health care utilization, which often can cost more than the insurance premiums collected. By underwriting this risk, the plan assumes the role of insurer.

Figure 1.1 illustrates the functions and mechanisms necessary for health care delivery in a managed care environment. The four key functions of financing, insurance, delivery, and payment constitute the quad-function model and are integrated in managed care to varying degrees.

Military Medical Care

The military medical care system is available, mostly free of charge, to active-duty military personnel of the U.S. Army, Navy, Air Force, and Coast Guard, as well as members of certain uniformed nonmilitary services such as the Public Health Service and the National Oceanographic and Atmospheric Association. This organized system offers comprehensive services, both preventive and treatment-oriented. Services are largely provided by salaried health care personnel. Various basic services are provided at dispensaries, sick bays aboard ships, first aid stations, medical stations, and base hospitals, and advanced medical care is provided in regional military hospitals.

Families and dependents of active-duty or retired career military personnel are treated at these hospitals or dispensaries or covered by *Tri-Care*, a program financed by the Department of Defense. This permits beneficiaries to receive care from both private and military medical care facilities.

The Veterans Administration (VA) health care system is provided to retired veterans who have served in the military, with priority given to those who are disabled. The VA system focuses on hospital care, mental health services, and long-term care and is one of the largest and oldest (dating back to 1930s) formally organized health care systems in the world. Its mission is to provide medical care, education and training, research, contingency support, and emergency management for the Department of Defense medical care system. It provides health care to more than 9.6 million individuals at over 1,100 sites, including 153 hospitals, 807 ambulatory and community-based clinics, 135 nursing homes, 209 counseling centers, 47 domiciliaries (residential care facilities), 73 home health care programs, and various contract care programs. The VA budget included $68.6 billion for veterans' medical care in 2017—an increase of 6% from 2016—and VA staff numbered over 360,000 in 2017 (Department of Veterans Affairs, 2017; National Center for Veterans Analysis and Statistics, 2007).

The VA system is organized into 21 *Veterans Integrated Service Networks (VISNs)*. Each VISN is responsible for coordinating the activities of hospitals and other facilities in its jurisdiction. Each VISN is allocated federal funds and is responsible for its equitable distribution among its hospitals and other providers as well as for improved efficiency and cost containment.

Subsystems for Special Populations

Special populations, or vulnerable populations, are persons with health needs but inadequate resources to address them, including individuals who are poor and uninsured, belong to a certain minority group or are of a certain immigration status, or live in geographically or economically disadvantaged communities. This population typically receives care through the nation's safety net, including public health insurance programs such as Medicare and Medicaid, and safety net providers such as community health centers, migrant health centers, free clinics, hospital emergency departments, and public hospitals. Many safety net providers offer comprehensive medical and enabling services according to individual needs—such as language assistance, transportation, nutrition and health education, social support services, and child care.

For example, federally qualified health centers have provided primary and preventive health services to rural and urban underserved populations for over 50 years. The Bureau of Primary Health Care (BPHC), under the Health Resources and Services Administration in the Department of Health and Human Services (DHHS), provides federal support for community health centers, including programs for migrant and seasonal farm workers and their families, homeless persons, public housing residents, and school-age children. These facilitate access to care for patients who are predominantly minority, low-income, uninsured, or enrolled in Medicaid, the public insurance program for the poor. In 2016, 1,367 community health organizations nationwide served 26 million people across 10,400 service sites and handled 104.1 million patient visits. Roughly 92% of this population had incomes under 200% of the federal poverty level, and 23% were uninsured (Bureau of Primary Health Care, 2017). Health centers have contributed to great improvements in health outcomes for the uninsured and for Medicaid populations and reduced disparities in health care and health status across socioeconomic and racial and ethnic groups (Politzer et al., 2003; Shi et al., 2001).

Medicare is one of the largest sources of public health insurance in the U.S., serving the elderly, the disabled, and those with end-stage renal disease. Managed by the Centers for Medicare and Medicaid Services (CMS) within the DHHS, Medicare offers coverage for hospital care, postdischarge nursing care, hospice care, outpatient services, and prescription drugs.

Medicaid is the third largest source of health insurance in the U.S., insuring approximately 19% of the U.S. population and providing coverage for low-income adults, children, the elderly, and the disabled (Kaiser

Family Foundation, 2016a). Medicaid is also the largest provider of long-term care to the elderly and the disabled, and has significantly expanded under the ACA.

In 1997, the government created the Children's Health Insurance Program (CHIP) to provide insurance to children in uninsured families. This program expanded coverage to children in families that have modest incomes but do not qualify for Medicaid. In 2016, the CHIP program spent $15.6 billion to cover approximately 5.9 million children (Kaiser Family Foundation, 2016b).

Although the U.S. offers government-funded health insurance, the safety net is by no means secure. The availability of safety net services varies by community. Vulnerable populations in communities without safety net providers often must forgo care or seek services from emergency departments where available. Safety net providers, in turn, face pressure from the increase in the number of poor and Medicaid-insured individuals in their communities.

Integrated Systems

Integrated delivery systems (IDSs), or health networks, were established through organizational integration beginning in the early 2000s. An IDS is a network of health care providers and organizations that provides coordinated health care to a population and is responsible for the health outcomes and health status of the population (Shortell et al., 1996). By owning or partnering with hospitals, physicians, and insurers, IDSs aim to deliver a range of services. The ACA encourages physicians and hospitals to integrate and coordinate services, which is expected to make health care more cost-effective and of higher quality.

An accountable care organization (ACO), a new model of integrated organization, is expected to respond to new payment incentives and be held accountable for better quality outcomes at lower cost under the new Medicare Shared Savings Program. Approximately 6 million Medicare beneficiaries receive care in an ACO, and since 2011 at least 744 organizations including those in the private sector have become ACOs. An estimated 23.5 million Americans are now served by an ACO. Medicare and commercial ACO initiatives demonstrate that ACOs can improve the quality of care, the patient experience, and even constrain costs (Yasaitis et al., 2016).

States are also turning to integrated Medicaid models to manage costs and encourage innovation in health care delivery. Medicaid ACOs are integrating primary care and behavioral health services, and some ACOs are exploring innovative financing models, such as cross-sectoral shared-savings models. So far, 42 states have implemented Medicaid managed care programs with risk-based reimbursements, and at least 10 states plan to expand managed care programs (Kaiser Family Foundation, 2015).

Due to the ACA and a focus on the triple aim of improved health, improved health care, and lower costs, health care is experiencing a paradigm shift to integrated, patient-centered care. The growing burden of chronic disease and the increasing number of people with complex health care needs require delivery systems that bring together various professionals and skills from the cure (health care) and care (long-term and social care) sectors.

The integration of primary care and behavioral health exemplifies this innovative team approach. Collaboration is challenging due to cultural and clinical differences between primary and behavioral health providers, but a team approach to care has proved to be a powerful means to develop this integrated model. Various health care professionals—including psychiatrists, physicians, nurse practitioners, social workers, psychologists, addiction counselors, care managers, community health workers, peers, medical assistants, nurse aides, and representatives from community agencies—comprise the integrated care team (SAMHSA-HRSA Center for Integrated Health Solutions, 2014).

Long-Term Care Delivery

Long-term care (LTC) consists of medical and nonmedical care for individuals with chronic health issues and disabilities that prevent them from performing regular daily tasks and includes both health care and support services for daily living. LTC is delivered in various settings, including patients' homes, assisted living facilities, and nursing homes. Most LTC services are provided by family members and friends without pay, and not covered by Medicare, so costs for LTC can impose a burden on families. Medicaid covers several levels of LTC services, but a person must be indigent to qualify. LTC insurance plans are also offered separately by insurance companies, but most people do not purchase them because premiums can be unaffordable. By 2020, it is estimated that over 12 million Americans will require LTC, which will impose a strain on the nation's financial resources (CMS, 2011).

Public Health System

The mission of the U.S. *public health system* is to improve and protect community health. The Institute of Medicine's[2] *Future of Public Health in the 21st Century* report outlined the need for a more robust public health infrastructure and a population-based health approach (Centers for Disease Control and Prevention [CDC], 2013). The National Public Health

---

2 The Institute of Medicine was renamed the National Academy of Medicine in 2015.

Performance Standards Program identifies 10 essential public health services that this system must deliver:

1. Monitor health status to identify and solve community health problems
2. Diagnose and investigate health problems and hazards
3. Inform, educate, and empower people about health problems and hazards
4. Mobilize the community to identify and solve health problems
5. Develop policies and plans to support individual and community health efforts
6. Enforce laws and regulations to protect health and safety
7. Provide people with access to necessary care
8. Ensure a competent, professional health workforce
9. Evaluate the effectiveness, accessibility, and quality of personal and population-based health services
10. Perform research to discover innovative solutions to health problems

Public health constituted 4.3% of total U.S. health care expenditures of $3.3 trillion in 2016 (CMS, 2017). Federal funding for preventing disease and improving community health varied widely by state in 2013, from $13.67 per capita in Indiana to $46.48 per capita in Alaska (Trust for America's Health & Robert Wood Johnson Foundation, 2014). To bolster public health efforts, the ACA created the Prevention and Public Health Fund to provide expanded, sustained national investments in prevention and public health, improve health outcomes, and enhance the quality of health care.

Expanded efforts are required in the fight against antibiotic resistance, obesity and heart disease, prescription drug overdose, and emerging health issues such as Chikungunya (an infectious disease) and the risks posed by e-cigarettes. Advanced information systems and data sharing have become more important in ensuring a strong public health system.

▶ Health Care Reform

A primary goal of health care reform efforts such as the ACA is to expand coverage and increase access to care. The ACA expanded Medicaid coverage in participating states to all nonelderly adults with incomes less than 138% of the federal poverty level (FPL), and subsidized insurance on the health care marketplace for small businesses and persons without employment-based insurance. As of November 2017, 33 states including the District of Columbia expanded their Medicaid programs in keeping with ACA provisions (Kaiser Family Foundation, 2017a). As of August 2016, 15 states operated their own exchanges. Other states used the federal exchange or operated an exchange with support from the federal government.

When the ACA's first open enrollment period began in 2013, 41 million Americans lacked insurance; by 2016, the number of uninsured Americans fell to 27 million (Commonwealth Foundation, 2017). The expansion of Medicaid increased coverage, improved access and families' financial security, and economically benefitted states and providers (Kaiser Family Foundation, 2017b). The Congressional Budget Office (CBO) reported that approximately 12 million people were covered by the exchanges in March 2016, 10 million of whom received subsidies to pay for insurance (CBO, 2017).

Another key provision of the ACA requires that private insurance plans cover recommended preventive services without any patient cost-sharing and, since this policy went into effect, an estimated 137 million people—55.6 million women, 53.5 million men, and 28.5 million children—have received no-cost coverage for preventive services (ASPE, 2015).

President Donald Trump and Republicans in Congress attempted to repeal and replace the ACA in 2017 but to date have been unable to pass a bill through the U.S. Senate. In 2017, the Senate voted to approve a "budget blueprint" to let Republicans repeal parts of the law. House Republicans announced their proposed replacement for the ACA, the American Health Care Act, but this failed amid a revolt among Republicans. The U.S. House of Representatives voted for the replacement by a narrow margin, sending the bill to the Senate for deliberation, but the repeal legislation failed to gain a simple majority in the Senate. Some Congress members suggested smaller bipartisan modifications to stabilize the ACA individual insurance marketplaces.

▶ Characteristics of the U.S. Health Care System

A nation's health care system is influenced by a host of factors, including politics, economics, technology, society and culture, physical environment, and demographic and other population characteristics. Together, these external forces have shaped the course of health care delivery in the U.S. This section summarizes the characteristics that distinguish the U.S. health care delivery system from those of other countries, with 10 primary differences listed below (**EXHIBIT 1.1**).

EXHIBIT 1.1 Main Characteristics of the U.S. Health Care System

- No central governing agency and little integration and coordination
- Technology-driven delivery system focusing on acute care
- High cost, unequal access, and average outcome
- Delivery of health care under imperfect market conditions
- Government as subsidiary to the private sector
- Fusion of market justice and social justice
- Multiple players and balance of power
- Quest for integration and accountability
- Access to health care services selectively based on insurance coverage
- Legal risks influencing practice behaviors

No Central Governing Agency; Little Integration and Coordination

The U.S. health care system stands in stark contrast to the health care systems of other developed nations, which have centrally controlled universal health care systems that authorize health care financing, payment, and delivery to all residents. The health care system in the U.S. is not centrally controlled; rather, it is financed publicly and privately and thus features various payment, insurance, and delivery mechanisms. Private financing, mostly through employers, accounts for about 55% of total U.S. health care expenditures, and the government finances the remaining 45% (CMS, 2017).

Centrally controlled health care systems are less complex and less costly, managing total expenditures with global budgets and with the ability to govern the availability and utilization of services. The U.S. has a large private infrastructure in which hospitals and physician clinics operate as private businesses, independently of the government. Even so, U.S. federal and state governments play an important role in health care delivery, determining public-sector expenditures and reimbursement for Medicaid and Medicare services. The government also establishes standards for participation through policy and regulation, and providers must comply with these standards to care for Medicaid and Medicare patients. Certification standards are also regarded as minimum quality standards in most health care industry sectors.

Technology Driven and Focused on Acute Care

The United States is a hotbed of research and innovation in medical technology. Scientific and technological advances often create a demand for new services, despite shrinking financial resources. Other factors also contribute to increased demand for expensive high technology care. Patients often assume the newest innovations represent the best quality care, and physicians often seek to use the newest technology. Hospitals compete for having the most modern medical equipment and face pressure to recoup capital investments made in technology. Legal risks for providers and health plans may also encourage the use of new technology.

Although technology has ushered in a new generation of clinical interventions, negative outcomes result from overuse. The use of new technology contributes to rising health care costs. Technological innovation has its place in medicine but, with limited resources, there is insufficient emphasis on primary care and public health, which lead to better population-level outcomes and are more cost-effective.

High in Cost, Unequal in Access, and Average in Outcome

Of all developed countries, the United States spends the most on health care services, which constituted nearly 17% of the gross domestic product [GDP] in 2016 (**FIGURE 1.2**), and many U.S. residents have limited access to even the most basic care.

Access is the ability of an individual to obtain health care when needed. In the U.S., access is restricted to persons who (1) have employer-based health insurance, (2) are covered under a government-sponsored health care program (including health coverage under the ACA), (3) can buy insurance with their own funds, (4) can pay for services privately, or (5) can obtain services through safety net providers. Health insurance is the primary—but not necessarily a sufficient—means for obtaining access to care. Despite expansion of health insurance, some people still face barriers to access. One-third

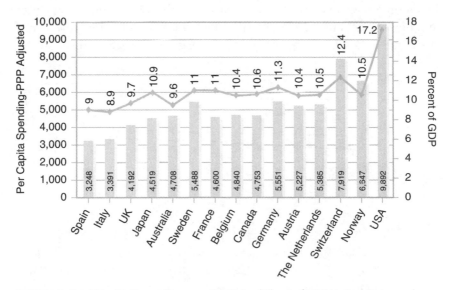

FIGURE 1.2 Total Health Expenditure per Capita and Share of GDP, United States and Selected Countries, 2016

Data from Organization for Economic Cooperation and Development. OECD health data. OECD Health Statistics [database], 2016. Accessed February 5, 2018.

of physicians do not take new Medicaid-insured patients (Decker 2012). For primary care—consistent basic and routine care—uninsured individuals cannot visit a physician without making out-of-pocket payments. Those who cannot afford to pay usually wait until developing health problems, when they may be cared for in a hospital emergency department.

Experts believe that inadequacy and disparity in access to primary care services are the main reasons that the U.S. lags behind other developed nations in population health. **FIGURE 1.3** shows the U.S. racial disparities in life expectancy, and **FIGURE 1.4** summarizes death rates among children in the Organization for Economic Cooperation and Development (OECD).

Imperfect Market Conditions

Under national health care programs, patients can select their providers, but true economic market forces are virtually nonexistent. In the U.S., health care delivery is largely in private hands, but health care is only partially governed by free market forces. Hence, the system is a quasi-market or an imperfect market system. The following key characteristics of free markets help explain why the U.S. health care system is not a true free market.

In a free market, many patients (buyers) and providers (sellers) act independently, and patients can choose providers based on price and quality of services. In reality, however, the payer is an MCO, Medicare, or Medicaid, not the patient. Prices are set by agencies outside the market and thus are not freely governed by the simple market forces of supply and demand.

A free health care market requires free competition among providers based on price and quality of services. Generally, free competition exists among providers in the U.S., but the consolidation of buying power into the hands of MCOs forces providers to form alliances and IDSs on the

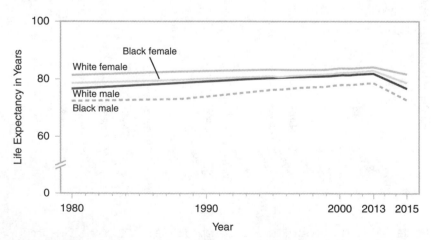

FIGURE 1.3 Life Expectancy at Birth

National Center for Health Statistics. Health, United States, 2016: In Brief. Hyattsville, MD. 2017, p 116. https://www.cdc.gov/nchs/data/hus/hus16.pdf

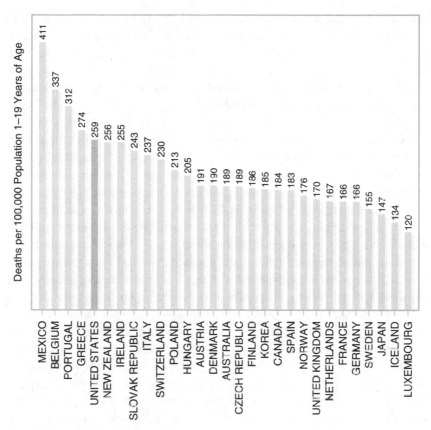

FIGURE 1.4 Death Rates Among Children 1–19 Years of Age, by OECD Country

Data from the year 2006 or most recent year. Doing Better for Children. Chapter 2: Comparative Child Well-being across the OECD; p. 51

supply side. In certain regions, a single medical system becomes the sole provider of major health care services. As the U.S. health care system continues to develop in this direction, it seems that only large metropolitan areas will have more than one large integrated system competing for the business of health plans.

Free markets work best when consumers are educated about products, but patients are not always well informed about their choices for health care. Direct-to-consumer advertising for pharmaceuticals and other products often complicates the decision of what is best for a patient. Choices of technologies, diagnostic methods, interventions, and medicines can be complex and require physician input. As an advocate, physicians can help educate their patients. Increasingly, consumers are taking initiative to educate themselves with resources on the Internet for gathering medical information, although such information is not necessarily reliable.

In a free market, patients are provided with information on the price and quality of services offered by each provider. In the U.S., however, pricing methods for health care confound free market mechanisms. Hidden costs make it difficult to gauge the full expense of services beforehand. *Item-based pricing*, for example, refers to the costs of ancillary services that tend to accompany surgeries and other major procedures. Patients may be informed of the cost ahead of time but cannot anticipate the additional cost of specialists and of supplies and facilities, and thus have difficulty ascertaining the total price before services are received. Package pricing and capitated fees can help overcome these challenges by bundling fees for packages of related services. *Package pricing* covers services bundled for an episode of care. This encompasses less than *capitation*, which covers all services that a health plan enrollee may need for a year.

Patients directly bear the cost of services received in a free market system. The purpose of insurance is to cover major expenses for unlikely events—but insurance covers basic and routine services, which undermines this principle. Coverage for minor events such as colds or coughs is equivalent to prepayment for such services. There is a moral hazard, namely, that enrollees typically use more services after purchasing insurance.

In a free market, demand for services is determined by market forces—when many individuals independently determine what to buy and when to buy products or services. But health care is different. First, decisions about utilizing health care are often determined by need, not by price-based demand. *Need* can be self-assessed or determined by a medical expert. Nevertheless, many factors discussed previously affect whether the person actually obtains care. Second, health care delivery can actually create demand. For example, practitioners with a financial interest in ordering further treatments may create artificial demand—commonly referred to as *provider-induced demand*.

Government as Subsidiary to the Private Sector

In most developed countries, the government plays a central role in health care delivery. But in the United States, the private sector has the dominant role. This can partially be explained by the American tradition of individual responsibility and a commitment to limiting government power. Government spending for health care is largely confined to filling in the gaps left unaddressed by the private sector, including public health functions such as clean water and sanitation, research and training support, and care for vulnerable populations.

Fusion of Market Justice and Social Justice

Market justice and social justice are contrasting theories governing how health care services are produced and distributed. The principle of *market justice* places the responsibility for fair distribution of health care on market forces in a free economy. Medical care and benefits are distributed according to people's willingness and ability to pay (Santerre & Neun, 1996, p. 7). In contrast, *social justice* emphasizes the well-being of the community over that of the individual; the inability to obtain medical services due to a lack of financial resources is considered unjust. In a system that blends public and private resources, the two theories often work well together, and both contribute their ideals to the overall system. For example, individuals who are employed and have middle-class incomes obtain employer-sponsored health insurance, whereas the most needy members of society depend on government-sponsored programs. At the same time, these two principles of justice create conflicts. For example, many small employers in the U.S. do not offer insurance, or else provide insurance that their employees cannot afford. Yet, these employees do not qualify for government assistance because their income exceeds a certain threshold. The ACA is intended to address this situation, but doing so may take years.

Multiple Players and Balance of Power

The U.S. health care system involves multiple players including physicians, administrators of health service institutions, insurance companies, large employers, and the government. Big business, labor, insurance companies, physicians, and hospitals form politically powerful special-interest groups represented before lawmakers by lobbyists. Each player has an economic interest to protect, but problems arise when players' interests are at odds. Providers seek to maximize government reimbursement for Medicare and Medicaid services, but the government strives to contain cost increases. Different interests produce counteracting forces in the U.S. health care system. One benefit is that they prevent any single entity from dominating the system. However, given so many conflicting interests, comprehensive, system-wide health care reform is nearly impossible, and cost containment is a challenge. Thus, health care reform is incremental or piecemeal and can be regressive as presidential administrations change. (Note: The ACA is an example of incremental, not comprehensive, reform that primarily addresses coverage.)

Quest for Integration and Accountability

Primary care in the U.S. makes for an ideal organizing hub for continuous, coordinated health care services. Although this model became popular as managed care was expanded, it is still undeveloped. Ideally, primary care integrates health care in comprehensive, coordinated, and continuous health care services through a seamless delivery—also referred to as a medical home or health home for patients. This model emphasizes the patient–provider relationship in improving the health of each person, thereby improving the health of the population. Key to this relationship is accountability. Provider accountability means providing quality care efficiently, while patient accountability means taking responsibility for one's health and using resources sensibly.

Access to Health Care Services Selectively Based on Insurance Coverage

The U.S. offers some of the best medical care in the world, yet this care is generally available only to individuals with insurance that provides adequate coverage or with sufficient resources to pay for services themselves. The uninsured have limited options for medical care. They can (1) pay physicians out of pocket at rates typically higher than those under insurance plans, (2) seek care from safety net providers, or (3) obtain treatment for acute illnesses at a hospital emergency department, for which hospitals do not receive direct payments unless patients can afford them. The Emergency Medical Treatment and Labor Act of 1986 requires screening and evaluation of all patients, provision of necessary stabilizing treatment, and hospital admission when necessary, regardless of ability to pay. Unfortunately, the misuse of emergency departments results in cost shifting, in which the costs of emergency room care to the uninsured are covered by patients with the ability to pay for services, privately insured individuals, employers, and the government (i.e., taxpayers).

Legal Risks Influence Practice Behaviors

As a society, Americans are quick to file lawsuits. With the prospects of great financial awards, many people bring alleged offenders to court at the slightest perceived harm. Private health care providers are susceptible to litigation, and medical malpractice lawsuits are a serious risk in the practice of medicine. For protection, most providers engage in *defensive medicine*—that is, prescribing additional diagnostic tests, scheduling checkup appointments, and maintaining abundant case documentation. Many such efforts are unnecessary and raise costs and inefficiency.

▶ Health Care Systems of Other Developed Countries

Three basic models for structuring national health care systems prevail in Western European countries and Canada. In Canada, health care is financed by the government through general taxes, but health care itself is delivered by private providers. In the quad-function model (see Figure 1.1), the Canadian system requires tighter consolidation of financing, insurance, and payment coordinated by the government, and delivery is characterized by detached private arrangements.

In Germany, health care is financed by government-mandated employer and employee contributions, and health care is also delivered by private providers. Private not-for-profit insurance companies—called sickness funds—collect the contributions and pay physicians and hospitals (Santerre & Neun, 2013). In this socialized health insurance system, insurance and payment functions are integrated, and financing is better coordinated with insurance and payment functions than in the U.S. Delivery is characterized by independent private arrangements, and the government has overall control.

In the United Kingdom, the infrastructure of health care delivery is managed by the government, as is the financing of a tax-supported national health insurance program. Most medical institutions are run by the government and most providers, including physicians, are government employees or organized in a publicly managed infrastructure. In the quad-function model, the British system requires tighter consolidation of all four functions, typically by the government.

Canada

In Canada, there have been several initiatives to integrate and coordinate care for chronically ill patients with complex health care needs. In 2004, as part of the 10-Year Plan to Strengthen Health Care, all provincial and territorial governments in Canada agreed to provide at least half of their populations with access to multidisciplinary primary care teams. By 2007, approximately three-fourths of family physicians were working in physician-led, multiprofessional practices (Marchildon & Mou, 2013). 60% of primary care physicians use computerized medical records throughout Canada (Health Council of Canada, 2013; Mossialos et al., 2015).

As of 2014, federal funding through the Canada Health Transfer was modified to be distributed to provinces on a per-capita basis, ending compensation from tax base variations that had benefited less wealthy provinces (Mossialos et al., 2015). The new funding policy seeks to improve equity, although it was criticized for reducing funding to less populated provinces where people are older and health care costs are higher (Marchildon & Mou, 2013). All provinces have sought to reduce generic drug prices, with several provinces greatly reducing these prices in recent years; in Ontario, in 2010, the price ceiling for a generic drug was lowered to 25% of the price of the corresponding brand-name drug, and British Columbia lowered its price ceiling to 20% in 2014 (Mossialos et al., 2015).

Primary care reform has been under way in Canada since 2000, when the federal government invested CA$800 million (US$647 million) over

6 years into the Primary Care Transition Fund. Provinces continue to reform their primary care systems, including provider payment methods, to incentivize movement to team-based practice, chronic disease management, and coordination of care with other providers, as well as to integrate primary care and public health (Hutchison et al., 2011; Mossialos et al., 2017; Sweetman & Buckley, 2014).

Moreover, there have been many initiatives to ensure quality of care. The federally-funded Canadian Patient Safety Institute is responsible for promoting best practices and developing tools, strategies, and standards for quality of care (Mossialos et al., 2017). Another federally funded institute, the Canadian Foundation for Healthcare Improvement, helps implement initiatives to improve performance and created an initiative to reduce inappropriate prescribing in long-term care facilities (Canadian Foundation for Healthcare Improvement, 2017).

Germany

Germany implemented the General Law on Patients' Rights in 2013, which includes measures to strengthen patients' rights, the most important of which is the incorporation into the Civil Code of rights, duties, and forms of etiquette pertaining to provider-patient relationships.

The federal cabinet passed the Bill of the First Act to Strengthen Long-Term Care in 2014, to support families who provide care to a family member at home and improve adult day care and short-term care by increasing the number of caregivers. Benefits and services are set to increase by 20% under this act. The Second Act to Strengthen Long-Term Care aims to redefine the need for care with the growing number of dementia patients and to expand long-term care eligibility, to include individuals with physical, mental, and psychological impairments (Backer, 2016).

The coalition agreement plan from 2013 includes proposals for measures to promote quality of care. The Federal Joint Committee was commissioned in 2014 to establish the Institute for Quality Assurance and Transparency in Health Care, and the Hospital Care Structure Reform Act introduced a focus on quality-related accreditation and payment of hospitals in 2016. In Germany, providers must also have a quality management system. All physicians are required to continue medical education, and drugs and procedures must receive health technology assessments before being reimbursed by sickness funds (Mossialos et al., 2017).

A new bill changes how Social Health Insurance contribution rates are determined and shared between employer and employee in an effort to contain indirect labor costs. Beginning in 2016, the general contribution rate (14.6%) was retained, but the special contribution rate for employees only (0.9%) and the supplementary premiums (and necessary specific social protection mechanisms) were abolished (Mossialos et al., 2017), replaced by a supplementary income-dependent contribution rate to be determined by each sickness fund on an individual basis. The average rate was 0.83% in 2015—that is, the insured paid less than they did in 2014 (Mossialos et al., 2017).

The Federal Cabinet passed the E-Health Act in 2015 to improve health care applications, providing deadlines to implement electronic applications and introducing related incentives and sanctions. Beginning in July 2018, statutory health insurance (SHI) physicians who do not participate in the national online claims data program will receive reduced pay (Busse et al., 2016).

United Kingdom

The purchasing and regulatory structures of the National Health Service (NHS) in England were significantly reformed under the Health and Social Care Act of 2012, which replaced 150 primary care trusts with clinical commissioning groups (of which there are now 211 in England) to make better use of resources in planning and purchasing decisions for a range of services. Clinical commissioning groups differ from primary care trusts in their governance. General practices must belong to a clinical commissioning group, whose governing body must be chaired by a general practitioner and include other clinicians alongside managers. Clinical commissioning groups controlled approximately half of the total NHS budget from 2013 to 2014.

NHS England was created to oversee clinical commissioning groups. Reforms have envisioned all hospitals becoming semi-autonomous foundation trusts; clinical commissioning groups would have greater freedom to commission different providers and enhance public scrutiny. But evaluating their impact on cost, health outcomes, and quality of care may be complex due to financial pressures on health care and social care services (National Audit Office, 2013).

The Five Year Forward View, published in 2014, outlined challenges facing the NHS and wide-ranging strategies to address them (NHS England, 2014). It covered themes from empowering patients and communities to testing new vanguard care models. To date, 50 vanguard sites have been established to test innovations in health care delivery including enhanced long-term care homes, vertically integrated hospital and community care, and networks for improved emergency care (NHS England, 2015). NHS England published Next Steps on the Five Year Forward View in 2017, which took stock of progress at the halfway point of the 5-year view and set priorities for future reforms (NHS England, 2017).

TABLE 1.1 presents selected features of the national health care programs and health outcomes of Canada, Germany, and the United Kingdom, as compared with the United States.

TABLE 1.1 Health Care Systems of Selected Industrialized Countries

	United States	Canada	United Kingdom	Germany
Type	Pluralistic	National health insurance	National health system	Socialized health insurance
Ownership	Private	Public/private	Public	Private
Financing	Voluntary, multipayer system (premiums or general taxes)	Single payer (general taxes)	Single payer (general taxes)	Employer–employee (mandated payroll contributions and general taxes)
Reimbursement (hospital)	Varies (DRGs, negotiated fee-for-service, per diem, capitation)	Global budgets	Global budgets	Per diem payments
Reimbursement (physicians)	RBRVS, fee-for-service	Negotiated fee-for-service	Salaries and capitation payments	Negotiated fee-for-service
Consumer copayment	Small to significant	Negligible	Negligible	Negligible
Life expectancy for women (years)	78.8	81.7	81.0	80.7
Infant mortality per 1,000 live births	5.8	4.8	3.9	3.3
Expenditures as a percentage of GDP (%)	17.2	10.6	9.7	11.3

Abbreviations: DRGs, diagnosis-related groups; RBRVS, resource-based relative value scale
Data from Organization for Economic Cooperation and Development. OECD health data. OECD Health Statistics [database], 2017, https://data.oecd.org/healthstat/life-expectancy-at-birth.htm. Accessed February 18, 2018.

▶ Systems Framework

A system is a set of interrelated, interdependent components designed to achieve some common goals, with logically coordinated components. While the various components of the health care delivery system in the United States are only loosely coordinated, the main components can be identified in the framework of a systems model (**FIGURE 1.5**). The systems framework shows how the structure of health care services in the U.S. is based on fundamental principles and provides a logical arrangement of the various components with a progression from inputs to outputs. The main elements are system inputs (resources), structure, processes, and outputs (outcomes). Outlook (future directions) is also a necessary element of a dynamic system. This framework has been used as the conceptual basis for organizing the chapters in this text.

System Foundations

The structure of the current health care system is not random, but rather explained by historical, cultural, social, and economic factors.

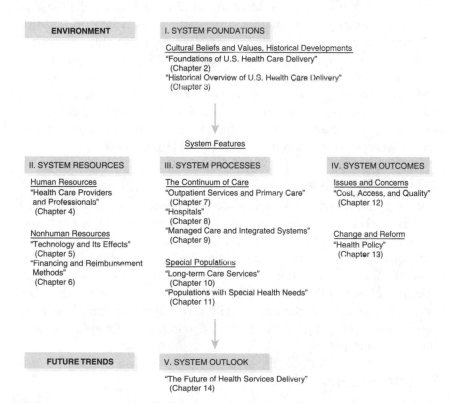

FIGURE 1.5 Systems Framework

As discussed elsewhere in this text, these factors also affect both forces shaping new trends and developments and those impeding change.

System Resources

Both human and nonhuman resources are essential for health care delivery. Human resources consist of the various types of workers directly engaged in the delivery of health care to patients. Such personnel— including physicians, nurses, dentists, pharmacists, other professionals trained at the doctoral level, and many kinds of allied health professionals—usually have direct patient contact. Numerous ancillary workers, such as those involved in billing and collection, marketing and public relations, and building maintenance, often play important but indirect supportive roles in health care delivery. Health care managers are needed to manage and coordinate the various types of services.

System Processes

System processes are carried out mainly through the health care delivery infrastructure, which consists of hospitals, clinics, long-term care providers, and other settings. Most health care services are delivered in non-institutional settings, mainly associated with outpatient care. Institutional health services (inpatient care) are predominantly associated with acute care hospitals. Managed care organizations are responsible for actual health care delivery, apart from their role in financing, insurance, and payment. Integrated systems deliver a range of health care services. Special institutional and community-based settings have been developed for long-term care and mental health, and the health care infrastructure must also support and accommodate special populations.

System Outcomes

System outcomes refer to critical issues and concerns surrounding what the health services system is able or unable to accomplish with regards to its primary objective—to provide cost-effective health services that meet quality standards to a nation. The aforementioned elements of the systems model—foundations, resources, and processes—play a critical role in achieving this objective. Access, cost, and quality are the main outcome criteria for evaluating a health care delivery system. Issues and concerns regarding these criteria can lead to initiatives for system reform through health policy.

System Outlook

Dynamic health care systems must look forward and consider future outcomes in the context of social, cultural, economic, and other forces.

▶ Conclusion

The United States has a unique health care delivery system, but it does not provide universal access, so not all Americans enjoy continuous, comprehensive health care. Health care delivery in the U.S. is characterized by a patchwork of subsystems developed through market forces or based on the need to care for certain populations. These components include managed care, the military medical care and VA systems, the system for vulnerable populations, and the emerging IDSs. Most countries with a national health care program have a private sector of varying size. The systems framework helps explain the roles of the various components of the U.S. health care delivery system in an organized fashion.

References

1. Assistant Secretary for Planning and Evaluation (ASPE). 2015. The Affordable Care Act is improving access to preventive services for millions of Americans. https://aspe.hhs.gov/pdf-report/affordable-care-act-improving-access-preventive-services-millions-americans. Accessed December 10, 2017.
2. Aventis Pharmaceuticals. 2002. *HMO-PPO digest: managed care digest series.* Bridgewater, NJ: Aventis Pharmaceuticals; pp. 1–88.
3. Backer G. 2016. Reform of the long-term care insurance in Germany. ec.europa.eu/social/BlobServlet?docId=16074&langId=en. Accessed March 29, 2018.
4. Bureau of Labor Statistics (BLS). 2016. Occupational employment and wages: healthcare practitioners and technical occupations. https://www.bls.gov/oes/2016/may/oes_nat.htm. Accessed March 28, 2018.
5. Bureau of Primary Health Care. 2011. *BPHC-UDS annual report.* Rockville, MD: Bureau of Primary Health Care, Health Resources and Services Administration.
6. Bureau of Primary Health Care. 2017. 2016 National Health Center Data. https://bphc.hrsa.gov/uds/datacenter.aspx. Accessed December 10, 2017.
7. Busse R, Blumel M, Quentin W, Spranger A. 2016. Health systems and policy monitor: Germany. http://www.hspm.org/countries/germany28082014/countrypage.aspx. Accessed February 2018.
8. Canadian Foundation for Healthcare Improvement. 2017. Building capacity. Enhancing leadership. Delivering improvement. http://www.cfhi-fcass.ca/AboutUs.aspx. Accessed February 2018.
9. Centers for Disease Control and Prevention (CDC). 2013. National Public Health Performance Standards Program. https://www.cdc.gov/nphpsp. Accessed June 7, 2015.
10. Centers for Medicare and Medicaid Services (CMS). 2011. Long term care facilities. https://www.cms.gov/Regulations-and-Guidance/Legislation/CFCsAndCoPs/LTC.html. Accessed August 2015.
11. Centers for Medicare and Medicaid Services (CMS). 2017. NHE fact sheet. https://www.cms.gov/research-statistics-data-and-systems/statistics-trends-and-reports/nationalhealthexpenddata/nhe-fact-sheet.html. Accessed December 2017.
12. Commonwealth Foundation. 2017. Effect of the Affordable Care Act on health care access. http://www.commonwealthfund.org/publications/issue-briefs/2017/may/effect-aca-health-care-access#/#1. Accessed December 10, 2017.

13. Congressional Budget Office. (CBO) 2017. Federal subsidies for health insurance coverage for people under age 65: 2016 to 2026. https://www.cbo.gov/publication/51385. Accessed December 10, 2017.

14. Decker SL. 2012. In 2011 nearly one-third of physicians said they would not accept new Medicaid patients, but rising fees may help. *Health Aff.* 31(8):1673–1679.

15. Department of Veterans Affairs. 2017. https://www.va.gov. Accessed February 3, 2018.

16. Health Council of Canada. 2013. *How Do Canadian primary care physicians rate the health system? Survey results from the 2012 Commonwealth Fund International Survey of Primary Care Doctors.* Toronto, Canada: Health Council of Canada.

17. Hutchison B, Levesque J-F, Strumpf E, Coyle N. 2011. Primary health care in Canada: systems in motion. *Milbank Q.* 89(2):256–288.

18. Kaiser Family Foundation. 2011. State health facts. https://www.kff.org/statedata/. Accessed March 19, 2018.

19. Kaiser Family Foundation. 2015. Medicaid enrollment in comprehensive risk-based managed care. https://www.kff.org/medicaid/state-indicator/medicaid -enrollment-in-comprehensive-risk-based-managed-care/?currentTimeframe=0 &sortModel= %7B%22colId %22:%22Location%22,%22sort%22:%22asc%22%7D. Accessed December 10, 2017.

20. Kaiser Family Foundation. 2016a. Total number of HMOs. https://www.kff.org/other /state-indicator/number-of-hmos/?currentTimeframe=0&sortModel=%7B%22colId %22:%22Location%22,%22sort%22:%22asc%22%7D. Accessed December 2017.

21. Kaiser Family Foundation. 2016b. Total CHIP spending. https://www.kff.org /medicaid/state-indicator/total-chip-spending/?currentTimeframe=0&sortMo del= %7B %22colId%22:%22Location%22,%22sort%22:%22asc%22%7D. Accessed December 2017.

22. Kaiser Family Foundation. 2017a. Status of state action on the Medicaid expansion decision. https://www.kff.org/health-reform/state-indicator/state-activity-around -expanding-medicaid-under-the-affordable-care-act/?currentTimeframe=0&sort Model=%7B%22colId%22:%22 Location %22,%22sort%22:%22asc%22%7D. Accessed December 10, 2017.

23. Kaiser Family Foundation. 2017b. The effects of Medicaid expansion under the ACA: Updated findings from a literature review. https://www.kff.org/medicaid/issue -brief/the-effects-of-medicaid-expansion-under-the-aca-updated-findings-from-a -literature-review-september-2017/. Accessed December 10, 2017.

24. Marchildon GP, Mou H. October 9, 2013. The funding formula for health care is broken. Alberta's windfall proves it. *Globe and Mail.* http://www.theglobeandmail .com/globe-debate/the-funding-formula-for-health-care-is-broken-albertaswindfall -proves-it/article14764089/. Accessed October 10, 2014.

25. Mossialos E, Djordevic A, Osborn R, Sarnak D. May 2017. International profiles of health care systems. Commonwealth Fund. http://www.commonwealthfund.org /~/media/files/publications/fund-report/2017/may/mossialos_intl_profiles_v5.pdf. Accessed February 2018.

26. Mossialos E, Wenzl M, Osborn R, Anderson C. 2015. 2014 international profiles of health care systems. Commonwealth Fund. Pub. no. 1802. http://www .commonwealthfund.org/~/media/files/publications/fund-report/2015/jan/1802 _mossialos_intl_profiles_2014_v7.pdf. Accessed May 2015.

27. National Audit Office. July 2013. *Managing the transition to the reformed health system.* United Kingdom: Department of Health; 1–46.

28. National Center for Health Statistics. 2007. *Health, United States,* 2007. Hyattsville, MD: Department of Health and Human Services.

29. National Center for Health Statistics. 2017. *Health, United States, 2016: With chartbook on long-term trends in health.* Hyattsville, MD: Department of Health and Human Services.
30. National Center for Veterans Analysis and Statistics. 2007. *FY07 VA information pamphlet.* Washington, DC: Department of Veterans Affairs.
31. NHS England. 2014. Five Year Forward View. https://www.england.nhs.uk /wp-content/uploads/2014/10/5yfv-web.pdf. Accessed February 2018.
32. NHS England. 2015. Five Year Forward View: Time to deliver. https://www.england .nhs.uk/wp-content/uploads/2015/06/5yfv-time-to-deliver-25-06.pdf. Accessed February 2018.
33. NHS England. 2017. Next steps on the NHS Five Year Forward View. https://www .england.nhs.uk/wp-content/uploads/2017/03/NEXT-STEPS-ON-THE-NHS-FIVE -YEAR-FORWARD-VIEW.pdf. Accessed February 2018.
34. Politzer RM, et al. 2003. The future role of health centers in improving national health. *J Public Health Policy.* 24(3):296–306.
35. SAMHSA-HRSA Center for Integrated Health Solutions. 2014. Essential elements of effective integrated primary care and behavioral health teams. https://www.integration .samhsa.gov/workforce/team-members/Essential_Elements_of_an_Integrated_Team .pdf. Accessed December 10, 2017.
36. Santerre RE, Neun SP. 2013. *Health economics: Theories, insights, and industry studies.* Chicago, IL: Irwin.
37. Shi L, et al. 2001. The impact of managed care on vulnerable populations served by community health centers. *J Ambul Care Manage.* 24(1):51–66.
38. Shortell SM, Gillies RR, Anderson D, Erickson K. 1996. *Remaking health care in America: Building organized delivery systems.* Hoboken, NJ: Jossey-Bass.
39. Sweetman A, Buckley G. 2014. Ontario's experiment with primary care reform. *University of Calgary School Public Policy Research Papers.* 7(11):1–37. https://www .policyschool.ca/wp-content/uploads/2016/03/ontario-health care-reform.pdf. Accessed March 28, 2018.
40. Trust for America's Health, Robert Wood Johnson Foundation. 2014. Investing in America's health: A state-by-state look at public health funding and key health facts. http://healthyamericans.org/assets/files/TFAH2014-InvestInAmericaRpt08.pdf. Accessed August 2014.
41. U.S. Bureau of the Census. 1998. *Statistical abstract of the United States: 1998.* 118th ed. Washington, DC: U.S. Bureau of the Census.
42. U.S. Bureau of the Census. 2007. Current populations report. In: *Income, poverty, and health insurance coverage in the United States: 2006.* Washington, DC: Government Printing Office; 60–233.
43. Yasaitis LC, Pajerowski W, Polsky D, Werner RM. 2016. Physicians' participation in ACOs is lower in places with vulnerable populations than in more affluent communities. *Health Aff (Millwood).* 35(8):1382–1390. doi: 10.1377/hlthaff .2015.1635.

CHAPTER 2
Foundations of U.S. Health Care Delivery

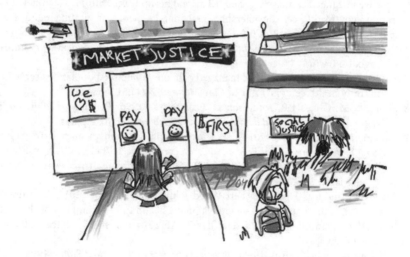

▶ Introduction

Curative medicine in the U.S. appears to yield diminishing returns on health improvement even as expenditures increase (Saward and Sorensen, 1980). Society benefits from the promotion of health and the prevention of disease, disability, and premature death. However, although curative medicine has been the focus of health care financing, progress has been slow toward an emphasis on health promotion, disease prevention, and health maintenance for individuals with chronic conditions. This is due to the U.S. health insurance system, cultural values, and medical practices that emphasize disease rather than health. Common definitions of health and measures of health status reflect these inclinations.

This chapter explores various aspects of health, major determinants of health, contrasting principles of market justice and social justice in health care delivery, and public health interventions for population health. Beliefs and values ingrained in American culture have been instrumental in laying the foundation of the current system, which is predominantly private, as opposed to a tax-financed national health care program. In recent years, however, societal values have shifted to a social justice mindset, and traditional values of self-reliance may be giving way to greater dependence on the government. Passage of the Affordable Care Act (ACA) presages a gradual shift away from market justice and toward social justice in the U.S. health care system.

▶ What Is Health?

In the United States, the concepts of health and health care have largely been governed by the medical model or, specifically, the biomedical model. Under the *medical model*, health is defined as the absence of illness or disease. This perspective emphasizes diagnosis and intervention to treat disease or symptoms. Optimal health exists when a person is free of symptoms and does not require treatment. Thus, *health care delivery* refers to the delivery of medical care or illness care. Prevention of disease and promotion of health are relegated to a secondary status; a measure often used to indicate lack of health in a population is mortality or death (see **FIGURE 2.1** for death rates by gender and cause in the United States).

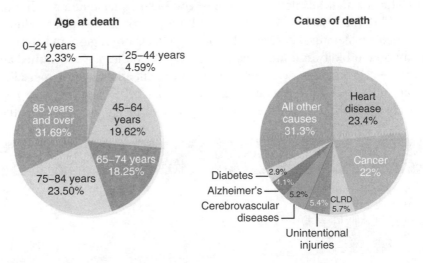

FIGURE 2.1 Age and Causes of Deaths for 2015

National Center for Health Statistics. Deaths: Final Data for 2015. https://www.cdc.gov/nchs/data/nvsr/nvsr66/nvsr66_06.pdf

Medical sociologists further define health as the state of optimal capacity of an individual to perform expected social roles and tasks, such as work, school, and household chores (Parsons, 1972). A person who is unable (as opposed to unwilling) to perform his or her social roles is considered sick—even though many people continue to engage in such obligations despite pain, cough, colds, and other disabilities, including mental distress. Hence, engagement in social roles does not necessarily signify optimal health.

The Society for Academic Emergency Medicine (SAEM) emphasizes both physical and mental health, defining health as "a state of physical and mental well-being that facilitates the achievement of individual and societal goals" (SAEM, 1992, p. 1386).

The World Health Organization's (WHO's) definition of health is most often cited as the ideal for health care delivery systems. The WHO (1948) defines *health* as "a complete state of physical, mental, and social well-being, and not merely the absence of disease or infirmity" (p. 100). This includes physical, mental, and social dimensions, and constitutes the biopsychosocial model of health. The WHO defines a *health care system* as all activities aimed at promoting, restoring, or maintaining health (McKee, 2001). Health care includes more than medical care.

In recent decades, there has been a growing interest in holistic or comprehensive health, which emphasizes the well-being of every aspect of what makes a person whole and complete. *Holistic medicine* seeks to treat the whole person (Ward, 1995). Holistic health incorporates the spiritual dimension in addition to the physical, mental, and social aspects of optimal health, and thus provides the most complete understanding of health (see **EXHIBIT 2.1** for key examples of health indicators). A growing volume of medical literature illustrates the healing effects of religion and spirituality on morbidity and mortality (Levin, 1994). Studies have identified an inverse association between religious involvement and all-cause mortality (McCullough et al., 2000). Religious and spiritual beliefs and practices positively influence physical, mental, and social well-being and may affect the

EXHIBIT 2.1 Indicators of Health

- Self-reported health status
- Life expectancy
- Morbidity (disease)
- Mental well-being
- Social functioning
- Functional limitations
- Disability
- Spiritual well-being

incidences, experiences, and outcomes of many medical problems (Bauer et al., 2017; Loureiro et al., 2017; Maugans, 1996; Rainville, 2017).

The spiritual dimension is often related to religious beliefs, values, and practices, and is described as meaning, purpose, and fulfillment in life, the hope and will to live, faith, and a relationship with God (Bauer et al., 2017; Loureiro et al., 2017; Marwick, 1995; Rainville, 2017; Ross, 1995; Swanson, 1995). The holistic health approach also incorporates alternative therapies into the predominant medical model.

Illness and Disease

The terms *illness* and *disease* are not synonymous, but are often used interchangeably as in this text. Illness is recognized by a person's perceptions and evaluation of how he or she feels. An individual may feel pain, discomfort, weakness, depression, or anxiety, whether or not a disease is present, but the presence or absence of a disease is determined by a medical professional's evaluation, not the patient's assessment. Certain diseases, such as hypertension (high blood pressure), are asymptomatic and do not always manifest in illness. In other words, a hypertensive person has a disease but may be unaware. It is possible to have disease without feeling ill or feel ill without having a disease.

Acute and Chronic Conditions

Diseases can be classified as acute, subacute, or chronic. An *acute condition* is relatively severe, episodic (of short duration), and often treatable (Timmreck, 1994, p. 26). It is subject to recovery, and treatment is generally provided in a hospital. Examples include a sudden interruption of kidney function or a myocardial infarction (heart attack).

A *subacute condition* lies between the acute and chronic extremes on the disease severity continuum, but also has acute features. Subacute conditions can be postacute, requiring further treatment after a stay in the hospital. Examples include ventilator and head trauma care.

A *chronic condition* is less severe but of long, continuous duration (Timmreck, 1994, p. 26). The patient may not fully recover. A chronic condition may be kept under control through appropriate medical treatment but, if left untreated, may lead to severe, life-threatening health problems. Examples include asthma, diabetes, and hypertension.

Quality of Life

The term *quality of life*, used in a denotative sense, indicates overall patient satisfaction with life during and after an encounter with the health care delivery system. The term is used in two ways: First, it indicates how satisfied a person is with his or her experiences while receiving services. Factors including comfort, dignity, privacy, security, degree of independence, decision-making autonomy, and attention to preferences are significant to most people, and are regarded as patient rights. Second, quality of life can refer to overall satisfaction with life and with self-perceptions of health, particularly after an intervention. Desirable processes during treatment and successful outcomes have a positive effect on an individual's ability to function and carry out social roles.

▶ Determinants of Health

Identification of *determinants of health* has contributed greatly to the understanding that a singular focus on care delivery is unlikely to improve population health. Because multiple factors determine health and well-being, a more balanced approach must emphasize health determinants at an individual level and policy interventions at the population level (**FIGURE 2.2**).

The major determinants of health (see examples in **EXHIBIT 2.2**) can be classified into four categories: environment, behavior and lifestyle, heredity, and medical care.

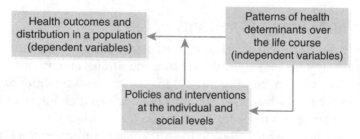

FIGURE 2.2   Schematic Definition of Population Health

Reproduced from Kindig D, Stoddart G. What is Population Health? *Am J Public Health*. 2003; 93 (3): 380-833

EXHIBIT 2.2   Examples of Health Determinants

- Physical activity
- Overweight/obesity
- Tobacco use
- Substance abuse
- Responsible sexual behavior
- Mental health
- Injury and violence
- Environmental quality
- Immunization
- Access to health care

Environment

Environmental factors encompass the physical, socioeconomic, socio-political, and sociocultural dimensions of life. Physical environmental factors such as air pollution, food and water contaminants, radiation, and toxic chemicals can significantly affect health; however, the influence of other environmental factors on health may not be so obvious. For example, socioeconomic status is related to health and well-being, and people with higher incomes often live in areas with less exposure to environmental risks and enjoy better access to care. Income inequality is associated with a variety of health indicators, such as life expectancy, age-adjusted mortality rates, and leading causes of death (Kaplan et al., 1996; Kawachi et al., 1997; Kennedy et al., 1996; Mackenbach, 1997; Peykari et al., 2015; Syden & Landberg, 2017). The greater the economic gap between the rich and the poor in a given geographic area, the worse the overall health of the population in that area.

The relationship between education level and health status is also well established. Less-educated Americans die earlier than their better-educated counterparts (Peykari et al., 2015; Syden & Landberg, 2017). One possible explanation is that better-educated people are more likely to avoid risky behaviors such as smoking and drug abuse (Peykari et al., 2015; Syden & Landberg, 2017).

The environment can also significantly influence developmental health. Good nurturing and stimulation during the first 3 years of life—a critical period for brain development—activate the brain's neural pathways and may permanently increase the number of brain cells. Early childhood development has an enormous influence on a person's future health.

Behavior and Lifestyle

Individual lifestyle, or *behavioral factors*, include diet, exercise, stress, risky or unhealthy behaviors, and other choices that may contribute to significant health problems. Heart disease, diabetes, stroke, sexually transmitted diseases, and cancer are some of the ailments directly linked to individual choice and lifestyle.

Heredity

Heredity is a key determinant of health because genetic factors predispose individuals to certain diseases. Little can be done to alter the genetic makeup a person has already inherited, but a healthy lifestyle and health-promoting behaviors can significantly influence the development and severity of inherited disease in those predisposed to it, as well as its risk for future generations.

Medical Care

Although environment, behavior and lifestyle, and heredity are more important determinants of health, well-being, and susceptibility to premature death, access to care is also a key factor influencing health. Both individual health and population health are closely related to access to adequate services for preventive and curative health. Nevertheless, medical care alone cannot ensure optimal health, and preventive interventions are not adequate unless individuals take responsibility for their health and well-being.

▶ Cultural Beliefs and Values

A value system helps define a society's ideals. The traditional cultural beliefs and values in the U.S. have been based on conservative principles of market justice, with social justice principles (discussed in the next section) taking a secondary place. In recent years, American society has become increasingly defined by various subcultures due to the steady influx of immigrants from different parts of the world. Such diversity promotes sociocultural variations in how people view their health and their attitudes and behaviors concerning health, illness, and death (Wolinsky, 1998, p. 39). Driven by these changing demographics, the foundational beliefs and values of U.S. culture are in a state of flux.

According to a survey conducted by the U.S. Census Bureau from 2009 to 2013, young adults today—labeled the millennial generation[1] by sociologists—differ greatly from previous generations, who are referred to as generation X and the baby boomers. A higher proportion of millennials are foreign born, one in four speaks a language other than English at home, and one in five lives in poverty even though a higher proportion have college degrees (U.S. Census Bureau, 2014). Millennials are more inclined toward social justice, for example, viewing the term *socialism* more positively and the term *capitalism* more negatively than the general population (Pew Research Center, 2011). A gradual transformation in traditional American beliefs and values is already changing the way Americans will receive care in the future.

▶ Distribution of Health Care

In a perfect world, health care production, distribution, and consumption have an equal impact on all members of a society. Unfortunately, no

---

1 The millennial generation, or millennials, commonly includes those persons born between 1982 and 2000, and numbers approximately 73 million people.

society has found a perfectly equitable method to distribute limited economic resources, and inequalities are inevitable. Societies, therefore, try to allocate resources according to guiding principles, guided by their values and belief systems. The fundamental question of distributive justice or equity is how a health care system can make essential services available to all members of society. This concern about equitable access to health care services is addressed by theories of *market justice* and *social justice*.

Market Justice

According to the principle of market justice, market forces can best achieve a fair distribution of health care services in a free economy. In such a system, medical care and benefits are distributed on the basis of people's willingness and ability to pay (Santerre & Neun, 1996, p. 7). People are entitled to purchase a share of available goods and services of interest. They must purchase these goods and services with financial resources acquired through their own legitimate efforts. This is how most goods and services are distributed in a free market. To give people something they did not earn is considered morally and economically wrong. Thus, the principle of market justice makes the following key assumptions:

- Health care, like any other economic good or service, can be governed by the free market forces of supply and demand.
- Individuals are responsible for their own achievements. When individuals pursue their own interests, the interests of society as a whole are best served (Ferguson & Maurice, 1970).
- People make rational choices in their decisions to purchase health care products and services to rectify their health problems and restore their health.
- People, in consultation with their physicians, know what is best for themselves. This implies that people place a certain degree of trust in their physicians.
- A free market, rather than the government, can allocate health care resources most efficiently and equitably.

Under a system characterized by market justice, health care production is determined by how willing and able customers are to purchase health care products and services at prevailing market prices. In a free market system, those with insufficient income or who are uninsured face financial barriers to access (Santerre & Neun, 1996, p. 7). Together, prices and ability to pay limit or ration the quantity and type of services consumed, and these limitations to access are referred to as *demand-side rationing* or price rationing. The key characteristics of market justice and their implications are summarized in **TABLE 2.1**.

TABLE 2.1 Comparison of Market Justice and Social Justice

Market Justice	Social Justice
Characteristics	
■ Views health care as an economic good	■ Views health care as a social resource
■ Assumes free market conditions for health services delivery	■ Requires active government involvement in health services delivery
■ Assumes that markets are more efficient in allocating health resources equitably	■ Assumes that the government is more efficient in allocating health resources equitably
■ Production and distribution of health care are determined by market-based demand	■ Medical resource allocation is determined by central planning
■ Medical care distribution is based on people's ability to pay	■ Ability to pay is inconsequential for receiving medical care
■ Access to medical care is viewed as an economic reward of personal effort and achievement	■ Equal access to medical services is viewed as a basic right
Implications	
■ Individual responsibility for health	■ Collective responsibility for health
■ Benefits are based on individual purchasing power	■ Everyone is entitled to a basic package of benefits
■ Limited obligation to the collective good	■ Strong obligation to the collective good
■ Emphasis on individual well-being	■ Community well-being supersedes that of the individual
■ Private solutions to social problems	■ Public solutions to social problems
■ Rationing based on ability to pay	■ Planned rationing of health care

Data from National Center for Health Statistics. Health, United States, 2016. Hyattsville, MD: U.S. Department of Health and Human Services; 2017:348

Market justice emphasizes individual, rather than collective, responsibility for health and proposes private, rather than government, solutions to social problems of health.

The principles of market justice work well in allocating economic goods when their unequal distribution does not affect the greater society. People live in different sizes and styles of homes, drive different types of automobiles, and spend money on different things based on individual success. However, market justice principles fail to rectify critical concerns such as crime, illiteracy, and homelessness, which significantly weaken the fabric of society. Recognizing the shortcomings of a free market system, many Americans suggest that health care is also a social concern.

Social Justice

The idea of social justice is at odds with the principles of capitalism and market justice. According to the principle of social justice, the equitable distribution of health care is a societal, rather than an individual, responsibility. This goal is best achieved when a central agency—usually the government—takes over the production and distribution functions. Social justice regards health care as a social good—not an economic good—to be collectively financed and available to all citizens regardless of individual ability to pay. Most industrialized countries long ago reached a consensus that health care is a social good (Reinhardt, 1994). Public health is also oriented towards social justice (Hart et al., 2017; Stoddard-Dare et al., 2017; Turnock, 1997). In a social justice system, the inability to obtain care due to a lack of financial resources is considered unjust. The principle of social justice is based on the following assumptions:

- Health care is different from most other goods and services.
- Responsibility for health is shared. Individuals are not totally responsible for their ill health because they do not control factors such as economic inequalities, unemployment, unsanitary conditions, or air pollution.
- Society has an obligation to the collective good. An unhealthy individual is a burden on society; a person carrying a deadly infection, for example, poses a threat to society. Society is obligated to eliminate (cure) the problem by providing health care to the individual, because this benefits society as a whole.
- The government, not the market, can make rational plans and better decide the quantity of health care to produce and how to make it available to all citizens.

In a social justice–based system, no country can afford to provide unlimited amounts of health care to all citizens. The government must limit the availability of certain services by deciding, for instance, how technology is distributed and who has access to certain high-tech services, even as basic services may be available to all. This concept is referred to as *planned rationing* or *supply-side rationing*. The main characteristics of social justice and their implications are summarized in Table 2.1.

Justice in the U.S. Health Care System

The current U.S. health care system is not a market justice–based system, because U.S. health care delivery does not follow principles of a free market system. A significant shift away from market justice began in 1965 with the creation of Medicare and Medicaid. Since then, the move toward social justice has been gradual, as most recently espoused in the ACA. Currently, less than half of health care financing in the U.S. comes from the government. The government also plays a major role in exercising control over the health care system through various policies for insurance, provider payment, availability of new drugs and procedures, use of information systems, medical research funding, quality initiatives, and other regulated areas.

In the U.S., the principles of market justice and social justice complement each other. Market justice drives private, employer-based health insurance, mainly for middle-income Americans. In contrast, social justice is the basis for publicly financed Medicaid, Medicare, and Children's Health Insurance Program coverage and worker's compensation programs. The two principles collide, however, when a significant number of uninsured are unable to afford insurance and are ineligible for Medicaid, Medicare, or other public programs.

▶ Strategies to Improve Health

Healthy People Initiatives

Since 1979, the United States has undertaken a series of 10-year plans outlining key national health objectives; TABLE 2.2 outlines the evolution of these *Healthy People* initiatives. These initiatives were founded on the integration of medical care with preventive services, health promotion, and education; integration of personal and community health care; and increased access to integrated care services. The *Healthy People* initiatives established benchmarks for and monitored progress towards the following goals: (1) to encourage collaborations across communities and sectors; (2) to empower individuals to make informed health decisions; and (3) to measure the impact of prevention activities (Office of Disease Prevention and Promotion, 2015a).

TABLE 2.2 Evolution of *Healthy People* Initiatives

Target Year	1990	2000	2010	2020
Overarching goals	▪ Decrease mortality: infants through adults ▪ Increase independence among older adults	▪ Increase span of healthy life ▪ Eliminate health disparities	▪ Increase quality and years of healthy life ▪ Eliminate health disparities	▪ Attain high-quality, longer lives free of preventable disease ▪ Achieve health equity; eliminate disparities ▪ Create social and physical environments that promote good health ▪ Promote quality of life, health development, and healthy behaviors across life stages
Number of topic areas	15	22	28	42
Number of objectives/measures	226	312	1,000	Approximately 1,200

Reproduced from Health People 2020. Office of Disease Prevention and Health Promotion. Retrieved from: https://www.healthypeople.gov/sites/default/files/healthy-people-overview.pdf

The current initiative, *Healthy People 2020*, launched in 2010 and building on the work of *Healthy People 2010*, takes into account achievements in the past decade, such as increased life expectancy and decreased death rate from coronary heart disease and stroke, and identifies areas for improvement in the next decade. The objectives of *Healthy People 2020* include identifying nationwide health priorities; increasing awareness and understanding of the determinants of health, disability, and disease; providing measurable objectives that apply at all levels; engaging multiple sectors to strengthen policies and improve practices driven by evidence and knowledge; and identifying critical research, evaluation, and data collection methods. *Healthy People 2020* will measure general health status, quality of life and well-being, determinants of health, and disparities (U.S. Department of Health and Human Services [DHHS], 2011).

The overarching goals of *Healthy People 2020* include the following:

- Attaining high-quality, longer lives free of preventable disease, injury, and premature death
- Achieving health equity, eliminating disparities, and improving the health of all groups
- Creating social and physical environments that promote good health for all
- Promoting quality of life, healthy development, and health behaviors across all life stages (Office of Disease Prevention and Promotion, 2015a)

The framework for *Healthy People 2020* is presented in **FIGURE 2.3**.

Four foundational health measures serve as indicators of progress toward achieving the aforementioned goals: general health status, quality of life and well-being, determinants of health, and disparities among the population (Office of Disease Prevention and Promotion, 2015a). Overall progress will include fewer adults smoking cigarettes, fewer children exposed to secondhand smoke, more adults being physically active, and fewer adolescents using alcohol or illicit drugs (DHHS, 2014; Greenberg et al., 2017).

The Healthy People Consortium is a group of organizations committed to promoting *Healthy People 2020*, and members work to ensure that the *Healthy People* initiatives meet the needs of their region, state, or community; share how their organization carries out the program; champion the goals and objectives; and participate in the program (Office of Disease Prevention and Health Promotion, 2015b).

The National Association of County and City Health Officials (NACCHO) established a partnership with *Healthy People 2020* to support and increase the use of the program among local health departments, nonprofit hospitals, and other organizations involved in community health

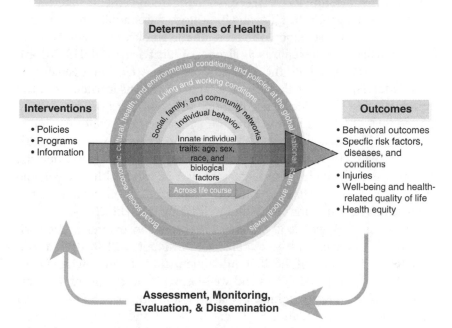

FIGURE 2.3 Action Model to Achieve *Healthy People 2020* Overarching Goals

assessment and improvement planning (NACCHO, 2015, 2017). NAC-CHO activities identify barriers and challenges, assess uptake at the local level, share examples of local use, promote use of the program through webinars and other means, offer training and technical assistance, and encourage collaborative efforts (DHHS, 2012).

In implementation, stakeholders in both public and private agencies play a crucial role. The *MAP-IT Guide* tool has been used to assemble partners, identify community needs, execute a plan, and evaluate progress. The *Healthy People 2020 state and territory coordinators* serve as liaisons to ensure that the state and/or territorial health plan aligns with the *Healthy People* goals and objectives. The *Healthy People 2020 Evidence-Based Resources Tool* allows users to search for interventions and resources by topic, objective, resource or intervention type, population, setting, and other characteristics. The *Stories from the Field* library of examples demonstrates how communities are implementing *Healthy People 2020* (DHHS, 2015a).

In terms of progress, the *Healthy People 2020* Leading Health Indicators (LHIs) are a subset of the *Healthy People* objectives chosen to communicate high-priority health issues and actions to address them. The 26 LHIs are organized into 12 topics. As of 2014, progress was made toward achieving the *Healthy People 2020* targets for the 26 LHIs, with 14 indicators (53.9%) either meeting their target or showing improvement. Noteworthy progress was made for the following indicators: fewer adults smoking cigarettes; fewer children exposed to secondhand smoke; more adults being active; and fewer adolescents using alcohol or illicit drugs (DHHS, 2015b).

Healthy People 2030, the fifth edition of the *Healthy People* program, addresses new challenges and builds on lessons learned from the initiatives' first four decades. Although progress has been made, the United States still lags behind other Organization for Economic Cooperation and Development (OECD) countries in key measures of health and well-being, including life expectancy, infant mortality, and obesity, despite spending the highest percentage of GDP on health. A challenge for *Healthy People 2030* is to guide the United States in achieving the population's potential for health and well-being (DHHS, 2017).

As *Healthy People 2030* is being developed, an overall framework with new objectives will be established. Although still in draft form, the overarching goals of the 2030 initiative include the following: (1) to attain healthy, purposeful lives and well-being; (2) attain health literacy, achieve health equity, eliminate disparities, and improve the health and well-being of all populations; (3) create social and physical environments that nurture the full potential for the health and well-being for all; (4) promote healthy development, healthy behaviors, and well-being throughout all life stages; and (5) engage with stakeholders and key constituents across sectors to take action and design policies to improve the health and well-being of all populations (DHHS, 2017).

Public Health

In contrast to individual health, *public health* focuses on improving population health and well-being. As an example of social justice, government plays the central role in developing and enhancing the public health infrastructure—at the national, state, and local levels—through tax dollars. Health indicators are developed to evaluate the effectiveness of the public health system, along with a national surveillance system to consistently track these indicators. Determinants of population health play a major role in evaluation.

Focus on Determinants

To improve the nation's health and minimize health disparities among its vulnerable populations, a framework embodying social and medical determinants must be developed. This framework, presented in **FIGURE 2.4**, places a balanced emphasis on both types of determinants, because it is the combination of these factors that shapes health and well-being. This

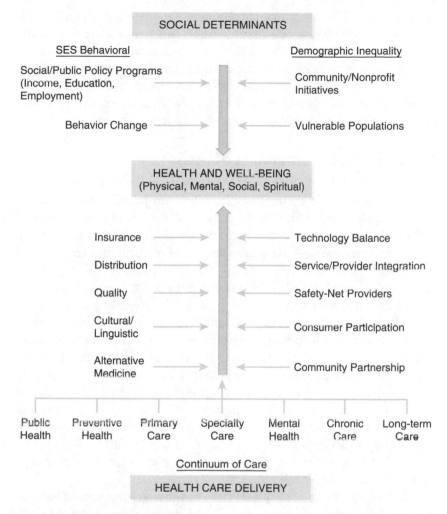

FIGURE 2.4 Social Determinants of Health

Secretary's Advisory Committee on Health Promotion and Disease Prevention Objectives for 2020. Phase I report recommendations for the framework and format of Healthy People 2010, p. 8, Exhibit A. http://www.healthypeople.gov/2010/hp2020/Advisory/PhaseI/PhaseI.pdf.

model synthesizes multiple influences and highlights points for intervention. In this model, health is not merely a state of being free of disease and disability, but it also includes the positive concept of well-being and encompasses the physical, mental, social, and spiritual aspects of health.

Social Determinants of Health

The framework presented in Figure 2.4 acknowledges the effects of demographics, socioeconomic status, individual behavior, and community inequalities and their influence on health. Personal demographics (e.g., race/ethnicity or age) directly affect vulnerability. Social and income inequalities also influence health disparities. Whether socioeconomic status is defined by education, employment, or income, both individual- and community-level socioeconomic status independently affect health. The health impact of individual behavior—such as smoking or exercise— is rarely isolated from its social and environmental contexts. Accordingly, the WHO Commission on Social Determinants of Health (2007) concluded that the social conditions in which people are born, live, and work are the single most important determinant of health status.

Medical Care Determinants of Health

Although social determinants affect health status, the medical care system focuses primarily on treating illness or poor health. Preventive care is an exception, and understanding the effects of care on health should include considering disparities in basic health care access and quality. The framework includes a broad spectrum of medical care services and health interventions. Whereas some services (preventive and primary care) contribute to overall health status, others are more influential in end-of-life situations (hospice and long-term care). As patients move across the spectrum, they may contend with fragmentation, poor continuity of care, and insufficient coordination of care for multiple health needs. In recent years, the Pan-American Health Organization (PAHO) and WHO updated their primary health care strategy to focus on improving countries' capacity to implement coordinated, effective, and sustainable strategies. Based on the concept of universal coverage and access to services, these strategies aim to sustainably improve population health and reduce health inequalities (PAHO, 2015, 2016). Services for mental health and chronic diseases are included in the primary health care framework (PAHO, 2015).

The relative value of health services in the spectrum should be evaluated when determining health policy. For example, should equal investments be made in each service, or are some investments better than others (e.g., primary care versus specialty care)? How can we optimize the medical system's potential for eliminating disparities using limited resources (e.g., focusing on primary care for all versus high-technology care for certain populations)? Other factors, such as quality of care, access to alternative therapies, and technology, also affect patient experience and health outcomes.

Social and Medical Points of Intervention

Considering that social and medical determinants respond to numerous forces, the framework highlights important points for health interventions. Dramatic reductions in health disparities can be attained through interventions in both the social and medical domains, according to four main strategies: (1) social or public policy interventions, (2) community-based interventions, (3) health care interventions, and (4) individual interventions.

Policy Interventions. Public policy directly guards the welfare of the nation through product safety regulations, screening food and water sources, enforcing safe work environments, and other ways. With fewer resources, however, vulnerable populations are uniquely dependent on social and public policy for programs that address basic nutritional, safety, social service, and health care needs.

One example of policy intervention is the Occupation Safety and Health Act of 1970, which created the Occupational Safety and Health Administration (OSHA) to protect employees from the potential dangers of an unsafe environment at the workplace. OSHA established the Injury and Illness Prevention Program, which requires employers to implement a system that ensures employees' compliance with a safe and healthy work environment. OSHA also provides on-site consultation to help small businesses establish occupational health and safety management systems (Autenrieth et al., 2015). This work is part of an overall effort to effectively identify workplace hazards and protect employees who otherwise may work in dangerous environments (Autenrieth et al., 2015; U.S. Department of Labor, 2011).

Health care reform also constitutes a policy intervention. The ACA, when it was enacted in 2010, made major changes to the U.S. health care and health insurance systems, significantly reducing the number and percentage of people without insurance. Coverage helps save lives, by encouraging early detection and prevention of serious medical conditions. More than 9.2 million people signed up for care on the national exchange in 2017, down by about 400,000 from 2016, but the fate of the ACA remains uncertain under the Trump administration. With the individual mandate to purchase health care insurance being repealed in 2019, the Congressional Budget Office (CBO) estimates that 13 million people will lose their insurance by 2027. An estimated 5 million of them previously bought health insurance as individuals either within or outside the ACA's marketplaces. Some will choose not to buy insurance, because the penalty has been lifted. Others, especially higher-income individuals ineligible for subsidies under the ACA, will likely drop their insurance because of increases in the average premiums predicted by the CBO. These premium increases will occur because, as the mandate is repealed, many young, healthy people will exit the health care markets, leaving behind a sicker, more costly insurance pool, and older individuals will be most affected (CBO, 2017).

Community-Based Interventions. Many sources of health disparities may be addressed at the community or local level. Neighborhood poverty, lack of health and social welfare resources, and lack of societal cohesion can contribute to inequalities in a community. Understanding the multidimensional risks and needs in a community can better equip the local agencies that are responsible for designing interventions to address health disparities in their communities; EXHIBIT 2.3 provides some examples of the interventions that may be developed. Community partnerships reflect the priorities of a population and are often managed by community members, and minimize cultural barriers and improve community buy-in to health improvement programs.

Addressing disparities using community approaches has several other advantages. Local businesses and other partners often have a stake in local health causes that help needy members of the community. Community leaders can play a central role in planning and managing strategies to improve health, and community solutions benefit from participatory decision-making in which community members are involved. Moreover, many community programs are run by nonprofit organizations, which are subsidized through federal, state, or local funds, and receive tax exemptions for their services. Thus, they offer services at lower cost than private health organizations, which are obligated to their shareholders to price services competitively.

For example, to counteract the rise in childhood obesity, many schools are beginning school-based nutritional programs. These multicomponent interventions involve administrators, food services staff, teachers, parents, and students. Teaching students proper nutrition in the classroom while educating parents makes the program more likely to succeed in curbing childhood obesity (Black et al., 2017).

Health Care Interventions. Health care interventions such as integrated electronic medical records systems can improve patient care and prevent safety events while simultaneously reducing waste in the health care system (Bae et al., 2017; Dorman & Miller, 2011; Hillestad et al.,

EXHIBIT 2.3 Strategies to Improve Health and Reduce Disparities

- Nutrition programs
- Work/environment safety efforts
- Community-based partnerships
- Culturally appropriate care
- Patient safety/medical error reduction
- Prevention-oriented effort
- Coordinated care for chronically ill persons

2005; Karafin et al., 2017; Kruse et al., 2017; Ratanawongsa et al., 2017; Sperl-Hillen et al., 2011). Electronic health records also promise to improve health care quality through better coordination and integration of care among providers. Coordinated, integrated care is particularly important in light of the increasing burden of chronic disease. For example, coordination of care and counseling for type 2 diabetes patients has been shown to improve blood glucose management.

Another example of a health care intervention is "value-based care." As health care delivery evolves rapidly worldwide and in the United States, there has been a rapid shift in reimbursement in the past few years, from a simple fee-for-service model to complex models that link payment to quality and value. Change in any large system can be difficult, but the transition to a value-based system is particularly challenging in health care, because both quality and cost are difficult to quantify. Professional societies and other medical groups are developing programs to define high-value care. Transitioning from a volume-based to a value-based care delivery and payment model of health care will be one of the most important efforts in health care delivery in the coming decade.

Value is defined as the quality of care achieved (numerator) divided by the cost of care (denominator) (Porter, 2010; Porter & Teisberg, 2006). In pragmatic terms, value is patient health outcomes achieved per dollar spent. Value is created through the quality of care delivered, not strictly by the volume of services provided (Institute for Healthcare Improvement, 2016). This value-based care movement recognizes what patients value in the context of defining health and health care outcomes and allocating limited resources.

The American Society of Clinical Oncology (ASCO) published a conceptual framework in 2015 to help physicians and patients make treatment decisions: the ASCO framework considers cost, along with more traditional clinical outcomes (Schnipper et al., 2015). In addition, the Centers for Medicare and Medicaid Services (CMS) has begun to change how hospitals and physicians are paid, with payments increasingly being tied to measures of quality (Burwell, 2015). The Medicare Access and CHIP Reauthorization Act (MACRA) eliminated the sustainable growth-rate (SGR) formula and directed the U.S. Department of Health and Human Services to develop infrastructure for quality measurement instead, as part of the government's attempt to transition from fee-for-service systems to reimbursement based on quality of care.

Individual-Level Interventions. Individual-level initiatives are critical in counteracting the effects of negative social determinants on health status. Altering individual health behaviors (e.g., reducing smoking and increasing exercise) is often the focus of individual-targeted interventions, and numerous theories have been promulgated to identify the complex pathways and barriers to changes or improvements in behavior. Integrating behavioral science into public health has been a valuable contribution, providing a toolbox of behavior-changing strategies for health.

▶ Conclusion

Health and health determinants are multifactorial. Medical care, while important, is only one factor that contributes to health and well-being. Factors such as physical, social, cultural, and economic environments; behaviors and lifestyles; and heredity all play roles in determining health and well-being for individuals and populations. Nowadays, health care delivery is primarily driven by the medical model, which emphasizes illness rather than wellness. Many efforts to improve health care delivery have failed to produce a proportionate impact on the improvement of health status. Applying holistic concepts of care, and integrating medical care with preventive and health promotion efforts, could significantly improve health, although it would require a fundamental change in how Americans think of health. It would also require individual responsibility for behavior and community partnerships to improve both personal and community health. Understanding the determinants of health, health education, community health assessment, and national initiatives such as *Healthy People 2020* is essential for accomplishing such goals.

Over the years, the U.S. health care system has gradually transitioned toward an emphasis on social justice, yet not all Americans enjoy equal access to care. To improve the nation's health and reduce disparities among its vulnerable populations, both the social and medical determinants of health must be addressed.

References

1. Autenrieth DA, et al. 2015. Client perceptions of occupational health and safety management system assistance provided by OSHA on-site consultation: Results of a survey of Colorado small business consultation clients. *J Occup Environ Hyg.* 12(11):804–817. doi: 10.1080/15459624.2015.1049270.
2. Bae J, Rask KJ, Becker ER. April 1, 2017. The impact of electronic medical records on hospital-acquired adverse safety events: Differential effects between single-source and multiple-source systems. *Am J Med Qual.* 1062860617702453. doi: 10.1177/1062860617702453.
3. Bauer AG, et al. 2017. Do black women's religious beliefs about body image influence their confidence in their ability to lose weight? *Prevent Chronic Dis.* 14:E98. doi: 10.5888/pcd14.170153.
4. Black AP, et al. 2017. How effective are family-based and institutional nutrition interventions in improving children's diet and health? A systematic review. *BMC Public Health.* 17(1):818-017-4795-5. doi: 10.1186/s12889-017-4795-5.

5. Burwell SM. 2015. Setting value-based payment goals: HHS efforts to improve US health care. *N Engl J Med*. 372(10):897–899.
6. Congressional Budget Office (CBO). 2017. Repealing the individual health insurance mandate: An updated estimate. https://www.cbo.gov/publication/53300. Accessed March 19, 2018.
7. Dorman T, Miller BM. 2011. Continuing medical education: The link between physician learning and health care outcomes. *Acad Med*. 86(11):1339.
8. Ferguson CE, Maurice SC. 1970. *Economic analysis*. Homewood, IL: Richard D. Irwin.
9. Greenberg AJ, et al. 2017. Public use of electronic personal health information: Measuring progress of the *Healthy People 2020* objectives. *Health Policy Technol*. 6(1):33–39. doi: 10.1016/j.hlpt.2016.08.003.
10. Hart M, et al. 2017. Twitter and public health (part 2): Qualitative analysis of how individual health professionals outside organizations use microblogging to promote and disseminate health-related information. *JMIR Public Health Surveill*. 3(4):e54. doi: 10.2196/publichealth.6796.
11. Hillestad R, et al. 2005. Can electronic medical record systems transform health care? Potential health benefits, savings, and costs. *Health Aff*, 24(5):1103–1117.
12. Institute for Healthcare Improvement. 2016. QCV100: An introduction to quality, cost, and value in health care. http://app.ihi.org/lms/home.aspx. Accessed December 11, 2017.
13. Kaplan GA, et al. 1996. Income inequality and mortality in the United States. *Br Med J*. 312(7037):999–1003.
14. Karafin MS, et al. 2017. National Heart, Lung, and Blood Institute Recipient Epidemiology and Donor Evaluation Study-III (REDS-III). Demographic and epidemiologic characterization of transfusion recipients from four US regions: Evidence from the REDS-III recipient database. *Transfusion*. doi: 10.1111/trf.14370.
15. Kawachi I, et al. 1997. Social capital, income inequality, and mortality. *Am J Publ Health*. 87:1491–1498.
16. Kennedy BP, et al. 1996. Income distribution and mortality: Cross sectional ecological study of the Robin Hood Index in the United States. *Br Med J*. 312(7037):1004–1007.
17. Kruse CS, et al. 2017. Impact of electronic health records on long-term care facilities: Systematic review. *JMIR Med Informatics*. 5(3):e35. doi: 10.2196/medinform.7958.
18. Levin JS. 1994. Religion and health: is there an association, is it valid, and is it causal? *Soc Sci Med*. 38(11):1475–1482.
19. Loureiro ACT, et al. 2017. The influence of spirituality and religiousness on suicide risk and mental health of patients undergoing hemodialysis. *Comprehen Psychiatry*. 80:39–45. doi: S0010-440X(17)30195-5.
20. Mackenbach JP. 1997. Socioeconomic inequalities in morbidity and mortality in Western Europe. *Lancet*. 349:1655–1660.
21. Marwick C. 1995. Should physicians prescribe prayer for health? Spiritual aspects of well-being considered. *JAMA*. 273(20):1561–1562.
22. Maugans TA. 1996. The SPIRITual history. *Arch Fam Med*. 5(1):11–16.
23. McCullough ME, et al. 2000. Religious involvement and mortality: A meta-analytic review. *Health Psychol*. 19(3):211–222.
24. McKee M. 2001. Measuring the efficiency of health systems. *Br Med J*. 323 (7308):295–296.
25. National Association of County and City Health Officials (NACCHO). 2015. *Healthy People 2020*—NACCHO partnership. http://www.naccho.org/topics/infrastructure /healthy-people/index.cfm. Accessed August 2, 2015.
26. National Association of County and City Health Officials (NACCHO). 2017. Health in all policies: Experiences from local health departments. https://www.naccho.org

/uploads/downloadable-resources/HiAP-Report_Experiences-from-Local-Health-Departments-Feb-2017.pdf. Accessed December 10, 2017.

27. Office of Disease Prevention and Promotion, Healthy People. 2015a. About *Healthy People*. https://www.healthypeople.gov/2020/About-Healthy-People. Accessed August 2, 2015.

28. Office of Disease Prevention and Health Promotion, Healthy People. 2015b. *Healthy People 2020. Healthy People* in action: Consortium members. https://www.healthypeople.gov/2020/healthy-people-in-action/Consortium-Members. Accessed August 2, 2015.

29. Pan-American Health Organization (PAHO). 2015. Primary health care strategy. World Health Organization. http://iris.paho.org/xmlui/handle/123456789/4031. Accessed March 28, 2018.

30. Pan-American Health Organization (PAHO). 2016. Inequities and barriers in health systems. http://www.paho.org/salud-en-las-americas-2017/?tag=primary-health-care-strategy. Accessed December 2017.

31. Parsons T. 1972. Definitions of health and illness in the light of American values and social structure. In: Jaco EG, ed. *Patients, physicians and illness: A sourcebook in behavioral science and health*. 2nd ed. New York, NY: Free Press.

32. Pew Research Center. 2011. Little change in public's response to "capitalism," "socialism." http://www.people-press.org/2011/12/28/little-change-in-publics-response-to-capitalism-socialism/?src=prc-headline. Accessed July 2015.

33. Peykari N, et al. 2015. Socioeconomic inequalities and diabetes: A systematic review from Iran. *J Diab Metab Disord*. 14:8-015-0135-4. eCollection 2015. doi: 10.1186/s40200-015-0135-4.

34. Porter ME. 2010. What is value in health care? *N Engl J Med*. 363(26):2477–2481.

35. Porter ME, Teisberg EO. 2006. *Redefining health care: Creating value-based competition on results*. Boston, MA: Harvard Business School Press.

36. Rainville G. 2017. The interrelation of prayer and worship service attendance in moderating the negative impact of life event stressors on mental well-being. *J Religion Health*. doi: 10.1007/s10943-017-0494-x.

37. Ratanawongsa N, et al. 2017. The challenges of electronic health records and diabetes electronic prescribing: Implications for safety net care for diverse populations. *J Diab Res*. 2017:8983237. doi: 10.1155/2017/8983237.

38. Reinhardt UE. 1994. Providing access to health care and controlling costs: The universal dilemma. In: Lee PR, Estes CL, eds. *The nation's health*. 4th ed. Sudbury, MA: Jones and Bartlett; 263–278.

39. Ross L. 1995. The spiritual dimension: Its importance to patients' health, well-being and quality of life and its implications for nursing practice. *Intl J Nurs Stud*. 32(5):457–468.

40. Santerre RE, Neun SP. 1996. *Health economics: Theories, insights, and industry studies*. Chicago, IL: Irwin.

41. Saward E, Sorensen A. 1980. The current emphasis on preventive medicine. In: Williams SJ, ed. *Issues in health services*. New York, NY: John Wiley & Sons; 17–29.

42. Schnipper LE, et al. 2015. American Society of Clinical Oncology statement: A conceptual framework to assess the value of cancer treatment options. *J Clin Oncol*. 33(23):2563–2577.

43. Society for Academic Emergency Medicine (SAEM), Ethics Committee. 1992. An ethical foundation for health care: An emergency medicine perspective. *Ann Emerg Med*. 21:1381–1387.

44. Sperl-Hillen J, et al. 2011. Comparative effectiveness of patient education methods for type 2 diabetes: A randomized controlled trial. *Arch Intern Med*. 171(22):2001–2010.

45. Stoddard-Dare P, et al. 2017. Paid sick leave and psychological distress: An analysis of U.S. workers. *Am J Orthopsychiatry.* doi: 10.1037/ort0000293.
46. Swanson CS. 1995. A spirit-focused conceptual model of nursing for the advanced practice nurse. *Issues Comprehen Pediatr Nurs.* 18(4):267–275.
47. Syden L, Landberg J. 2017. The contribution of alcohol use and other lifestyle factors to socioeconomic differences in all-cause mortality in a Swedish cohort. *Drug Alcohol Rev.* 36(5):691–700. doi: 10.1111/dar.12472.
48. Timmreck TC. 1994. *An introduction to epidemiology.* Sudbury, MA: Jones and Bartlett.
49. Turnock BJ. 1997. *Public health: What it is and how it works.* Gaithersburg, MD: Aspen.
50. U.S. Census Bureau. 2014. New Census Bureau statistics show how young adults today compare with previous generations in neighborhoods nationwide. http://www .census.gov/newsroom/press-releases/2014/cb14-219.html. Accessed June 2015.
51. U.S. Department of Health and Human Services (DHHS). 2011. About *Healthy People.* http://www.healthypeople.gov/2020/about/default.aspx. Accessed December 10, 2011.
52. U.S. Department of Health and Human Services (DHHS). 2012. Office of Disease Prevention and Promotion, Healthy People. Using *Healthy People 2020* to achieve your goals: Implementation, action, and new tools. Presentation. http://www .healthypeople.gov/sites/default/files/HP_Stakeholder%20Webinar_110712_508 _PPT.pdf. Accessed December 2012.
53. U.S. Department of Health and Human Services (DHHS), Office of Disease Prevention and Health Promotion. 2014. *Healthy People 2020* leading health indicators: Progress update. http://www.healthypeople.gov/sites/default/files/LHI -ProgressReport-ExecSum_0.pdf. Accessed Aug.2014.
54. U.S. Department of Health and Human Services (DHHS). 2015a. Implementing *Healthy People 2020* in state and territorial health agencies. http://www.astho .org/Programs/Prevention/Healthy-People-2020-Overview-Slide-Deck/. Accessed December 10, 2017.
55. U.S. Department of Health and Human Services (DHHS). 2015b. *Healthy People 2020* leading health indicators: Progress update. https://www.healthypeople.gov/sites /default/files/LHI-ProgressReport-ExecSum_0.pdf. Accessed December 10, 2017.
56. U.S. Department of Health and Human Services (DHHS). 2017. *Healthy People 2030* draft framework. https://www.healthypeople.gov/2020/About-Healthy-People /Development-Healthy-People-2030/Draft-Framework. Accessed December 10, 2017.
57. U.S. Department of Labor. 2011. Injury and illness prevention programs. https://www.dol .gov/osha/regs/unifiedagenda/fall2010/1218-AC48.htm. Accessed December 10, 2011.
58. Ward B. 1995. Holistic medicine. *Austral Fam Phys.* 24(5):761–762, 765.
59. WHO Commission on Social Determinants of Health. 2007. *A conceptual framework for action on the social determinants of health.* Geneva, Switzerland: World Health Organization. http://www.who.int/social_determinants/resources/csdh_framework _action_05_07.pdf. Accessed June 2015.
60. Wolinsky F. 1998. *The sociology of health: Principles, practitioners, and issues.* 2nd ed. Belmont, CA: Wadsworth.
61. World Health Organization (WHO). 1948. *Preamble to the Constitution.* Geneva, Switzerland: World Health Organization.

CHAPTER 3

Historical Overview of U.S. Health Care Delivery

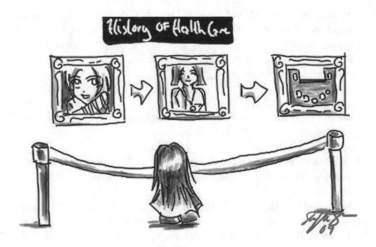

▶ Introduction

Knowledge of the history of health care is essential for understanding the main characteristics of the medical delivery system as it exists today. For example, the system's historical foundations explain why a government-run national health care system has not materialized in the United States. This is unlike what exists in Canada and Great Britain, for instance. Instead, the United States has predominantly a private health care industry that also receives a fairly substantial amount of financing from the government.

Traditionally held American cultural beliefs and values, the social fabric of the American society, technological advances, economic constraints, political opportunism, and ecological forces are the main historical factors that have continued to shape U.S. health care delivery; examples are provided in **EXHIBIT 3.1**. The ebb and flow of the same forces will shape health care's future direction.

The agents of change just mentioned often interact in a complex manner. For example, President Barack Obama's political agenda trumped economic constraints and led to the enactment of the Affordable Care Act (ACA; nicknamed "Obamacare") in 2010 through ideological and political maneuvering. Historically, the beliefs and values espoused by the majority of Americans—such as capitalism, self-reliance, and limited government—have been primarily responsible for shielding the U.S. health care system from a major overhaul. Conversely, social, political, and economic forces led to certain compromises, as seen in the creation of Medicare and Medicaid and other public programs to extend health care to certain defined groups of people. The growing political clout of

---

EXHIBIT 3.1 Major Forces of Change in U.S. Health Care Delivery

- Cultural beliefs and values
  - Self-reliance
  - Welfare assistance for the needy
- Social makeup
  - Demographic shifts
  - Immigration
  - Health status
  - Urbanization
- Technological advances
  - Scientific research
  - New treatments
  - Training of health professionals
  - Facilities and equipment
  - Information technology
- Economic constraints
  - Health care costs
  - Private and public health insurance
  - Family incomes
- Political opportunism
  - President's agenda
  - Political party ideology
  - Political maneuvers
  - Power of interest groups
  - Laws and regulations
- Ecological forces
  - New diseases
  - Drug-resistant infections
  - Global travel and transport

the elderly population in the United States, for example, was instrumental in the addition of a prescription drug benefit to Medicare in 2003.

Advancements in science and technology have played a major role in shaping the U.S. health care delivery system. As a result, medical practice in the United States is highly specialized, while basic and routine primary care is given only secondary importance.

This chapter traces the evolution of health care delivery through four recognizable historical periods, each demarcating a major change in the structure of the medical delivery system. The first phase is the *preindustrial era*, which lasted from the middle of the 18th century until the latter part of the 19th century. The second phase is the *postindustrial era*, which began in the late 19th century. The third phase—called the *corporate era*—includes developments that started around 1970 and continue into the 21st century. The fourth phase, which is still in its infancy, is characterized by health care reform—namely, the passage of the ACA and its potential repeal and replacement.

▶ Medical Services in Preindustrial America

From colonial times to the late 1800s, medical education and practice were far more advanced in Great Britain, France, and Germany than they were in the United States. The practice of medicine in the United States had a strong domestic—rather than professional—character because medical procedures were rather primitive. The nation had only a handful of hospitals. There was no health insurance, private or public. Therefore, health care had to be purchased using personal funds, and health care was delivered in a free market. The main characteristics of health care delivery during this period are summarized in **EXHIBIT 3.2**.

Medical Training

Until around 1870, medical training was largely received through individual apprenticeship with a practicing physician rather than through university education. It is ironic that many of the preceptors under whom medical students apprenticed were themselves poorly trained (Rothstein, 1972, p. 86). Only a small number of medical schools existed at that time. To train a larger number of students than was possible through apprenticeship, American physicians began opening medical schools, albeit mainly to supplement their incomes by collecting student fees that were paid directly to the physicians.

These physicians did not have classroom facilities at their disposal, however, nor did they have the authority to confer the doctor of medicine (MD) degree. Hence, they had to affiliate with local colleges to use

EXHIBIT 3.2 Health Care Delivery in Preindustrial America

- Medical training and education were not grounded in science.
- Primitive medical procedures were practiced.
- Intense competition existed because any tradesman could practice medicine.
- People relied on family members, neighbors, and publications for domestic remedies.
- Physicians' fees were paid out of personal funds.
- Health care was delivered in a free market.
- Hospitals were few in number and located only in big cities.
- Hospitals had poor sanitation and unskilled staff.
- Almshouses served the destitute and disruptive elements of society and provided some basic nursing care.
- State governments operated asylums for patients with untreatable, chronic mental illness.
- Pesthouses quarantined people with contagious diseases.
- Dispensaries delivered outpatient charity care in urban areas.

their facilities and confer degrees. As part of this approach, four or more physicians would get together to form a faculty. Medical schools were inexpensive to operate and often quite profitable. It is estimated that 42 such schools were in operation in the United States in 1850 (Rothstein, 1972, p. 91).

Medical education at this point was still seriously lacking in science. The 2-year MD degree required attending courses for 3 to 4 months during the first year and then essentially repeating the same coursework during the second year. Because fees were paid only as the student passed each course, low standards and a less-than-rigorous curriculum were necessary to attract and retain students. Even the best medical schools admitted students without a high school diploma. Training in the biological sciences was considered useful but not essential. Laboratories were nonexistent. Library facilities were inadequate, and clinical observation and practice were not part of the curriculum (Starr, 1982).

Medical Practice

The early practice of medicine can be regarded more as a trade than as a profession, because medical education was not grounded in science. It most assuredly lacked the prestige it has today. First, it did not require a rigorous course of study, clinical practice, residency training, board exams, and licensing, without all of which it is impossible to practice medicine today. Second, medical procedures were primitive because medical science was still in its infancy. Bleeding, use of emetics, and purging with enemas and purgatives were popular forms of clinical therapy in early medicine.

Treatment of mentally ill patients was even more inhumane compared to current practices. Mental illness was often viewed as aberrant behavior, for which the treatment was to apply penal methods to restore sanity. Dr. Benjamin Rush (1749–1813), known as the father of American psychiatry, believed that mental illness was caused by irritation of the blood vessels in the brain. His treatment methods included bleeding, purging, hot and cold baths, and mercury (National Library of Medicine, 2014).

Surgery was limited because anesthesia had not yet been developed, and antiseptic techniques were not known. The stethoscope and x-rays had not been discovered. The clinical thermometer was not in use, and the microscope was not available for medical diagnosis. Physicians mainly relied on their five senses and experience to diagnose and treat medical problems. Hence, in most cases, physicians did not possess technical expertise any greater than that possessed by family members at home and experienced neighbors in the local community.

One of the main consequences of nonprofessional medicine was that anyone—trained or untrained—could practice as a physician. The clergy, for example, often combined medical services and religious duties. The generally well-educated clergymen and government officials were actually more learned in medicine than many physicians (Shryock, 1966, p. 252). Tradesmen such as tailors, barbers, commodity merchants, and those engaged in numerous other trades also practiced the healing arts by selling herbal prescriptions, nostrums, elixirs, and cathartics. The red-and-white striped poles (symbolizing blood and bandages) outside barber shops today are reminders that barbers also functioned as surgeons at one time, using the same blade to cut hair, shave beards, and perform bloodletting.

This system of free entry into medical practice created intense competition. Physicians did not enjoy the status, influence, and income that they do today. Indeed, many physicians found it necessary to engage in a second occupation because income from their medical practice alone was inadequate to support a family. It is estimated that most physicians' incomes in the mid-1800s put them in the lower echelon of the middle class (Starr, 1982, p. 84).

In the small communities of rural America, a spirit of strong self-reliance prevailed. Families and communities treated the sick using folk remedies that were passed on from one generation to the next. It was common for people to consult published books and pamphlets on home remedies (Rosen, 1983, p. 2). The market for physicians' services was also limited by affordability. Most families simply could not afford the cost because they had to pay for services out of pocket, without the help of health insurance. Also, most Americans resided in small rural communities, and summoning a physician could require traveling for several hours, and sometimes an entire day, which resulted in loss of work and income.

Medical Institutions

Before the 1880s, the United States had only a few isolated hospitals, which were found in large cities such as New York, Boston, New Orleans, St. Louis, and Philadelphia. In France and Great Britain, in contrast, general hospital expansion began long before the 1800s (Stevens, 1971, pp. 9–10). In Europe, medical professionals were closely associated with hospitals and readily adopted new advances in medical science. The situation was much different in the United States, where hospitals were characterized by deplorable sanitary conditions and poor ventilation. Unhygienic practices prevailed because nurses were generally unskilled and untrained. It was far more dangerous to receive care in a hospital than at home. Hospitals had a popular image as houses of death and institutions of welfare. People went to hospitals only because of dire circumstances, not by personal choice.

The forerunner of today's hospitals and nursing homes in the United States was the *almshouse* (also called a *poorhouse*). Almshouses existed in almost all cities of moderate size and were run by the local government. The almshouse was not a health care institution in the true sense, but rather a place where the destitute and disruptive elements of society were confined. The inmates, as they were called, included many of the elderly, the homeless, orphans, the ill, and the disabled of the community. They were given food, shelter, and some basic nursing care if needed. In many cases, the almshouse was an infirmary, old-age facility, mental asylum, homeless shelter, and orphanage all rolled into one institution. Living conditions in these institutions were squalid, and they were a far cry from today's health care facilities. Thus the early health care institutions emerged mainly to take care of indigent people who could not be cared for by their own families.

An *asylum*—commonly referred to as a *lunatic asylum*—was the forerunner of today's inpatient psychiatric facilities. Although almshouses were used to accommodate some mental patients, asylums were built by state governments for patients with untreatable, chronic mental illness. Actually, asylums were established out of humanitarian considerations; they were intended to prevent aimlessly wandering people with serious mental illness from being put in jail (Norris, 2017). Attendants in these asylums employed physical and psychological techniques in an effort to return patients to some level of rational thinking. Dr. Benjamin Rush, for example, invented a tranquilizer chair[1] and a spinning gyrator for psychiatric patients that induced vertigo, perspiration, and nausea.

---

1 The online *Psychology Dictionary* describes it as a heavy wooden chair in which the patient would be strapped across his or her chest, abdomen, knees, and ankles, with his or her head inserted into a wooden box (https://psychologydictionary.org/tranquilizer-chair/).

Another type of institution, the *pesthouse*, was operated by local governments to isolate people who had contracted a contagious disease such as cholera, smallpox, typhoid, or yellow fever. Their main function was to contain the spread of communicable disease and protect the inhabitants of a city.

Dispensaries were established as outpatient clinics to provide free care to those who could not afford to pay. They provided basic medical care and dispensed drugs to ambulatory patients (Raffel, 1980, p. 239). Around 1900 in the United States, approximately 100 dispensaries were located in large cities (Madison, 1990). Generally, young physicians and medical students desiring clinical experience staffed the dispensaries (as well as hospital wards) on a part-time basis for little or no income (Martensen, 1996). The dispensary can be regarded as the forerunner of today's more than 1,200 free and charitable clinics where services are delivered mainly by trained volunteer staff to the poor, the homeless, and the uninsured.

▶ Medical Services in Postindustrial America

The postindustrial era was marked by the growth and development of a medical profession that benefited from urbanization, new scientific discoveries, and reforms in medical education. American physicians formed professional organizations that acted as a powerful force in resisting proposals for a national health care program. The private practice of medicine, free from employment by hospitals and corporations, became firmly entrenched as physicians organized into a cohesive profession, opted for specialization, and gained power and prestige. The hospital emerged as a repository for high-tech facilities and equipment. Private and public health insurance took roots. Notable developments of this era are summarized in **EXHIBIT 3.3**.

Medical Profession

Notably, much of the transformation in U.S. medicine occurred in the aftermath of the American Civil War (1861–1865), as the country transitioned from a rural agricultural economy to a system of industrial capitalism. Urban development attracted increasingly more Americans to the growing towns and cities. In 1840, only 11% of the U.S. population lived in urban areas; by 1900, that share had increased to 40% (Stevens, 1971, p. 34).

Urbanization created increased reliance on the specialized skills of paid professionals, as this trend distanced people from family-based care. At the same time, urbanization led to the concentration of medical practice in cities and towns, where office-based practice began

EXHIBIT 3.3 Notable Developments During the Postindustrial Era

- Urbanization
- Scientific discoveries and their applications in medicine
  - Advanced science-based treatments
  - Rising health care costs
  - Imbalance between specialists and generalists
- Medical education reform
- Power and prestige of physicians
- Organized medicine
  - Control over medical training
  - Powerful political interest group
  - Support of licensing laws
  - Opposition to national health insurance proposals
  - Support of private entrepreneurship in medical practice
- Hospitals became true medical care institutions
- Reform of mental health care
- Growth of private health insurance
- Creation of Medicare and Medicaid

to replace house calls. Closer geographic proximity to their patients enabled physicians to see more patients in a given amount of time. Their greater productivity, in turn, produced higher incomes for the physicians.

As medicine became increasingly driven by science and technology, lay people could no longer deliver legitimate medical care. Science-based medicine also created an increased demand for the advanced services that only trained professionals could provide. Developments in bacteriology, antiseptic surgery, anesthesia, immunology, and diagnostic techniques, along with a growing array of new drugs, helped bring medical practice into the category of a legitimate profession. **EXHIBIT 3.4** summarizes some of the groundbreaking early scientific discoveries in medicine made during this era.

The preoccupation with science and technology in the American culture brought numerous benefits, but also produced some undesirable effects. For example, an overemphasis on the use of technology in medical care delivery created a bias toward specialization in medical training, which ultimately ended up creating far too many specialists in relation to generalists. Technology and specialization also increased the cost of medical care, but without significantly improving the health status of Americans. In contrast, other developed nations emphasized primary care in which, apart from delivering routine and basic care, a primary care physician and trained nurses ensured the continuity, coordination, and appropriateness of medical services received by a patient.

EXHIBIT 3.4 Groundbreaking Medical Discoveries

- The discovery of anesthesia was instrumental in advancing the practice of surgery. Nitrous oxide (laughing gas) was first employed as an anesthetic around 1846 for tooth extraction by Horace Wells, a dentist. Later, ether and chloroform were used as anesthetics. Before the anesthetic properties of certain gases were discovered, strong doses of alcohol were used to dull the sensations. The surgeon who could do procedures, such as limb amputations, in the shortest length of time was held in high regard.
- Around 1847, Ignaz Semmelweis, a Hungarian physician practicing in a hospital in Vienna, implemented the policy of hand washing. Thus an aseptic technique was born. Semmelweis was concerned about the high death rate from puerperal fever among women after childbirth. Even though the germ theory of disease was unknown at this time, Semmelweis surmised that there might be a connection between puerperal fever and the common practice by medical students of not washing their hands before delivering babies and right after doing dissections. Semmelweis's hunch was right.
- Louis Pasteur is generally credited with pioneering the germ theory of disease and microbiology around 1860. Pasteur demonstrated sterilization techniques, such as boiling to kill microorganisms and withholding exposure to air to prevent contamination.
- Joseph Lister is often referred to as the father of antiseptic surgery. Around 1865, he used carbolic acid to wash wounds and popularized the chemical inhibition of infection (antisepsis) during surgery.
- Advances in diagnostics and imaging can be traced to the discovery of x-rays in 1895 by Wilhelm Roentgen, a German professor of physics. Radiology became the first machine-based medical specialty. Some of the first training schools in x-ray therapy and radiography in the United States attracted photographers and electricians to become doctors in roentgenology (a term derived from the inventor's name).
- Alexander Fleming discovered the antibacterial properties of penicillin in 1929.

The American Medical Association

The American Medical Association (AMA) historically played a critical role in galvanizing the medical profession and in protecting the interests of physicians. The concerted activities of physicians through the AMA have been collectively referred to as *organized medicine* to distinguish them from the uncoordinated actions of individual physicians competing in the marketplace (Goodman & Musgrave, 1992, pp. 137, 139). Although it was founded in 1847, the AMA did not attain real strength until it delegated regional control by organizing its members into county and state medical societies. It first consolidated its power by controlling medical education. The AMA also vigorously pursued its objectives by supporting states in the establishment of medical licensing laws that made it illegal to practice medicine without a state-issued license.

In the postindustrial era, employment of physicians by hospitals and insurance companies was frowned upon. Physicians who attempted to seek salaried employment in a corporate setting were chastised by the medical profession and pressured into abandoning such practices. Independence from corporate control promoted private entrepreneurship and put American physicians in an enviable strategic position in relation to organizations such as hospitals and insurance companies.

Thanks to the AMA's concerted activities, physicians' incomes grew dramatically, and the supremacy of the profession was fully realized. The sphere of physicians' influence expanded into nearly all aspects of health care delivery. For example, laws were passed that prohibited individuals from obtaining certain classes of drugs without a physician's prescription. In addition, health insurance paid for treatments only when they were rendered or prescribed by physicians.

Educational Reform

Advances in medical science necessitated the reform of medical education, which started around 1870 when medical schools began affiliating with universities. In 1871, Harvard Medical School completely revolutionized the system of medical education. The academic year was extended from 4 to 9 months, and the length of medical education was increased from 2 to 3 years. Following the European model, laboratory instruction and clinical courses such as chemistry, physiology, anatomy, and pathology were added to the curriculum.

Johns Hopkins University took the lead in further reforming medical education when it opened its medical school in Baltimore, Maryland, in 1893. For the first time, medical education became a graduate training program requiring a college degree—not a high school diploma—as an entrance requirement. Johns Hopkins also pioneered the practice of complementing classroom education with residency training in its own teaching hospital. Standards at Johns Hopkins became the model of medical education in other leading institutions around the country. Even so, in the early 1900s, fewer than half of the medical schools provided acceptable levels of training.

In 1910, a widely acclaimed report was published by Abraham Flexner under the auspices of the Carnegie Foundation for the Advancement of Teaching. The *Flexner Report,* as it came to be known, was based on an inspection of medical schools. It found widespread inconsistencies in medical education. By this time, the AMA had gained a firm foothold in medical training by creating the Council on Medical Education. It pushed for state laws that required graduation from a medical school accredited by the AMA as the basis for a license to practice medicine

(Haglund & Dowling, 1993). Educational standards were formalized, and schools that did not meet the proposed standards were forced to close.

As a note of interest, Howard University School of Medicine (1869) and the Meharry Medical College (1876) were established at the end of the American Civil War specifically to prepare black physicians to practice medicine.

Development of Hospitals

As had already occurred in Europe, the growth of hospitals in the United States came to symbolize the institutionalization of health care (Torrens, 1993). The hospital became the center around which other medical services were organized.

Advancements in medical science created the need to centralize expensive facilities and equipment in a medical institution, reflecting the reality that physicians could no longer afford to have the needed equipment and facilities in their own offices. The hospital became the center for advanced technology used in medical diagnosis and treatment and for the training of various types of health care personnel. The expansion of surgery also became centered in the hospital. Alongside these developments came remarkable progress in sanitation practices. The professionalization of nursing promoted healing and improved patient recovery. As a result of these changes, the growing appeal of hospital services in communities, sick patients' increasing need for hospital care, and the increasing professionalization of medical practice became closely intertwined. Physicians began to play a dominant role in hospital affairs, even though they were not employees of the hospitals. Employment of physicians as hospitalists is a recent phenomenon.

Reform of Mental Health Care

At the turn of the 20th century, federal policy in the United States promoted education and research in psychiatry. By the 1960s, the concept of community mental health was born, and deinstitutionalization became a major thrust of mental health reform. This trend coincided with not only a better understanding of mental health, but also the availability of new drug therapies. Thus, the core of mental health care shifted from mental asylums to community-based mental health services. The deinstitutionalization movement further intensified after the U.S. Supreme Court's 1999 decision in *Olmstead v. L.C.*, which directed the states to provide community-based services, wherever appropriate, to people with mental illness. Today, mental institutions deliver services mainly for those with severe and persistent mental illness (Patrick et al., 2006).

▶ History of Health Insurance

There are several reasons why private health insurance (also called *voluntary health insurance*) took root and expanded in the United States. Much later, the struggle to meet the medical needs of the elderly and the poor in an environment of rising health care costs prompted the U.S. Congress to create the publicly financed Medicare and Medicaid programs in the 1960s.

Worker's Compensation

The first broad-coverage health insurance in the United States emerged in the form of worker's compensation. This system was originally designed to make cash payments to workers for wages lost because of job-related injuries and disease. Later, compensation for medical expenses and death benefits for survivors were added.

Between 1910 and 1915, worker's compensation laws made rapid progress in the United States (Stevens, 1971, p. 136). In view of its widespread acceptance, some reformers believed that because Americans had been persuaded to adopt compulsory insurance against industrial accidents, they could also be persuaded to adopt compulsory insurance against sickness. Worker's compensation served as a trial balloon for the idea of government-sponsored health insurance. However, the growth of private health insurance, along with other key factors discussed here, prevented any proposals for a national health care program from taking hold in the United States.

Emergence and Rise of Private Health Insurance

During the early 1900s, medical treatments and hospital care became a more entrenched part of American life. At the same time, they became increasingly more expensive. Because people could not predict their future needs for medical care or its costs, some kind of insurance was needed to spread an individual's financial risk over a large number of people. Between 1916 and 1918, 16 state legislatures, including those in New York and California, attempted to enact legislation compelling employers to provide health insurance, but their efforts were unsuccessful (Davis, 1996).

First Hospital Plan and the Birth of Blue Cross

The dire economic conditions of the Great Depression set the stage for innovation in health insurance to cover hospitalization costs. On the one hand, hospitals were vulnerable to economic instability when they relied too much on philanthropic donations. On the other hand, individual patients faced not only loss of income from illness but also burdensome debt from medical care costs when they needed hospitalization.

In 1929, the blueprint for modern health insurance was conceived when Justin F. Kimball began a hospital insurance plan for teachers at Baylor University Hospital in Dallas, Texas. Within a few years, it became the model for Blue Cross plans around the country (Raffel, 1980, p. 394). At first, other independent hospitals copied Baylor and started to offer single-hospital plans. Within a few years, plans sponsored by groups of hospitals became more popular because they offered consumers a choice of hospitals. The American Hospital Association supported these hospital plans and became the coordinating agency that united the plans into the Blue Cross network. The Blue Cross plans were nonprofit; that is, they had no shareholders to receive profit distributions. Later, control of the plans was transferred to a completely independent body, the Blue Cross Commission, which subsequently became the Blue Cross Association (Raffel, 1980, p. 395).

Hospital insurance quickly grew in popularity. In 1946, Blue Cross plans in 43 states served 20 million members. Within a few years, lured by the success of the Blue Cross plans, commercial insurance companies also started offering hospital insurance. Between 1940 and 1950 alone, the proportion of the U.S. population covered by hospital insurance increased from 9% to 57% (Anderson, 1990, p. 128). Private health insurance had received the AMA's endorsement, but the AMA had also made it clear that health insurance plans should include only hospital care, not physicians' fees.

First Physician Plan and the Birth of Blue Shield

In 1939, the California Medical Association started the first Blue Shield plan, which was designed to pay physicians' fees. By endorsing hospital insurance and by actively developing the first plans that covered physicians' services, the medical profession protected its own financial interests. The AMA ensured that private health insurance would be preserved, and the organization remained adamantly opposed to government-run national health insurance.

Starting in 1974, Blue Cross and Blue Shield plans began to merge. Now, in nearly every state, Blue Cross and Blue Shield plans are joint corporations or have close working relationships (Davis, 1996).

Employment-Based Health Insurance

Three main factors explain how health insurance in the United States became employer based:

- During the World War II period, the U.S. Congress imposed wage freezes in an attempt to control wartime inflation. In response, many employers started offering health insurance to their workers to compensate for the loss of raises in their salaries.

■ In 1948, the U.S. Supreme Court ruled that employee benefits were a legitimate part of union–management negotiations. Health insurance, in turn, became an important component of collective bargaining between unions and employers.

■ In 1954, Congress amended the Internal Revenue Code to make employer-paid health coverage nontaxable. In economic value, employer-paid health insurance was equivalent to getting additional salary without having to pay taxes on it, which provided an incentive to obtain health insurance as an employer-furnished benefit.

In subsequent years, employment-based health insurance expanded rapidly, and private health insurance became the primary vehicle for the delivery of health care services in the United States.

Failure of National Health Insurance in the United States

Industrialization of Western Europe meant that a large segment of the populations worked as hired laborers, in countries such as England, and later in Germany. Unification of Germany under Otto von Bismarck led to rapid industrialization, but labor unrest threatened political stability. Universal health insurance for all citizens was seen as a means to obtain workers' loyalty and thwart any labor uprisings.

By 1912, national health insurance had spread throughout Europe, but political conditions in the United States were quite different. Unlike the situation in European countries, the American government was highly decentralized and engaged in little direct regulation of social welfare. Despite this fact, Theodore Roosevelt ran for the U.S. presidency in 1912 on a platform of social reform—and, perhaps not surprisingly, was defeated by Woodrow Wilson. Even so, the Progressive movement favoring national health insurance remained alive for several more years.

The entry of the United States into World War I in 1917 dealt a political blow to the national health care movement, as anti-German feelings were aroused and the U.S. government denounced German social insurance. Opponents of national health care disparaged it as a Prussian menace that was inconsistent with American values (Starr, 1982, pp. 240, 253). Any subsequent attempts to introduce national health insurance were met with the stigmatizing label of *socialized medicine*—a term that has since become synonymous with any large-scale government-sponsored expansion of health insurance. The traditional American values based on capitalism, self-determination, distrust of big government, and reliance on the private sector to address social concerns stood as a bulwark against broad-based government interventions. Conversely, during times of national distress, such as the Great Depression, pure necessity may have legitimized the advancement of social programs, such as Social Security and unemployment compensation.

The AMA played a leading role in opposing national health care, seeing it as a potential threat to the private practice of medicine. For example, the AMA was instrumental in the demise of several bills related to national health insurance that were introduced in Congress in the early 1940s during Franklin Roosevelt's presidency. In 1946, Harry Truman became the first president to make a direct appeal for a national health care program (Anderson, 1990, p. 119). Initial public reaction to Truman's plan was positive, but when a government-controlled medical plan was compared with privately obtained insurance, polls showed a drastic decline in public support. The AMA was once again vehement in denouncing the plan. Other powerful health care interest groups, such as the American Hospital Association, also opposed the proposal. In 1948, Truman was reelected while promising national health insurance, which actually came as a surprise to many political observers. This time, the AMA launched what was to become one of the most expensive lobbying efforts in U.S. history. Its campaign directly linked national health insurance with communism until the idea of socialized medicine was firmly implanted in the public's minds. By 1950, national health insurance was a dead issue, and it remained so for several decades.

In 1993, President Bill Clinton made national health insurance one of his top priorities, but his proposal was largely rejected by the American people. Defeat of the Clinton plan furnished another lesson on the power of beliefs and values prevalent in the United States. As a matter of principle, Americans have endorsed tax-supported health insurance to help needy citizens, but they also have been unwilling to pay, in the form of higher taxes, for what a universal health insurance program could realistically cost. Moreover, Americans have been uneasy about more government regulation and interference with employment-based private health insurance. **EXHIBIT 3.5** provides a summary of the main historical reasons for the failure of national health insurance in the United States.

Creation of Medicare and Medicaid

Before 1965, private health insurance was the only widely available source of payment for health care, and it was available primarily to middle-class working people and their families. The elderly, the unemployed, and the poor had to rely on their own resources, on limited public programs, or on charity from hospitals, clinics, and individual physicians.

The earlier debates over national health insurance had made one thing clear: Most Americans did not desire government intervention in how they received health care, with one exception—they would be less opposed to reform initiatives for the underprivileged classes. In principle, the poor were considered a special class who could be served through a government-sponsored program. The elderly—those

EXHIBIT 3.5 Reasons Why National Health Insurance Has Historically Failed in the United States

- Unlike in Europe, national health care failed to get an early footing because of labor and political instability in the United States.
- The decentralized American system gave the U.S. federal government little direct control over social policy.
- The German social insurance system was denounced during World War I. Since then, the term "socialized medicine" has been used as a synonym for "national health insurance."
- The AMA opposed national health care initiatives.
- Middle-class Americans have traditionally espoused beliefs and values that are consistent with capitalism, self-determination, and distrust of big government.
- Middle-class Americans have been averse to higher taxes to pay for the increased cost of a national health care program.

65 years of age and older—were another group that started to receive increased attention in the 1950s. On their own, most of the poor and the elderly could not afford the increasing cost of health care. Also, because the health status of these population groups was significantly worse than that of the general population, their medical needs were more critical. The elderly, in particular, had a higher incidence and prevalence of disease than did younger age groups. Despite their greater need for health care, fewer than half of all elderly persons were covered by private health insurance. Even if they could afford it, many of them were unable to obtain private health insurance because of their poor health status. At the same time, the growing elderly middle class was becoming a politically active force.

A bill introduced in Congress by Aime Forand in 1957 started the momentum for including necessary hospital and nursing home care as an extension of Social Security benefits (Stevens, 1971, p. 434). The AMA, however, undertook a massive campaign to portray a government-run plan as a threat to the physician–patient relationship. The bill stalled initially, but public hearings around the country, which were packed by the elderly, produced an intense grassroots support to push the issue onto the national agenda (Starr, 1982, p. 368). Compromise legislation, the Medical Assistance Act, also known as the Kerr-Mills Act, was passed and went into effect in 1960. Under this act, federal grants were given to the states so they could extend health services under their welfare programs to low-income elderly persons. However, enrolling the elderly in a welfare program became controversial, as liberal congressional representatives voiced their opposition by claiming that it was a source of humiliation to the elderly (Starr, 1982, p. 369). Within 3 years, the program was declared ineffective because many states did not even implement it (Stevens, 1971, p. 438).

In 1964, health insurance for the aged and the poor became a top priority of President Lyndon Johnson's Great Society programs. Eventually, Congress approved a three-part program that provided publicly financed health insurance to all elderly individuals, regardless of their incomes. Part A and Part B of Medicare (also known as *Title 18* of the Social Security Act of 1965) became the first two layers. *Part A* of Medicare was designed to use Social Security funds to finance hospital insurance and short-term nursing home coverage after discharge from a hospital. *Part B* of Medicare was designed to cover physicians' bills through government-subsidized insurance, for which the elderly would pay a small portion of the premiums. The *Medicaid* program (*Title 19* of the Social Security Act of 1965) was the third layer. It covered the eligible poor and was based on the earlier Kerr-Mills Act program. It would be financed through federal matching funds to the states in accordance with each state's per capita income.

Although adopted together, Medicare and Medicaid reflected sharply different traditions. Medicare enjoyed broad grassroots support and, being attached to Social Security, had no class distinction. Medicaid, in contrast, carried the stigma of public welfare. As a federal program, Medicare had uniform national standards for eligibility and benefits; the state-administered Medicaid programs, however, varied across states in terms of eligibility and benefits. Medicare covered anyone age 65 or older, whereas Medicaid became a *means-tested program*, which confined eligibility to people below a predetermined income level. Consequently, many of the poor did not qualify because their incomes exceeded the means-test limits.

Initially created to cover only the elderly, Medicare was expanded in 1973 to cover two other categories of people: (1) nonelderly disabled people receiving Social Security for at least 24 months and (2) people with end-stage renal disease who needed dialysis or a kidney transplant. In 1997, Medicare added coverage options under *Part C*, and in 2003 a prescription drug benefit (*Part D*) was passed into law. The main distinctions between Medicare and Medicaid are summarized in **EXHIBIT 3.6**.

Soon after their inception, Medicare and Medicaid became instrumental in covering millions of Americans. By 1970, 20.4 million individuals received health care through Medicare and another 17.6 million through Medicaid. The increased coverage, however, came at a high price—namely, unrelenting government regulations and uncontrolled public expenditures.

The Medicare and Medicaid programs are financed by the government, but most beneficiaries receive health care services from private hospitals, physicians, and other providers. As a major payer of health care services, the government has implemented numerous regulations that govern the delivery of services and reimbursement to providers. As a result, the regulatory powers of government have increasingly encroached on the private sector. In 1977, the Health Care Financing

EXHIBIT 3.6 Comparisons Between Medicare and Medicaid

Medicare	Medicaid
■ Covers all elderly persons, nonelderly disabled persons on Social Security, and nonelderly persons with end-stage renal disease	■ Covers only the very poor
■ No income/means test	■ Income criteria established by states (means test)
■ No class distinction	■ Public welfare
■ Part A for hospitalization and short-term nursing home stay; Part B for physician and other outpatient services; Part C for managed care; and Part D for prescription drugs	■ All services are covered under one program
■ Nationally uniform federal program	■ Program varies from state to state
■ Title 18 of the Social Security Act	■ Title 19 of the Social Security Act
■ Part A financed through a payroll tax paid by employees, employers, and the self-employed; Part B subsidized through general taxes, but the participants pay part of the premium cost; cost-sharing in Parts C and D	■ Financed by the states, with matching funds from the federal government according to each state's per capita income

Administration (now called the Centers for Medicare and Medicaid Services) was created to manage Medicare and Medicaid separately from the Social Security Administration.

The creation of Medicare and Medicaid had a drastic impact on both federal and state budgets, but the federal government bore the brunt of this burden. As shown in **TABLE 3.1**, the U.S. gross domestic product—representing total economic consumption—grew at an average annual rate of 7.6% between 1965 and 1970. By comparison, total state and local government expenditures for health care grew at a rate of 12.5%. In the case of the federal government, however, health care expenditures increased at an average annual rate of 30%. Hence, the federal government bore most of the expenditures for Medicare and Medicaid.

TABLE 3.1 Average Annual Percent Increase in Gross Domestic Product and Federal and State Expenditures Between 1965 and 1970

	Total (%)	Health Care (%)
Gross domestic product	7.6	—
Federal government expenditures	11.3	30.0
State and local government expenditures	13.6	12.5

Data from National Center for Health Statistics. Health, United States, 1995, p. 235.

▶ Medical Services in the Corporate Era

The latter part of the 20th century and the beginning of the 21st century have been marked by the growth and consolidation of large business corporations and tremendous advances in global communications, transportation, and trade. These developments have changed the way health care is delivered in the United States and, indeed, around the world. The rise of medical corporations, the information revolution, and globalization have been interdependent phenomena.

Corporatization of Health Care Delivery

Corporatization here refers to the ways in which health care delivery in the United States has become the domain of large organizations. Since the 1990s, managed care has become the primary source for health insurance and the delivery of medical services to the majority of Americans. The emergent managed care organizations (MCOs) wielded their immense purchasing power to obtain health care services at discounted prices and used the strength accorded by their consolidation to implement various types of controls to reduce the rising costs of health care. To counteract this imbalance, providers began to consolidate as well, and larger, integrated health care organizations began forming. Large *integrated delivery systems* (IDSs) can provide a full array of health care services, including hospital inpatient care, surgical services in both inpatient and outpatient settings, primary care and multispecialty outpatient services, home health care, long-term care, and specialized rehabilitation services. Together, MCOs and IDSs have corporatized the delivery of health care in the United States. At the same time, though, they have made the health care system extremely complex.

In a health care landscape increasingly dominated by corporations, individual physicians have struggled to preserve their autonomy. As a matter of survival, many physicians had to consolidate into larger group practices, form strategic partnerships with hospitals, or start their own specialty hospitals. A growing number of physicians have become employees of hospitals and other large medical corporations.

Information Revolution

The delivery of health care is being transformed in unprecedented and irreversible ways by telecommunications. For example, telemedicine and e-health have been on the rise. *Telemedicine* came to the forefront in the 1990s with technological advances in the distant transmission of image data. This technology has made it possible to provide health care at a distance, such as real-time transmission of video examinations as well as telesurgery. *E-health* refers to health care information and services offered over the Internet by professionals and nonprofessionals alike (Maheu et al., 2001). These services include medical information from reliable sources such as the prestigious National Institutes of Health and the world-renowned Mayo Clinic through their websites, online purchase of health care products, online consultations with physicians, and online interactions with other consumers about health-related matters. The Internet revolution has put more decision-making power into the hands of patients and their surrogates about what they may think is best for them. Access to expert information is no longer strictly confined to the physician's domain, which in some ways has led the patient to be less dependent on health care professionals.

Globalization

Globalization refers to various forms of cross-border economic activities. It is driven by the global exchange of information, the production of goods and services more economically in developing countries, and the increased interdependence of mature and emerging world economies. It confers many advantages, but also has some downsides.

From the standpoint of cross-border trade in health services, Mutchnick and colleagues (2005) identified four different modes of economic interrelationships:

- Cross-country telemedicine and outsourcing of certain medical services have been made possible by advanced telecommunications technology. For example, teleradiology (the electronic transmission of radiological images over a distance) enables physicians in the United States to transmit radiological images overseas, where they are interpreted and reported back either the same or the next day. The radiologists residing overseas are licensed and credentialed in the United States.

- Consumers travel abroad to receive medical care (sometimes referred to as medical tourism). For example, countries such as India and Thailand offer surgeries in state-of-the-art medical facilities to foreigners at a fraction of what it would cost to have the same procedures done in the United States or Europe.
- Foreign direct investment in health services enterprises has become common. For example, Chindex International, a U.S. corporation, provides medical equipment, supplies, and clinical care in China. American providers such as Johns Hopkins Medicine International, the Cleveland Clinic, and Duke University's Global Health Institute support innovation and delivery of quality medical services through collaborative arrangements with other countries.
- Health professionals are choosing to move to other countries that offer high demand for their services and better economic opportunities than their native countries. Migration of physicians from developing countries helps alleviate at least some of the shortage in underserved locations in the developed world. On the downside, the developing world pays a price when emigration leaves these countries with shortages of trained professionals.

▶ Era of Health Care Reform

Health care reform refers to major changes through government policy to expand health insurance to the uninsured. Recent efforts to reform health care were based on government intervention in the financing and delivery of health care. Most notably, the ACA represents the most sweeping reform undertaken since the creation of Medicare and Medicaid in 1965. At the time of the highly controversial ACA's passage, the presidency and the majority membership in both the U.S. House of Representatives and Senate were in the hands of the Democratic Party, and the legislation failed to win a single vote from Republicans. Perhaps surprisingly, the AMA supported the legislation. Since its heyday in political activism, the AMA has become a much weaker organization, supported by only 17% of U.S. doctors (Scherz, 2010).

After the ACA's enactment, more than half of the states and some private parties filed lawsuits challenging the constitutionality of the legislation. In 2012, the U.S. Supreme Court rendered a 5–4 decision, which was split over the two main parts of the ACA. First, the law's mandate requiring all Americans to have health insurance was upheld as constitutional. In part, the majority opinion read, "The Affordable Care Act's requirement that certain individuals pay a financial penalty for not obtaining health insurance may reasonably be characterized as a tax" (Liptak, 2012). Thus, the Court's decision on this issue was based on Congress's power to impose new taxes—in this case, for not having health insurance. In the second part of the Court's decision, it struck down as unconstitutional the federal government's attempt to coerce states into expanding their Medicaid programs by threatening to eliminate federal funding for those states that chose not to expand Medicaid coverage under the ACA (Anderson & Health Policy Institute of Ohio, 2012).

In 2014, in *Burwell v. Hobby Lobby Stores, Inc.*, the U.S. Supreme Court ruled against a controversial ACA requirement that forced certain employers to provide contraceptives that might be deemed to induce abortions. In a 5–4 decision, the Court ruled that in the case of a closely held corporation, the owners of which may have deeply held religious convictions against providing drugs or devices that may destroy an embryo, the ACA violated the Religious Freedom Restoration Act of 1993. Hobby Lobby had claimed that it faced annual fines of $475 million for failure to comply with the ACA (Liptak, 2014). The Court argued that the ACA imposed a substantial burden on religious liberty.

Health Care Reform in a Flux

Even before the ACA was fully implemented, health policy researchers Nardin and colleagues (2013) had stated:

> Our finding… runs counter to the common perception that the ACA will cover virtually all legal residents. The ACA will leave tens of millions uncovered. It will do little to alter racial disparities in coverage.… The ACA, whatever its merits, will fall well short of its stated goal of providing affordable care for all Americans.

This insight largely proved correct, even though the number of uninsured was markedly reduced under the ACA, particularly among low-income people who became newly eligible for Medicaid[2] and those who became eligible for tax credits to purchase private health insurance through government-established exchanges. Nevertheless, in 2017, health care reform once again became an issue for national debate.

---

2 Thirty-one states and the District of Columbia expanded their Medicaid programs, as intended under the ACA.

Inability to obtain health insurance and affordability remained thorny issues even after the ACA's implementation. With each passing year, fewer insurers have participated in the exchanges where people can buy private insurance, and the cost of insurance has been rising sharply. In the market for employer-based health insurance, fewer small employers with less than 50 workers were able to offer insurance to their workers. For example, 59% were able to offer health insurance in 2012; by 2017, only 50% could do so (Claxton et al., 2017). The cost of insurance and worker contributions toward that cost have also risen dramatically. For example, between 2012 and 2017, total employment-based health insurance costs rose 19%, whereas worker contributions increased by 32% for family coverage (Claxton et al., 2017).

Despite the issues just pointed out, and promises by politicians to reform the system, the U.S. Congress failed to pass a broad health care reform bill in 2017. However, the Tax Cuts and Jobs Act of 2017, passed and signed into law in December 2017, effectively repealed the mandate in the ACA that required all Americans to have health insurance. The mandate to either have health insurance or pay a tax penalty was one of the main anchors of the ACA, although this provision did not actually promote the expected growth in the purchase of health insurance. The second main anchor of the ACA, requiring employers to offer health insurance to the workers, could not be repealed through the tax law.

At the time of this text's writing, it was unclear how Congress would address the lingering issues with health insurance, in terms of both coverage and cost. With a partially repealed ACA, however, the urgency to address health care reform in 2018 had only intensified.

▶ Conclusion

In a little more than 100 years, health care delivery has come a long way in the United States, evolving from a primitive and family-oriented craft to a technology-driven service and the largest industry in the country. In the process, many medical procedures and services have become increasingly unaffordable. Both private and public health insurance have become firmly entrenched mechanisms to pay for costly health care. Medicare, Medicaid, and other public programs, however, cover only those individuals who meet established criteria for eligibility. Efforts to create a national health insurance program have repeatedly failed.

The late 20th century and early 21st century have been characterized as the corporate era in the delivery of medical care. Corporatization has put the delivery of health care into the hands of large managed care and integrated health care organizations, and it has turned the delivery of medical care into a complex enterprise. The information revolution has created advanced telecommunication technologies, whose application in medical care has made the distant delivery of certain health care services possible. E-health has given consumers access to health care information over the Internet. Globalization has added a worldwide dimension to the delivery of medical care through telemedicine, outsourcing, and foreign direct investment in health care delivery.

An era of health care reform was inaugurated in the United States with the passage of the Affordable Care Act in 2010. However, contrary to the promises made by its supporters, the law failed to provide affordable coverage to millions of Americans, although it did significantly reduce the number of uninsured. One major anchor of the ACA—the mandate to have health insurance or pay a penalty tax—was repealed under the Tax Cuts and Jobs Act of 2017. In contrast, nagging concerns regarding coverage and costs have not been resolved and remain in a state of flux.

References

1. Anderson D, Health Policy Institute of Ohio. 2012. The Supreme Court's ruling on the Affordable Care Act: A review of the decision and its impact on Ohio. http://www.healthpolicyohio.org/wp-content/uploads/2014/02/scotus_brief.pdf. Accessed April 2018.
2. Anderson OW. 1990. *Health services as a growth enterprise in the United States since 1875*. Ann Arbor, MI: Health Administration Press.
3. Claxton G, et al. 2017. *Employer health benefits: 2017 annual survey*. Chicago, IL: Henry J. Kaiser Family Foundation.
4. Davis P. 1996. The fate of Blue Shield and the new blues. *S Dakota J Med*. 49(9):323–330.
5. Goodman JC, Musgrave GL. 1992. *Patient power: Solving America's health care crisis*. Washington, DC: CATO Institute.
6. Haglund CL, Dowling WL. 1993. The hospital. In: Williams SJ, Torrens PR, eds. *Introduction to health services*. 4th ed. New York, NY: Delmar; 133–176.
7. Liptak A. June 28, 2012. Supreme Court upholds health care law, 5–4, in victory for Obama. *The New York Times*. http://www.nytimes.com/2012/06/29/us/supreme-court-lets-health-law-largely-stand.html. Accessed January 9, 2018.
8. Liptak A. June 30, 2014. Supreme Court rejects contraceptives mandate for some corporations. *The New York Times*. http://www.nytimes.com/2014/07/01/us/hobby-lobby-case-supreme-court-contraception.html. Accessed April 2015.
9. Madison DL. 1990. Notes on the history of group practice: The tradition of the dispensary. *Med Group Manage J*. 37(5):52–54, 56–60, 86–93.
10. Maheu MM, et al. 2001. *E-health, telehealth, and telemedicine: A guide to start-up and success*. San Francisco, CA: Jossey-Bass.
11. Martensen RL. 1996. Hospital hotels and the care of the "worthy rich." *JAMA*. 275(4):325.
12. Mutchnick IS, et al. 2005. Trading health services across borders: GATS, markets, and caveats. *Health Aff: Web Exclusive*. 24(suppl 1):W5-42–W5-51.
13. Nardin R, et al. June 6, 2013. The uninsured after implementation of the Affordable Care Act: A demographic and geographic analysis. *Health Aff Blog*. http://healthaffairs

.org/blog/2013/06/06/the-uninsured-after-implementation-of-the-affordable-care
-act-a-demographic-and-geographic-analysis/. Accessed June 28, 2015.

14. National Library of Medicine. 2014. Diseases of the mind: Highlights of American psychiatry. https://www.nlm.nih.gov/hmd/diseases/benjamin.html. Accessed January 7, 2018.

15. Norris C. 2017. A history of madness: Four venerable Virginia lunatic asylums. *Virginia Mag History Biography.* 125(2):138–182.

16. Patrick V, et al. 2006. Facilitating discharge in state psychiatric institutions: A group intervention strategy. *Psychiatric Rehab J.* 29(3):183–188.

17. Raffel MW. 1980. *The U.S. health system: Origins and functions.* New York, NY: John Wiley & Sons.

18. Rosen G. 1983. *The structure of American medical practice 1875–1941.* Philadelphia, PA: University of Pennsylvania Press.

19. Rothstein WG. 1972. *American physicians in the nineteenth century: From sect to science.* Baltimore, MD: Johns Hopkins University Press.

20. Scherz H. May 7, 2010. Why the AMA wants to muzzle your doctor. *Wall Street Journal.* http://online.wsj.com/article/SB10001424052748703961104575226323909364054.html. Accessed October 2011.

21. Shryock RH. 1966. *Medicine in America: Historical essays.* Baltimore, MD: Johns Hopkins University Press

22. Starr P. 1982. *The social transformation of American medicine.* Cambridge, MA: Basic Books.

23. Stevens R. 1971. *American medicine and the public interest.* New Haven, CT: Yale University Press.

24. Torrens PR. 1993. Historical evolution and overview of health services in the United States. In: Williams SJ, Torrens PR, eds. *Introduction to health services.* 4th ed. New York, NY: Delmar.

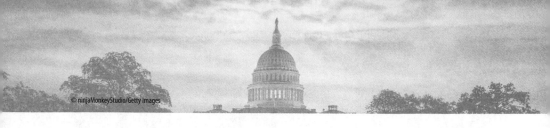

CHAPTER 4

Health Care Providers and Professionals

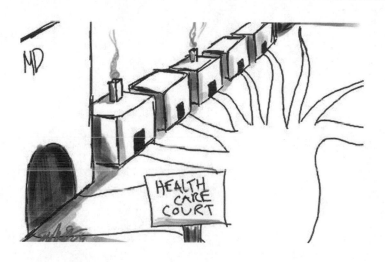

▶ Introduction

The U.S. health care industry is the largest employer in the nation, employing about 13.6% of the nation's total labor force (U.S. Bureau of Labor Statistics, 2016). The health care sector of the U.S. economy will continue to grow because of (1) growth in the overall population, mainly due to immigration; (2) aging of the population, as the baby boomers continue to turn age 65 years and older through 2029; and (3) increased life expectancies.

Health professionals are among the most well-educated and diverse of all labor force groups. Almost all of the practitioner groups are now represented by professional associations, and health services professionals work in a variety of health care settings. According to 2016 data (TABLE 4.1), the

TABLE 4.1 Persons Employed at Health Services Sites

Site	1994		2001		2016	
	Number of Persons (in thousands)	Percentage Distribution	Number of Persons (in thousands)	Percentage Distribution	Number of Persons (in thousands)	Percentage Distribution
All health services sites	10,587	100.0	12,211	100.0	17210	100.0
Offices and clinics of physicians	1,404	13.3	1,387	11.4	1,611	9.4
Offices and clinics of dentists	596	5.6	672	5.5	897	5.2
Offices and clinics of chiropractors	105	1.0	120	1.0	135	0.78
Hospitals	5,009	47.3	5,202	42.6	6990	40.6
Nursing care facilities	1,692	16.0	1,593	13.0	1786	10.4
Other health services sites	1,781	16.8	3,273	26.5	5791	33.6

Data from U.S. Bureau of Labor Statistics. Labor Force Statistics from the Current Population Survey. 2016. http://www.bls.gov/cps/cpsaat18.htm 2016 data retrieved from https://www.bls.gov/cps/cpsaat18.htm

majority of health professionals are employed by hospitals (40.6%), followed by nursing care facilities (10.4%), and physicians' offices and clinics (9.4%) (U.S. Bureau of Labor Statistics, 2016).

The demand for health services professionals closely follows demographic trends (mentioned previously), advances in research and technology, disease and illness trends, and changes in health insurance and the delivery of services. Advances in scientific research contribute to new methods of preventing, diagnosing, and treating illness. New sophisticated medical techniques and machines are constantly being introduced, creating the need to update skills. Specialization in medicine has contributed to the proliferation of various types of medical technicians. In addition, the trend in diseases from acute to chronic conditions has created a greater need for health services professionals who are formally prepared to address health risks and their consequences and prevention. Recent expansion of health insurance coverage under the Affordable Care Act (ACA) will lead to greater utilization of health care services and, in turn, a greater demand for health care professionals. Delivery of health care through managed care and a greater emphasis on prevention in the ACA will require more primary care providers.

This chapter provides an overview of the large array of health services professionals. It summarizes their training and practice requirements, major roles, practice settings in which they are generally employed, and critical issues concerning their professions. Emphasis is placed on physicians, who play a leading role in the delivery of health care. Nonphysician practitioners with advanced training also fill a critical role in the delivery of primary care services. In addition, the chapter describes the imbalance between primary and specialty care services, the maldistribution of practitioners, and the looming personnel shortages.

▶ Physicians

Physicians play a central role in health care services by evaluating a patient's health condition, diagnosing abnormalities, and prescribing treatment. Some physicians are engaged in medical education and research to find new and better ways to control and cure health problems.

All states require physicians to be licensed before they can practice medicine. The licensure requirements include graduation from an accredited medical school that awards a doctor of medicine (MD) or doctor of osteopathic medicine (DO) degree, successful completion of a licensing examination administered by either the National Board of Medical Examiners or the National Board of Osteopathic Medical Examiners, and completion of a supervised internship/residency program (Stanfield, 1995, pp. 102–104). *Residency* is graduate medical education in a specialty that takes the form of paid on-the-job training, usually in a hospital. Most physicians serve a 1-year rotating internship after graduation before entering a residency, which may last 2 to 6 years.

The number of active physicians, both MDs and DOs, has steadily increased in the United States, rising from 14.1 to 27.2 physicians per 10,000 people from 1950 to 2016 (TABLE 4.2). Of the 192 medical schools in the United States, 163 teach allopathic medicine (defined in the next section) and award the MD degree, and 29 teach osteopathic medicine and award the DO degree.

Similarities and Differences Between MDs and DOs

Both MDs and DOs use traditional methods of treatment, including drugs and surgery. The two differ mainly in their philosophies and approaches to treatment. *Osteopathic medicine*, practiced by DOs, emphasizes the musculoskeletal system (e.g., the correction of joints or tissues). In their treatment plans, DOs stress preventive medicine such as diet and the environment as factors that might influence natural resistance. They take a holistic approach to patient care. In contrast, MDs are trained in *allopathic*

TABLE 4.2   Active Physicians: Type and Number per 10,000 Population

Year	All Active Physicians	Doctors of Medicine	Doctors of Osteopathy	Active Physicians per 10,000 Population
1950	219,900	209,000	10,900	14.1
1960	259,500	247,300	12,200	14.0
1970	326,500	314,200	12,300	15.6
1980	457,500	440,400	17,100	19.7
1990	589,500	561,400	28,100	23.4
1995	672,859	637,192	35,667	25.6
2000	772,296	727,573	44,723	27.8
2012	826,001	763,000	63,000	28.3
2016	877,616	810,043	67,534	27.2

Data are from the National Center for Health Statistics 2014. Health, United States (p. 291); 2015. Health, United States (p. 292). Hyattsville, MD: U.S. Department of Health and Human Services.

medicine, which views medical treatment as an active intervention to produce a counteracting reaction in an attempt to neutralize the effects of disease. MDs, particularly generalists, may also use preventive medicine along
with allopathic treatments. Approximately one-third of MDs and more
than one-half of DOs are generalists (U.S. Bureau of Labor Statistics, 2017).

Generalists and Specialists

Whereas most DOs are generalists, most MDs are specialists. In the United
States, physicians trained in family medicine/general practice, general
internal medicine, and general pediatrics are considered primary care physicians or *generalists* (Rich et al., 1994). Primary care physicians typically
provide preventive services (e.g., health examinations, immunizations,
mammograms, Pap smears) and treat frequently occurring and less severe
problems. Referrals are often made to specialists for problems that occur
less frequently or require complex diagnostic or therapeutic approaches.

Physicians in non-primary care specialties dealing with particular
diseases or organ systems are referred to as *specialists.* Specialists must be
certified in an area of medical specialization, which commonly requires
additional years of advanced residency training followed by several years
of practice. A specialty board examination is often required as the final
step for becoming a board-certified specialist. The most common medical
specialties include anesthesiology, cardiology, dermatology, specialized
internal medicine, neurology, obstetrics and gynecology, ophthalmology,
pathology, pediatrics, psychiatry, radiology, and surgery. These specialties can be divided into six major functional groups: (1) the subspecialties
of internal medicine; (2) a broad group of medical specialties; (3) obstetrics and gynecology; (4) surgery of all types; (5) hospital-based radiology,
anesthesiology, and pathology; and (6) psychiatry (Cooper, 1994).

Hospitalists

The specialty of a *hospitalist* is organized around the site of care—that is,
the hospital—instead of a specific organ, disease, or age. Hospitalists are
involved in inpatient medicine, and their roles parallel those of primary
care physicians in an outpatient setting, in that they manage the care of
hospitalized patients. This specialty has long served a significant role in
urban hospitals in Canada and the United Kingdom.

The hospitalist specialty appeared in the U.S. health care system to a
significant extent after managed care began to dominate the health care
system and place an emphasis on cost-efficiency. Hospitalists seek to
decrease overall cost and length of stay for patients, while maintaining
referring-physician satisfaction. Most practicing hospitalists train under

various primary care concentrations such as general internal medicine, family practice, or general pediatrics.

Differences Between Primary and Specialty Care

Primary care can be distinguished from specialty care by the time, focus, and scope of services provided to patients. The five main areas of distinction are as follows:

1. In linear time sequence, primary care is first-contact care and is regarded as the portal of entry to the health care system (Kahn et al., 1994). Specialty care, when needed, generally follows primary care.

2. In managed care and integrated delivery environments, primary care physicians serve as gatekeepers—an important role in controlling costs, utilization rates, and the rational allocation of resources. In the gatekeeping model, specialty care requires referral from a primary care physician.

3. Primary care is longitudinal, and primary care providers follow a patient through the course of treatment and coordinate various activities, including initial diagnosis, treatment, referral, consultation, monitoring, and follow-up. Specialty care is episodic and, therefore, more focused and intense.

4. Primary care focuses on the whole person. The patient may have multiple health issues—a condition referred to as comorbidity. Primary care seeks to balance the patient's multiple health issues, including referrals to specialists when needed. Specialty care deals with particular diseases or organ systems of the body and is limited in scope to episodes of illness, specific organ systems, or the disease process. Specialty care is also associated with secondary and tertiary levels of services.

5. The difference in scope between primary and specialty care is reflected in how providers are trained. Primary care medical students spend a significant amount of time in ambulatory care settings, familiarizing themselves with a variety of patient conditions and problems. Students in medical subspecialties spend significant time in inpatient hospitals, where they are exposed to state-of-the-art medical technology to diagnose and treat diseases and perform surgeries.

Work Settings and Practice Patterns

Physicians work in a variety of settings including hospitals, where they are employed as medical residents, staff physicians, or hospitalists, and the public sector, in places such as federal government agencies, public health clinics, community and migrant health centers, schools, and prisons. Most physicians, however, are office-based practitioners in private clinics, where they work as partners or salaried employees under contractual arrangements. TABLE 4.3 shows that in 2013, physicians in general family practice were involved in the highest proportion of ambulatory care visits in the United States (18.9%), followed by those in internal medicine (13.7%) and pediatrics (10.2%).

Imbalance and Maldistribution of Physicians

In 2016 there were, on average, 271.6 active physicians per 100,000 people in the United States, ranging from a high of 443.5 in Massachusetts to a low of 186.1 in Mississippi. States with the highest number of physicians per 100,000 people are concentrated in the Northeast (Association of American Medical Colleges [AAMC], 2017).

Looming Shortages and the Affordable Care Act

There is much debate about the U.S. physician workforce. Key factors affecting the adequacy of the physician workforce include growth in the insured population due to health care reform law, an aging U.S. population, an aging health care workforce, workforce diversity, and the economy. Another important factor, the evolution of health care technology, increases the likelihood of diagnosis and the breadth of treatable ailments (Alliance for Health Reform & Robert Wood Johnson Foundation, 2011).

The ACA, enacted in March 2010, is expected to add 32 million previously uninsured persons to the pool of insured patients by 2019—and they will need physicians. This growth of the insured population is one of

TABLE 4.3 Ambulatory Visits by Generalists and Specialists in the United States, 2013

Obstetrics/gynecology	6.3%
Pediatrics	10.2%
Internal medicine	13.7%
General/family practice	18.9%
Specialists	50.9%

National Center for Health Statistics. Health, United States, 2016. Hyattsville, MD; 2017:289–290.

the key factors expected to worsen the current shortage of physicians for at least another decade. By 2025, the deficit could grow by 25% (AAMC, 2008). Health professional shortages vary across fields of practice. To fill the need for health care providers, the ACA establishes grant programs for education and training for primary care, direct care, oral health specialists, geriatric education centers, behavioral health, cultural competency, nursing, nurse practitioners, public health, and underrepresented minorities (American Public Health Association, 2011).

Another factor influencing the physician shortage is the aging of the U.S. population and demands from the complex chronic care needs of older persons. The first baby boomers turned 65 in January 2011, becoming eligible for Medicare, and a total of 78 million baby boomers will turn 65 by 2030. Providers for this population are already in short supply. In recent years, the greatest growth in utilization of health care services has been among those 75 years of age and older. Geriatricians—that is, primary care physicians for this population—number a mere 6,830 and are spread thinly, with just one for every 1,900 seniors age 75 or older. According to an Institute of Medicine[1] study, the United States will need 36,000 geriatricians by 2030 to meet the needs of the elderly.

The physician workforce itself is aging, with sources suggesting that one-third of current physicians will retire in the next 10 years. Nearly 40% of doctors are above 55 years of age, and younger professionals have different practice patterns than their predecessors. For example, health professionals between the ages of 25 and 40 tend to work fewer hours than previous generations did.

The United States has approximately 80 primary care physicians per 100,000 people—on average, 68 primary care physicians per 100,000 rural residents, and 84 primary care physicians per 100,000 urban residents. With this unequal distribution, many areas have relative primary care shortages, especially rural communities and areas of measurable social deprivation (American Academy of Family Physicians, 2013).

Both the literature and practice examples suggest promising strategies that employers and policymakers can implement to address the needs and challenges of the evolving health care workforce. Workforce assessment is a critical first step for employers to map the demographics of their workforce, identify skills gaps, plan for leadership succession, and facilitate the transfer of knowledge from mature workers to entry-level hires.

Transitioning to a team-oriented approach to organizing health care jobs may also allow health care professionals with varying strengths and abilities to stay on the job longer. Peer mentoring and job shadowing are

---

1 The Institute of Medicine was renamed the National Academy of Medicine in 2015.

other techniques that can enhance the skills of new workers while keeping mature workers productive for longer.

Another strategy is to employ community health workers to take over certain duties from primary care providers. Health workers frequently come from the neighborhoods they serve. Most provide health education, make follow-up calls, and visit patients in their homes. Because their role is nonclinical, they are easier to train and less costly to hire, but limited in versatility.

Geographic Maldistribution

Physicians often concentrate in larger numbers in metropolitan and suburban areas rather than in rural and inner-city areas. The former generally offer better prospects for living standards, professional interaction, access to modern facilities and technology, and professional growth.

The demand for physicians' services is primarily determined by the population's health care needs. The actual delivery of services, however, is based on people's ability to pay for them, mainly through health insurance. The need-based model assumes an even distribution of physicians, whereas demand factors favor the distribution of physicians mostly in metropolitan and suburban areas, where most of the well-insured populations live. Together with physician preferences, the demand factor leaves rural areas and inner cities with provider shortages.

Specialty Maldistribution

Besides the geographic maldistribution of physicians, an imbalance exists between primary and specialty care in the United States. From 1965 to 1992, the number of primary care physicians increased by only 13%, whereas the number of specialists increased by 121% (Rivo & Kindig, 1996). In the U.S., approximately 38% of physicians are generalists, while the remaining 62% are specialists (National Center for Health Statistics, 2017). In other industrialized countries, generalists typically constitute over 50% of the physician workforce.

Specialty maldistribution has become ingrained in the U.S. health care delivery system for three main reasons: medical technology, reimbursement methods and remuneration, and specialty-oriented medical education. By comparison, the need for primary care physicians is determined mainly by general population demographics. The population grows at a slower rate than technological advancements, so the gap between the primary care and specialty care physician workforce numbers continues to expand.

In the United States, the higher incomes of specialists relative to primary care physicians have contributed to the imbalance between the primary care and specialty physicians workforces. In addition, specialists have more predictable hours and enjoy higher prestige, both among their colleagues and by society in general (Rosenblatt & Lishner, 1991; Samuels & Shi, 1993). High status and prestige are especially accorded to tertiary care and specialties employing high technology. Unsurprisingly, these considerations influence the career decisions of many medical students.

The imbalance between generalists and specialists has several undesirable consequences. Having too many specialists has contributed to the high volume of intensive, expensive, and invasive medical services as well as to the rise in health care costs (Greenfield & Nelson, 1992; Rosenblatt, 1992; Schroeder & Sandy, 1993; Wennberg et al., 1993). In addition, having more surgeons increases the demand for initial contacts and follow-up visits with surgeons. Seeking care directly from specialists is often less effective than with primary care physicians, who often provide early intervention before complications develop (Starfield, 1992; Starfield & Simpson, 1993). Notably, a health care workforce with higher numbers of primary care professionals is associated with lower overall mortality and death rates from cardiovascular disease and cancer (Shi, 1992, 1994). Primary care physicians have also been the major providers for minorities, the poor, and people in underserved areas (Ginzberg, 1994; Starr, 1982). Hence, underserved populations suffer the most from shortages of primary care physicians.

▶ Dentists

Dentists are the major providers of dental care. Their main role is to diagnose and treat problems related to the teeth, gums, and tissues of the mouth. All dentists must be licensed to practice. Licensure requirements include graduation from an accredited dental school that awards a doctor of dental surgery (DDS) or doctor of dental medicine (DMD) degree, along with successful completion of both written and practical examinations.

Eight dental specialty areas are recognized by the American Dental Association: orthodontics (straightening teeth), oral and maxillofacial surgery (operating on the mouth and jaws), pediatric dentistry (dental care for children), periodontics (treating gums), prosthodontics (making artificial teeth or dentures), endodontics (root canal therapy), public health dentistry (community dental health), and oral pathology (diseases of the mouth). TABLE 4.4 describes the distribution of these specialties. The growth of dental specialties is influenced by technological advances, such as implant dentistry, laser-guided surgery, orthognathic surgery to restore facial form and function, new metal combinations for prosthetic devices, new bone graft materials in tissue-guided regeneration techniques, and new materials and instruments.

TABLE 4.4 Specialties for Dentists, 2016	
Dentists	153,500
Orthodontists	5,200
Oral surgeons	5,380
Dentists, all other	5,400
Total	169,480

Occupational employment and wages: national employment matrix. www.bls.gov. Accessed February 11, 2018.

Many dentists are involved in the prevention of dental decay and gum disease, including regular cleaning of teeth and educating patients on proper dental hygiene. Hence, dental offices generally employ dental hygienists and assistants to perform many preventive and routine care services. Dentists also spot symptoms that require treatment by a physician.

Most dentists practice in private offices, alone, or in groups. Dental offices operate as private businesses, and dentists often perform business tasks such as staffing, financing, purchasing, leasing, and work scheduling. Some dentists work at dental clinics in private companies, retail stores, franchised dental outlets, or managed care organizations (MCOs). Group dental practices—which typically offer lower overhead and increased productivity—have slowly grown. The federal government also employs dentists, mainly in the Department of Veterans Affairs and the U.S. Public Health Service hospitals and clinics.

Employer-sponsored dental insurance has increased the demand for dental care by enabling a greater segment of the population to afford it. The demand for dentists will continue to increase as populations with high dental needs increase, such as the elderly, the handicapped, the homebound, and patients with human immunodeficiency virus (HIV) infection. Other factors contributing to the increased demand for dentists include greater awareness of the importance of dental care for general health, the widespread appeal of the cosmetic and aesthetic dentistry, and the inclusion of dental care in many publicly funded programs (e.g., Head Start, Medicaid, community and migrant health centers, maternal and infant care).

▶ Pharmacists

The traditional role of pharmacists has been to dispense medicines prescribed by physicians, dentists, and podiatrists and to provide consultation on the proper selection and use of medicines. All states require a license to practice pharmacy. Since 2005, the bachelor of pharmacy degree has been phased out, and instead a PharmD degree requiring 6 years of postsecondary education has become the standard. Licensure requirements include graduation from an accredited pharmacy program as well as successful completion of a state board examination and practical experience or completion of a supervised internship. The 2016 annual salary of pharmacists ranged between $87,120 and $157,950.

Most pharmacists are generalists—dispensing drugs and advising providers and patients—but some become specialists. Pharmacotherapists specialize in drug therapy and work closely with physicians. Nutrition-support pharmacists determine and prepare drugs for nutritional therapy. Radiopharmacists or nuclear pharmacists produce radioactive drugs for patient diagnosis and therapy.

Most pharmacists hold salaried positions and work in community pharmacies that are independently owned or are part of a national drugstore, supermarket, or department store chain. Pharmacists are also employed by hospitals, MCOs, home health agencies, clinics, government health services organizations, and pharmaceutical manufacturers (**TABLE 4.5**).

The role of pharmacists has expanded over the last two decades from the preparation and dispensing of prescriptions to drug product education and expertise on specific drugs, drug interactions, and generic drug substitution. In about half of U.S. states, pharmacists have authority to initiate or modify drug treatment, as long as they have collaborative agreements with physicians. Pharmacists play a critical role in informing consumers, especially those with chronic conditions, about prescription drugs and their potential misuse. This education and counseling role is broadly referred to as *pharmaceutical care*. Including pharmacists in the health care team is particularly important in the hospital and community to ensure appropriate prescriptions and medication adherence.

TABLE 4.5 Sites of Employment for Pharmacists, 2016

Retail	134,610
Hospitals	71,390
Internet pharmacists, wholesalers, physician offices	11,080
Other	3,300
Total	231,460

Occupational employment and wages: national employment matrix. www.bls.gov. Accessed February 11, 2018.

▶ Other Doctoral-Level Health Professionals

In addition to physicians, dentists, and some pharmacists, some other health professionals have doctoral education, including optometrists, psychologists, podiatrists, and chiropractors. **TABLE 4.6** identifies the numbers of these professionals in 2016.

Optometrists provide vision care, such as examination, diagnosis, and correction of vision problems. They must be licensed to practice. Licensure requirements include possession of a doctor of optometry (OD) degree and successful completion of a written and a clinical state board examination. Most optometrists work in solo or group practices, while others work for the government, MCOs, optical stores, or vision care centers as salaried employees.

Psychologists provide patients with mental health care. They must be licensed or certified to practice. The ultimate recognition is the diplomate in psychology, which requires a doctor of philosophy (PhD) or doctor of psychology (PsyD) degree, a minimum of 5 years of postdoctoral experience, and the successful completion of a professional psychology examination administered by the American Board of Examiners. Psychologists may specialize in several areas, such as clinical, counseling, developmental, educational, engineering, personnel, experimental, industrial, psychometric, rehabilitation, school, and social domains (Stanfield, 1995, pp. 280–282). Considering the prevalence of mental health problems, the demand for psychologists for all age groups is likely to continue to increase for the foreseeable future.

Podiatrists treat patients with diseases or deformities of the feet by performing surgical operations, prescribing medications and corrective devices, and administering physiotherapy. They must be licensed. Licensure requirements include graduation from an accredited program that awards a doctor of podiatric medicine (DPM) degree and successful completion of a national examination administered by the National

TABLE 4.6 Employment Levels of Doctoral-Level Health Professionals in the United States, 2016

Optometrists	40,200
Psychologists	166,600
Podiatrists	11,000
Chiropractors	47,400

Occupational employment and wages: national employment matrix. www.bls.gov. Accessed February 11, 2018.

Board of Podiatry. Most podiatrists work in private practice, although some are salaried employees of health services organizations.

Chiropractors provide treatment to patients through chiropractic (Greek for "done by hand") manipulation, physiotherapy, and dietary counseling, typically helping patients with neurologic, muscular, and vascular disturbances. Chiropractic care is based on the belief that the body is a self-healing organism; thus chiropractors do not prescribe drugs or perform surgery. Chiropractors must be licensed to practice. Licensure requirements include graduation from a 4-year accredited program that awards a doctor of chiropractic (DC) degree and successful completion of an examination by the state chiropractic board. Most chiropractors work in a private solo or group practice. Due to a largely sedentary work environment in the United States and the limitations of modern Western medicine, chiropractors can play a significant role in addressing musculoskeletal disorders.

▶ **Nurses**

Nurses constitute the largest group of health care professionals. The nursing profession developed around hospitals after World War I and primarily attracted women. Before World War I, more than 70% of nurses worked in private duty, in patients' homes, or for private-pay patients in hospitals. Federal funding for nursing education increased after World War II, in the Nursing Training Act of 1964, the Health Manpower Act of 1968, and the Nursing Training Act of 1971. However, state funding remains the primary source of support for nursing schools.

Nurses are the main caregivers for sick and injured patients and address physical, mental, and emotional needs. All states require that nurses be licensed to practice. Licensure requirements include graduation from an approved nursing program and successful completion of a national examination. Educational preparation distinguishes between two levels of nurses: registered nurses and licensed practical nurses. Registered nurses (RNs) must complete an associate's degree (ADN), a diploma program, or a bachelor of science in nursing (BSN) degree. ADN programs take about 2 to 3 years to complete and are offered by community and junior colleges; diploma programs take 2 to 3 years to complete and are offered by hospitals; and BSN programs take 4 to 5 years to complete and are offered by colleges and universities (Stanfield, 1995, pp. 126–199). Licensed practical nurses (LPNs)—called licensed vocational nurses (LVNs) in some states— must complete a state-approved program in practical nursing and pass a national written examination. Most LPN programs last about 1 year and include both classroom study and supervised clinical practice.

Nurses work in a variety of health care settings, and many still do private-duty nursing in patients' homes. They are often classified according to work settings—for example, hospital nurses, long-term care nurses, public health nurses, private-duty nurses, office nurses, and occupational health or industrial nurses. Head nurses supervise other nurses; for example, RNs supervise LPNs.

With hospitals now treating much sicker patients than in the past, patient-to-nurse staffing ratios have increased, and caregiving by nurses has become more intensive. The remarkable growth in alternative settings for care has created new employment opportunities for nurses. The growing opportunities for RNs in supportive roles such as case management, utilization review, quality assurance, and prevention counseling have also increased the demand for their services. The current national shortage of nurses is likely to increase (Sochalski, 2002). Slow growth in wages, low job satisfaction, and inadequate career mobility pose major impediments to attracting and retaining nurses (Sochalski, 2002). Many U.S. hospitals turn to developing countries (such as the Philippines and China) for their nursing supply, and this trend is likely to continue.

Advanced-Practice Nurses

The term *advanced-practice nurse* (APN) refers to nurses who have education and clinical experience beyond that required of an RN. There are four areas of specialization for APNs (Cooper, 1998): clinical nurse specialists (CNSs), certified registered nurse anesthetists (CRNAs), nurse practitioners (NPs), and certified nurse-midwives (CNMs). NPs and CNMs are also classified as nonphysician practitioners; they are discussed in the next section. Besides being direct caregivers, APNs perform other activities such as collaborating and consulting with other health care professionals, educating patients and other nurses, collecting data for clinical research projects, and participating in the development and implementation of total quality management programs, critical pathways, case management, and standards of care (Grossman, 1995). There are 206,800 APNs in the United States according to the 2012 National Sample Survey of Registered Nurses.

The main difference between CNSs and NPs is that CNSs work in hospitals, whereas NPs mainly work in primary care settings. CNSs can specialize in specific fields such as oncology, neonatal health, cardiac care, or psychiatric care.

▶ Nonphysician Practitioners

The term *nonphysician practitioner* (NPP)—also called nonphysician clinician, midlevel provider, and physician extender—refers to clinical professionals who practice in many areas in which physicians practice but who do not possess an MD or a DO degree. NPPs receive less advanced training than physicians but more advanced training than RNs, and typically include physician assistants (PAs), NPs, and CNMs. In many instances of primary care, they can substitute for physicians. They do not, however, engage in the entire range of primary care nor deal with complex cases requiring physician expertise (Cooper, 1998). Hence, NPPs often work in close consultation with physicians.

NPs work predominantly in primary care, whereas PAs are evenly divided between primary care and specialty care. In 2017, there were 203,800 NPs, 106, 200 PAs, and 11,826 CNMs in the U.S. (U.S. Bureau of Labor Statistics, 2017).

PAs are members of a health care team who work in a dependent manner with a supervising physician (1986, p. 3). PAs may perform procedures only under physician supervision. They assist onsite or offsite physicians in the delivery of care to patients and perform services including evaluation, monitoring, diagnostics, therapeutics, counseling, and referral (Fitzgerald, 1995).

In 2017, there were 229 accredited PA training programs in the United States, which were steadily growing in enrollment (Accreditation Review Commission on Education for the Physician Assistant, 2017). PA programs award bachelor's degrees, certificates, associate degrees, or master's degrees. In most states, PAs have the authority to prescribe medications.

NPs are individuals who have successfully completed a program of study leading to competence as RNs in an expanded role. NPs constitute the largest group of NPPs and have experienced the most growth (Cooper, 1998); since 1997, however, enrollment in NP preparatory programs has gradually declined. The training of NPs may take place in a certificate program (at least 9 months in duration) or in a master's degree program (2 years of full-time study). States vary in NP licensure and accreditation requirements. Most NPs are now trained in master's-level or post-master's–level nursing programs. In addition, NPs must complete clinical training in direct patient care. The primary function of NPs is to promote wellness and health through patient education, and they spend time with patients to help them understand the need to take responsibility for their own health; hence, they are an important adjunct to the practice of primary care physicians. They also provide service in nursing homes (Brody et al., 1976). NPs have the authority to prescribe medications in almost all states.

CNMs are RNs with additional training from a nurse-midwifery program in areas such as maternal and fetal procedures, maternal and child nursing, and patient assessment (Endicott, 1976). CNMs deliver babies, provide family planning education, and manage gynecologic and obstetric care. They often substitute for obstetricians/gynecologists in prenatal and postnatal care, but refer abnormal or high-risk patients to obstetricians or jointly manage care of such patients. During childbirth, patients cared for by CNMs are less likely to have continuous electronic monitoring, induced labor, or anesthesia, which are associated with lower cesarean section rates and less use of resources including length of hospital stay, operating room costs, and use of anesthesia staff (Rosenblatt et al., 1997).

Value of NPP Services

Efforts to establish the roles of NPs, PAs, and CNMs as nonphysician health care providers began in the late 1960s, when it was recognized that they could improve access to primary care, especially in rural and underserved areas. Their work helps alleviate some problems created by the geographic maldistribution of physicians. Indeed, NPPs can provide both high-quality and cost-effective medical care. Compared to physicians, NPPs spend more time with patients and establish better rapport. NPs often have better communication and interviewing skills than physicians— skills that are particularly important in community and migrant health centers in assessing patients who are predominantly of minority origin and often have little education (Brody et al., 1976). Clients report greater satisfaction with NPs because NPs are more likely to perform comprehensive examinations. CNMs are considered effective in providing access to obstetric and prenatal services in rural and poor communities.

Before NPPs can be used to their full potential, however, issues to be resolved include legal restrictions on practice, reimbursement policies, and relationships with physicians. The lack of autonomy to practice is a noteworthy barrier facing midlevel providers, as many states require physician supervision. NPPs also face financial barriers in reimbursement, which is generally indirect—that is, made to the physicians with whom they practice.

▶ Allied Health Professionals

In the early 20th century, the health care provider workforce consisted of physicians, nurses, pharmacists, and optometrists. The growth in technology and specialized interventions placed greater demands on physicians and nurses and limited the time they could spend with patients.

Such time constraints created a need to train other professionals as adjuncts to or substitutes for physicians and nurses. Allied health professionals receive specialized training, and their clinical interventions are meant to complement the work of physicians and nurses. Through their assistance, physicians and nurses are relieved of time pressures and can attend to functions that require their expertise and keep abreast of the latest advances in their disciplines.

Allied health includes many areas and constitutes approximately 60% of the U.S. health care workforce. An *allied health professional* is a person who has received a certificate or associate's, bachelor's, or master's degree; doctoral-level training; or post-baccalaureate training in a health care-related science and who has responsibility for the delivery of health or related services. These services may be associated with the identification, evaluation, and prevention of diseases and disorders; dietary and nutritional services; rehabilitation; or health system management. Furthermore, allied health professionals differ from those with a degree in medicine (MD or DO), dentistry, optometry, podiatry, chiropractic, or pharmacy; a graduate degree in health administration; a degree in clinical psychology; or a degree equivalent to one of these. Allied health professionals can be divided into two broad categories: technicians and/or assistants and therapists and/or technologists.

Technicians and Assistants

Typically, technicians and assistants receive less than 2 years of postsecondary education and are trained to perform procedures. They require supervision from therapists or technologists to ensure care plan evaluation in the treatment process. Technicians and assistants include physical therapy assistants, certified occupational therapy assistants, medical laboratory technicians, radiological technicians, and respiratory therapy technicians.

Technologists and Therapists

Technologists and therapists receive more advanced training, including education in evaluating patients, diagnosing problems, and developing treatment plans. They must also be trained to evaluate the appropriateness and potential side effects of therapy treatments and to teach procedural skills to technicians.

Some key allied health professionals are graduates of programs accredited by their respective professional bodies. For example, such programs train physical therapists (PTs), who provide care for patients with movement dysfunction. The bachelor's degree program has been phased out for PTs, replaced by master's degree (MPT or MSPT) or doctoral degree (DPT) programs in physical therapy. Passing an examination administered by the American Physical Therapy Association is also required for licensure.

Occupational therapists (OTs) help people improve their ability to perform tasks in their daily living and work environments. OTs help rehabilitate individuals with conditions that are mentally, physically, developmentally, or emotionally disabling. OT interventions help people live independently or be more productive at their workplace. The minimum requirements for entering the OT profession are possessing a bachelor's or master's degree in occupational therapy and passing a certification examination administered by the National Board for Certification in Occupational Therapy.

Dietitians, or nutritionists and dietetic technicians, ensure that institutional foods and diets are prepared according to nutritional standards. Dietitians are registered by the Commission on Dietetic Registration of the American Dietetic Association.

Dispensing opticians fit eyeglasses and contact lenses. They are certified by the American Board of Opticianry and the National Contact Lens Examiners.

Speech/language pathologists treat patients with speech and language problems, whereas audiologists treat patients with hearing problems. The American Speech-Language-Hearing Association is the credentialing association for audiologists and speech/language pathologists.

Social workers help patients and families cope with problems from long-term illness, injury and rehabilitation, and other issues. Bachelor's and master's degree programs in social work in the United States are accredited by the Council on Social Work Education.

▶ Public Health Professionals

The field of public health employs diverse health professionals. Public health professionals focus on the whole community, rather than on the individual, and work to address issues such as access to health care, infectious disease control, environmental health issues, and violence and injury issues. Public health professionals include physicians, researchers, administrators, lawyers, environmentalists, and social scientists. In addition to education in their primary profession, many public health professionals possess a graduate degree from a school of public health. As of 2017, there were 64 accredited schools of public health in the United States. The five core disciplines in public health education are biostatistics, epidemiology, health services administration, health education /behavioral science, and environmental health (Association of Schools and Programs of Public Health, 2017).

▶ Community Health Workers

Health care providers are increasingly using a team-based approach to deliver care. Indeed, the complexity of health problems of many Americans, combined with the specialization of health professionals, makes health care teamwork and team training essential. This is especially true for addressing risk factors for chronic conditions and for treating people with multiple chronic diseases, including one-fourth of Americans and two-thirds of people age 65 or older (Graffunder & Sakurada, 2016).

Community health workers (CHWs) are integral to many health care systems. Their roles vary and include both the socially oriented tasks of natural helpers and the clinical tasks of physician extenders. As natural helpers, CHWs play an important role in connecting public and primary care to their communities. As primary health care becomes patient-centered and community-oriented, the natural helper roles—which emphasize trust, rapport, understanding, and the ability to communicate with the community—take on an increased significance.

In some states, the community health worker is a more formal member of the integrated primary health care team. In this role, the CHW provides structured linkages between the community, the patient, and the health care system. In essence, CHWs act as the missing piece of the primary health care puzzle. They connect health care services to the community and, when functioning as full members of the health care team, help ground and contextualize primary care practices in the community. Such community-oriented primary care leads to increased patient satisfaction, better community acceptance, and improved health outcomes. The most effective CHWs are strongly embedded in their communities; they have clear supervision within the health care system, clearly defined roles in the health care system, and rigorous training and a defined system of advancing their education and roles within the health care system (Herman, 2011).

CHWs often receive brief training and minimal supplies, and many work on the periphery of health care service areas, usually at a distance from health facilities. For these reasons, key to success is strong management and supportive supervision through the implementation of clear reporting structures and frequent consultations between CHWs and other professionals who lead integrated health care teams (Campbell et al., 2004). Without strong management, CHWs could exceed the limits of their training and have poorly-defined job ownership and accountability.

To work effectively, CHWs must be integrated into the mainstream health care delivery system. In the patient-centered medical home (PCMH) model, a health care team guided by a clinical primary care provider such as a personal physician or nurse practitioner, provides continuous, comprehensive, and coordinated care in a culturally and linguistically sensitive manner throughout a patient's lifetime. CHWs can fill essential roles of care in this model.

In 2011, the Centers for Disease Control and Prevention (CDC) and the Division for Heart Disease and Stroke Prevention published *Addressing Chronic Disease Through CHWs: A Policy and Systems-Level Approach*; this report recommended that states integrate CHWs in high-risk communities to prevent chronic disease. Likewise, the Institute of Medicine (IOM) has recommended including CHWs in the strategic plan to prevent, control, and reduce the impact of hypertension (CDC, 2014). The ACA identified the need to encourage CHW engagement in health promotion and improving health for medically underserved populations. Moreover, the CDC has called for stronger support for CHW programs to help eliminate health disparities related to the prevention and management of diabetes (CDC, 2014; IOM, 2001).

In today's complex health care system, patient care can no longer be delivered within the silos of individual health professions. The health care workforce must be redesigned to accommodate the growing number of patients entering the health care system. As primary care teams develop within the PCMH movement, primary care practices will become the hub of access to care. To meet patients' needs, health care policymakers, researchers, and clinicians must examine the feasibility and value of integrating CHWs into primary care while preserving their role as community advocates in community-related activities and initiatives (Franklin et al., 2015).

▶ Health Services Administrators

Health services administrators are employed at the top, middle, and entry levels of various organizations that deliver health services. Top-level administrators provide leadership and strategic direction, work closely with governing boards, and are responsible for the long-term success of an organization. They are responsible for the operational, clinical, and financial outcomes of the organization. Middle-level administrators may have leadership roles in major centers such as outpatient, surgical services, or nursing services, or they may be departmental managers in charge of diagnostics, dietary, rehabilitation, social services, environmental services, or medical records. They are involved in major planning and coordinating functions, organizing human and physical resources, direction and supervision of other employees, operational and financial controls, and decision making. Midlevel administrators often have direct responsibility for implementing changes, enhancing efficiency, and developing new procedures based on changes in the health care delivery system. Entry-level administrators may function as assistants to midlevel managers and supervise a small number of operatives. Their main function may be to oversee and assist with operations critical to the efficient operation of a departmental unit.

Health services administration is taught at the bachelor's and master's degree levels in a variety of settings, with programs leading to several different degrees. There are academic programs in schools of medicine, public health, public administration, business administration, and allied health sciences. Bachelor's degrees prepare students for entry-level positions, while midlevel and senior-level positions require a graduate degree. The most common degrees held by health services administrators are the master of health administration (MHA) or master of health services administration (MHSA), master of business administration (MBA, with a health care management emphasis), master of public health (MPH), and master of public administration (or affairs; MPA) (Pew Health Professions Commission, 1998). The U.S. graduate schools of public health that are accredited by the Council on Education for Public Health help train health services administrators in MHA/MHSA and MPH programs.

Growth of the elderly population, along with the current shortage of qualified administrators, is creating opportunities for long-term care management. Training of nursing home administrators has been greatly influenced by government licensing regulations. Passing a national examination administered by the National Association of Boards of Examiners of Long-Term Care Administrators is a standard requirement; however, the educational qualifications for a license vary significantly from one state to another. Although the basic academic qualification required by most states is a bachelor's degree, acquiring adequate skills in nursing home administration requires a degree that specializes in long-term care administration or health care management (Singh, 2005).

▶ Patient-Centered Care

As the health care system emphasizes high-value delivery, the terms "population health" and "patient-centered care" have become common. (**FIGURE 4.1** illustrates the evolution of health care from an individual-focused to a population-focused approach.) Patient-centered care refers to care that is respectful of and responsive to individual patient preferences, needs, and values, in which patient values guide all clinical decisions (IOM, 2001). Population health refers to the health outcomes of a group of individuals, including the distribution of outcomes within the group. Population health outcomes are the product of multiple determinants of

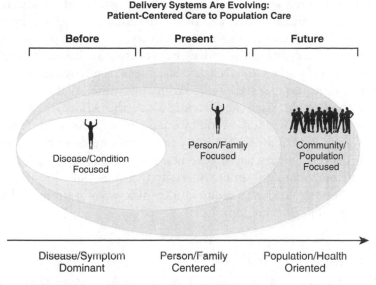

Delivery Systems Are Evolving:
Patient-Centered Care to Population Care

Before   **Present**   **Future**

Disease/Condition
Focused

Person/Family
Focused

Community/
Population
Focused

Disease/Symptom
Dominant

Person/Family
Centered

Population/Health
Oriented

FIGURE 4.1 Evolution of the Focus of Health Care Delivery

health, including medical care, public health, genetics, behaviors, social factors, and environmental factors (IOM, 2013). Already many disruptive innovations that have a transformative influence on the health care system are emerging—for example, novel payment strategies, new delivery mechanisms such as accountable care organizations, and the rapid expansion of health information technology (Blumenthal, 2011). This new environment is transforming the volume-driven payment model to reward value, improve the patient experience, and promote population health.

In a patient-centered care model, providers manage and coordinate care and are accountable for disease prevention and wellness. Accountable systems of care serve as organized, vertically integrated networks that employ and contract with physician offices or community health centers. They are responsible for facilitating cross-sector care management and health information exchange, and for integrating health care services over the continuum of care for their patients and populations. Such accountable systems of care also link the provider network to community services systems and social and economic resources, including public health and behavioral health services, by addressing the social and economic determinants of health and upstream risk factors for the community.

▶ Conclusion

Health services professionals in the United States constitute the largest proportion of the health care labor force. The growth and development of these professions are influenced by demographic trends, research and technology advances, disease and illness trends, and the changing environment of health care financing and delivery. Physicians play a leading role in the delivery of health services, but are maldistributed by specialty and geography in the United States. Shortages of physicians and other health care professionals are foreseen in the future, as the number of insured people has risen significantly since the Affordable Care Act was implemented. In addition to physicians, many other health services professionals contribute significantly to health care delivery, including nurses, dentists, pharmacists, optometrists, psychologists, podiatrists, chiropractors, nonphysician providers, and various allied health professionals. These professionals require different levels of training and work in a variety of health care settings.

References

1. Accreditation Review Commission on Education for the Physician Assistant. 2017. Accredited physician assistant programs. https://www.physicianassistantedu.org/accredited-physician-assistant-programs/. Accessed December 10, 2017.
2. Alliance for Health Reform, Robert Wood Johnson Foundation. 2011. Health care workforce: Future supply vs. demand. http://www.allhealthpolicy.org/wp-content/uploads/2017/03/Health_Care_Workforce_104.pdf. Accessed December 11, 2017.
3. American Academy of Family Physicians. 2013. Geographic distribution of primary care physicians affects health care. https://www.aafp.org/news/government-medicine/20130620geodistpolicy.html. Accessed December 11, 2017.
4. American Academy of Physician Assistants. 1986. *PA Fact Sheet.* Arlington, VA: American Academy of Physician Assistants.
5. American Public Health Association. 2011. The Affordable Care Act's public health workforce provisions: Opportunities and challenges. https://www.apha.org/~/media/files/pdf/topics/aca/apha_workforce.ashx. Accessed December 11, 2017.
6. Association of American Medical Colleges (AAMC), Center for Workforce Studies. 2008. The complexities of physician supply and demand: Projections through 2025. https://www.aamc.org/download/426242/data/. Accessed March 28, 2018.
7. Association of American Medical Colleges (AAMC). 2017. State physician workforce data book. https://members.aamc.org/eweb/upload/2017%20State%20Physician%20Workforce%20Data%20Report.pdf. Accessed December 2017.
8. Association of Schools and Programs of Public Health. 2017. About ASPPH. https://www.aspph.org/about/. Accessed December 2017.
9. Blumenthal D. 2011. Implementation of the federal health information technology initiative. *N Engl J Med.* 365(24):2426–2431.
10. Brody SJ, et al. 1976. The geriatric nurse practitioner: A new medical resource in the skilled nursing home. *J Chronic Dis.* 29(8):537–543.
11. Campbell M, et al. 2004. Improving multiple behaviors for colorectal cancer prevention among African American church members. *Health Psychol.* 23(5):492–502.
12. Centers for Disease Control and Prevention (CDC). 2014. Community health workers/promotores de salud: Critical connections in communities. http://www.cdc.gov/diabetes/projects/pdfs/comm.pdf. Accessed December 11, 2017.

13. Cooper RA. 1994. Seeking a balanced physician workforce for the 21st century. *JAMA*. 272(9):680–687.
14. Cooper RA. 1998. Current and projected workforce of nonphysician clinicians. *JAMA*. 280(9):788–794.
15. Endicott KM. 1976. In: Health Resources Administration, U.S. Public Health Service, *Health in America: 1776–1976*. DHEW Pub. No. 76616. Washington, DC: U.S. Department of Health, Education, and Welfare; 138–165.
16. Fitzgerald MA. 1995. The midlevel provider: Colleague or competitor? *Patient Care*. 29(1):20.
17. Franklin CM, et al. 2015. Interprofessional teamwork and collaboration between community health workers and healthcare teams: An integrative review. *Health Serv Res Manag Epidemiol*. 2:2333392815573312. doi: 10.1177/2333392815573312.
18. Ginzberg E. 1994. Improving health care for the poor. *JAMA*. 271(6):464–467.
19. Graffunder C, Sakurada B. April 6, 2016. Preparing health care and public health professionals for team performance: The community as classroom. https://nam.edu/wp-content/uploads/2016/05/Preparing-Health-Care-and-Public-Health-Professionals-for-Team-Performance-The-Community-as-Classroom.pdf. Accessed December 11, 2017.
20. Greenfield S, Nelson EC. 1992. Recent developments and future issues in the use of health status assessment measures in clinical settings. *Med Care*. 30(5 suppl):MS23–MS41.
21. Grossman D. 1995. APNs: pioneers in patient care. *Am J Nurs*. 95(8):54–56.
22. Herman AA. 2011. Community health workers and integrated primary health care teams in the 21st century. *J Ambul Care Manage*. 34(4):354-61. doi: 10.1097/JAC.0b013e31822cbcd0.
23. Institute of Medicine (IOM). 2001. *Crossing the quality chasm: A new health system for the 21st century*. Washington, DC: National Academy Press.
24. Institute of Medicine (IOM). 2013. Working definition of population health. http://nationalacademies.org/hmd/~/media/Files/Activity%20Files/PublicHealth/PopulationHealthImprovementRT/Pop%20Health%20RT%20Population%20Health%20Working%20Definition.pdf. Accessed March 28, 2018.
25. Kahn NB, et al. 1994. AAFP constructs definitions related to primary care. *Am Fam Physician*. 1994;50(6):1211–1215.
26. National Center for Health Statistics. 2017. *Health, United States, 2016: With chartbook on long-term trends in health*. Hyattsville, MD: National Center for Health Statistics.
27. Pew Health Professions Commission. November 10, 1998. Pew Commission urges increased action to cut U.S. physician supply. *PT Bull*. p. 10.
28. Rich EC, et al. Preparing generalist physicians: The organizational and policy context. *J Gen Intern Med*. 1994;9(1 suppl):S115–S122.
29. Rivo ML, Kindig D. 1996. A report on the physician work force in the United States. *N Engl J Med*. 334(13):892–896.
30. Rosenblatt RA. 1992. Specialists or generalists: On whom should we base the American health care system? *JAMA*. 267(12):1665–1666.
31. Rosenblatt RA, Lishner DM. 1991. Surplus or shortage? Unraveling the physician supply conundrum. *Western J Med*. 154(1):43–50.
32. Rosenblatt RA, et al. 1997. Interspecialty differences in the obstetric care of low-risk women. *Am J Public Health*. 87(3):344–351.
33. Samuels ME, Shi L. 1993. *Physician recruitment and retention: A guide for rural medical group practice*. Englewood, CO: Medical Group Management Press.

34. Schroeder S, Sandy LG. 1993. Specialty distribution of U.S. physicians: The invisible driver of health care costs. *N Engl J Med*. 328(13):961–963.
35. Shi L. 1992. The relation between primary care and life chances. *J Health Care Poor Underserved*. 3(2):321–335.
36. Shi L. 1994. Primary care, specialty care, and life chances. *Intl J Health Serv*. 24(3):431–458.
37. Singh DA. 2005. *Effective management of long-term care facilities*. Sudbury, MA: Jones and Bartlett.
38. Sochalski J. 2002. Nursing shortage redux: Turning the corner on an enduring problem. *Health Aff*. 21(5):157–164.
39. Stanfield PS. 1995. *Introduction to the health professions*. Sudbury, MA: Jones and Bartlett.
40. Starfield B. 1992. *Primary Care: Concepts, evaluation, and policy*. New York, NY: Oxford University Press.
41. Starfield B, Simpson L. 1993. Primary care as part of US health services reform. *JAMA*. 269:3136–3139.
42. Starr P. 1982. *The social transformation of American medicine: The rise of a sovereign profession and the making of a vast industry*. New York, NY: Basic Books.
43. U.S. Bureau of Labor Statistics. 2016. Labor force statistics from the current population survey. https://www.bls.gov/cps/cpsaat18b.htm. Accessed December 10, 2017.
44. U.S. Bureau of Labor Statistics. 2017. Occupational outlook handbook, nurse anesthetists, nurse midwives, and nurse practitioners. https://www.bls.gov/ooh/healthcare/nurse-anesthetists-nurse-midwives-and-nurse-practitioners.htm. Accessed December 10, 2017.
45. Wennberg JE, et al. Summer 1993. Finding equilibrium in U.S. physician supply. *Health Aff*. pp. 89–103.

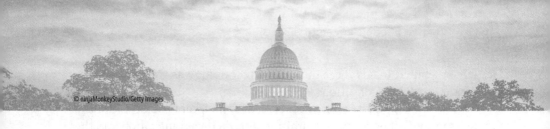

CHAPTER 5
Technology and Its Effects

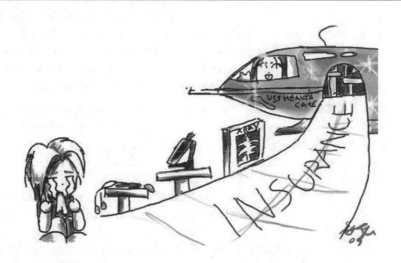

▶ Introduction

Medical technology has brought numerous benefits to modern civilization. These benefits, however, have come at a price—a price that society has to pay. Research and development (R&D) and the production of new technology are costly, although sophisticated advanced diagnostic procedures have reduced health complications and disability. New medical cures have increased longevity, and new drugs have helped stabilize chronic conditions and given an improved quality of life to many. The fact that life expectancy almost doubled from 1900 to 1965 was a result of advances in social conditions—improved sanitation, nutrition, and living conditions—rather than advances in medical treatment. The continuing increase in longevity since then, however, is largely attributed to advances in medical technology as well as to better nutrition and living conditions.

With the rising costs of medical care, at some point society will have to face the conflict between a commitment to medical innovation and the adoption of new technology on the one hand and cost containment on the other hand. Reining in medical spending in the United States so that it is on par with the spending in other advanced nations has remained an elusive dream, despite various efforts to contain rising costs.

Canadians and residents of other industrialized nations in Europe, who have enjoyed universal health insurance for several decades, have been able to place limits on the availability and use of costly technology through supply-side rationing. In contrast, the notion of medical rationing has not proved palatable to Americans. Hence, the idea of extending health care to all Americans has presented a major predicament.

During the postindustrial era, developments in science and technology were instrumental in drastically changing the nature of health care delivery. Since then, the ever-increasing proliferation of new technology has continued to profoundly alter many facets of health care delivery. Following are some of the major changes triggered by technology:

- New technology has raised consumer expectations about what may be possible. Patients' expectations have considerable influence on their health care–seeking behavior, leading to greater demand for and utilization of the latest and best that technology can offer.
- Technology influences the organization and financing of medical services. Specialized services that previously could be offered only in hospitals are now available in outpatient and community settings.
- The introduction of advanced technology has influenced the scope and content of medical training and shaped the practice of medicine, fueling a trend toward specialization in medicine at the expense of public health, preventive medicine, and primary care.
- Although some medical technology may reduce costs, as a whole technology has contributed to health care cost escalation. For both the consumer and the provider, the cost of excessive treatment has generally been of little concern as long as a third party—either an insurance plan or the government—pays for it.
- Technology has raised complex moral and ethical dilemmas in medical research and decision making. For example, when critically ill patients are put on life support with little hope of full recovery, health care resources may be wasteful.

Economic globalization has also enveloped biomedical knowledge and technology. This is particularly true for the developed and developing nations where leading physicians have access to the same scientific knowledge through medical journals and the Internet. Most drugs and medical devices available in the United States are also available in many other parts of the world.

▶ What Is Medical Technology?

Medical technology refers to the practical application of scientific knowledge to improve people's health and to create efficiencies in the delivery of medical care. Medical science has greatly benefited from developments in other applied sciences, such as chemistry, physics, engineering, and pharmacology. For example, advances in organic chemistry made it possible to identify and extract the active ingredients found in natural plants to produce drugs and anesthetics. Developments in electrical and mechanical engineering led to such medical advances as radiology, cardiology, and encephalography (Bronzino et al., 1990, p. 11). Magnetic resonance imaging (MRI), a technology that had its origins in basic research on the structure of the atom, was later transformed into a major diagnostic tool (Gelijns & Rosenberg, 1994). The disciplines of computer science and communication systems have found applications in health information technology and telemedicine (Tan, 1995, p. 4).

Nanomedicine is an emerging area of medical technology that requires manipulation of materials at the atomic and molecular levels. Scientists are working on the use of nano[1] materials as means for accurate diagnosis and treatment of diseases, such as cancer.

In its narrow sense, medical technology includes sophisticated machines, pharmaceuticals, and biological therapies. In a broader sense, it also covers medical and surgical procedures used in rendering medical care, ultramodern facilities and settings of care delivery, health information systems, and management and operational systems that make health care delivery more efficient (**EXHIBIT 5.1**).

▶ Health Information Technology

Information technology (IT) has become an integral part of health care delivery. IT involves computer applications that transform massive amounts of data into useful information. This technology is indispensable for managing the vast array of information that is used in patient care delivery, quality improvement, cost containment, billing and collections, and other aspects of operating health care organizations. Most large health care organizations have information systems departments and managers who are charged with maintaining and improving the flow of information. In addition, IT applications are increasingly being used to link health care

---

1 A nanometer is one-billionth of a meter.

EXHIBIT 5.1   Examples of Medical Technology

- Diagnostic equipment
  - Computed tomography (CT) scanner
  - Magnetic resonance imaging (MRI)
- Equipment and devices to render treatment
  - Lithotripter
  - Heart and lung machine
  - Kidney dialysis machine
  - Pacemaker
- Pharmaceuticals
- Medical procedures
  - Open-heart surgery
  - Tissue transplants
  - Hip and knee replacements
- Facilities and organizational systems
  - Medical centers and systems
  - Laboratories
  - Managed care networks
  - Health information systems
  - Patient care management
  - E-health and e-therapy
  - Telemedicine
  - Distance education
  - Electronic medical records

organizations to agencies outside those organizations. For example, it is a common practice to electronically transmit billing information to payers.

Major Categories

Specific IT system applications in health services delivery fall into five main areas.

First, *clinical information systems* are IT applications that support patient care delivery. Electronic medical records, for example, can quickly provide reliable information necessary to guide clinical decision making and to produce timely reports on the quality of care delivered. Computerized physician-order entry enables physicians to transmit orders electronically from the patient's bedside or physician's office. Telemedicine is based on integrated applications of telecommunications and information technologies. *Health informatics* is the term now used for IT applications that are designed to improve clinical efficiency, accuracy, and reliability.

Second, *administrative information systems* are designed to assist in carrying out financial and administrative support activities such as payroll, patient accounting, staff scheduling, materials management, budgeting and cost control, and office automation.

Third, *decision support systems* provide information and analytical tools to support managerial decision making. Such tools are used to forecast patient volume, project staffing requirements, evaluate financial performance, analyze utilization, conduct clinical research, and improve quality and productivity.

Fourth, *clinical decision support systems* (CDSSs) are interactive software systems designed to help clinicians with decision-making tasks, such as determining a diagnosis or recommending a treatment for a patient (O'Sullivan et al., 2014). Their use, however, is not yet widespread.

Finally, Internet and e-health applications enable patients and practitioners to access information, facilitate interaction between consumers or between patients and providers, add certain conveniences for both physicians and patients, and enable the possibility of *virtual visits* online between a patient and physician.

Electronic Health Records

Electronic health records (EHRs) are IT applications that replace the traditional paper medical records. In the United States, use of EHRs in health delivery organizations is well under way, but little progress has been made in the development of information-sharing networks. EHR networks make it possible to access individual records online from many separate, interoperable automated systems within an electronic network. The ability to share and access patient information by various users is referred to as *interoperability*. Some evidence indicates that EHR use produces improved patient care by enabling physicians to have timely access to patient records, alerting them to a potential for medical errors, and making critical lab values available when needed (King et al., 2014). On the downside, using EHRs may be time consuming, resulting in decreased productivity (Palmer, 2014). Also, the U.S. health care system has a long way to go in achieving interoperability because a significant number of physicians who use EHRs still do not get all the needed information electronically (Hsiao et al., 2015).

According to the Institute of Medicine[2] (2003), a fully developed EHR system includes four key components:

- Collection and storage of health information on individual patients over time, where health information is defined as information pertaining to the health of an individual or health care provided to an individual
- Immediate electronic access to individual- and population-level information by authorized users

---

2 The Institute of Medicine was renamed the National Academy of Medicine in 2015.

- Provision of knowledge and decision support that enhance the quality, safety, and efficiency of patient care (health informatics)
- Support of efficient processes for health care delivery

HITECH and MACRA Laws

U.S. health policy has promoted incentives to increase the use of EHRs by health care providers. For example, the Health Information Technology for Economic and Clinical Health (HITECH) Act of 2009 provides financial incentives for adopting and making meaningful use of EHRs. *Meaningful use* refers to specific criteria related to quality, safety, efficiency, and other aspects of use that providers are required to meet. Subsequently, the Medicare Access and CHIP Reauthorization Act of 2015 (MACRA) combined certain quality and efficiency criteria into a Merit-based Incentive Payment System (MIPS). For those providers who meet the performance criteria in 2017, their payments will be adjusted upward in 2019.

The Health Insurance Portability and Accountability Act

To alleviate concerns about the confidentiality of patient information, the Health Insurance Portability and Accountability Act (HIPAA) of 1996 restricted the legal use of personal medical information for three main purposes: health care delivery to the patient, operation of the health care organization, and reimbursement. The HIPAA legislation mandated strict controls on the transfer of personally identifiable health data between two entities, provisions for disclosure of protected information, and criminal penalties for violation (Clayton, 2001). It also established certain patient rights, such as the right of patients to inspect and have copies of their protected health information, to request corrections to the records, and to restrict who may obtain the information. The HITECH law strengthened the civil and criminal enforcement of HIPAA by including increased penalties for violations.

The Internet, E-Health, and E-Therapy

The Internet has continued to revolutionize certain aspects of health care delivery. *E-health* refers to "all forms of electronic health care delivered over the Internet, ranging from informational, educational, and commercial 'products' to direct services offered by professionals, nonprofessionals, businesses, or consumers themselves" (Maheu et al., 2001). The use of e-health has grown as many providers have created secure Internet portals to enable patients to access their EHRs; allow patient–provider email messaging; and use mobile apps for smartphones and tablets (Ricciardi et al., 2013).

E-therapy has emerged as an alternative to face-to-face therapy for behavioral health support and counseling (Skinner & Latchford, 2006). Also referred to as online therapy, e-counseling, teletherapy, or cyber-counseling, *e-therapy* refers to professional therapeutic interactions that occur online between qualified mental health professionals and their clients. A growing body of evidence indicates that e-therapy is effective for a variety of psychosocial problems (Barak et al., 2008). The main difference between e-health and e-therapy is that the former is a self-help approach for obtaining Web-based information; the latter involves interaction with a health care professional.

By accessing self-help information from the Internet, patients have become more active participants in their own health care. Of course, while information empowers patients, it also has the potential to create conflict between patients and their physicians. Using the right source can provide valid and up to date information to both consumers and practitioners. For instance, departments of the U.S. government offer a wealth of research-based information.

The Internet is not merely a source of information, but also offers new ways to create efficiency. In practice settings, the Internet is being used to register patients, direct them to alternative care sites, transmit diagnostic results, and order pharmaceuticals and other products. In addition, by accessing patient information through the Internet from their homes or hospital lounges, physicians can get a head start on their hospital rounds (Morrissey, 2002).

Telemedicine and Remote Monitoring

Telemedicine, or distance medicine, employs telecommunications technology for medical diagnosis and patient care when the provider and the client are separated by distance. It also enables a generalist to consult a specialist when a patient's illness and diagnosis are complex. Areas of specialized medical services in telemedicine include teleradiology, telepathology, and telesurgery. General adoption of telemedicine has been slow, however. Some of the main barriers have been licensure of physicians and other providers across state borders, concerns about legal liability, and lack of reimbursement for services provided via telemedicine. Also, the cost-effectiveness of most telemedicine applications remains unsubstantiated. Diagnostic and consultative teleradiology, in contrast, is almost universally reimbursed and has proved to be cost-effective (Field & Grigsby, 2002).

Remote in-home patient monitoring programs that monitor vital signs, blood pressure, and blood glucose levels are proving to be cost-effective (Haselkorn et al., 2007). Likewise, remote monitoring of cardiac implantable electronic devices, such as pacemakers and cardioverter defibrillators, has shown a high level of patient acceptance and satisfaction (Morichelli et al., 2014). Remote monitoring may also reduce hospital utilization (White-Williams et al., 2015).

Tele-ICU is a relatively new development in telemedicine. It links intensivists[3] and other critical care professionals to a system network that enables remote monitoring of intensive care units (ICUs). The system provides real-time patient assessment capabilities and communication with bedside teams through ongoing virtual rounds (Goran, 2012). Studies show that tele-ICU programs are linked to lower patient mortality, shorter lengths of stay, and increased patient safety (Lilly et al., 2014).

▶ Diffusion and Utilization of Medical Technology

The development and dissemination of technology is called *technology diffusion*. This factor determines which new technology will be developed, when it will be made available for use, and where it can be accessed.

In general, high-tech procedures are more readily available in the United States than they are in most other countries, and little is done to limit the expansion of new medical technology. For example, compared with most hospitals in industrialized countries, American hospitals perform a far greater number of catheterizations, angioplasties, and heart bypass surgeries. The United States also has more high-tech equipment available for its population than most countries do. For example, in 2015, the United States had 39.0 MRI units per 1 million population, compared with 33.6 units in Germany, 14.5 units in Australia, 9.5 units in Canada, and 7.2 units in the United Kingdom. Only Japan had more MRI units: 51.7 per 1 million population (Organization for Economic Cooperation and Development[4] [OECD], 2017). To control medical costs, most nations have tried to limit—mainly through central planning (supply-side rationing)—the diffusion and utilization of high-tech procedures. For instance, the National Institute for Health and Clinical Excellence (NICE) of Great Britain decides whether the National Health Service should make certain medical technologies available (Milewa, 2006). Consequently, nations that employ central planning generally have "waiting lines" for specialized services. For example, in Canada, in 2017, patients could expect to wait 10.8 weeks for an MRI, 4.1 weeks for a CT scan, and 3.9 weeks for an ultrasound (Barua, 2017). The rationing of medical technology through central planning curtails costs, but it also restricts access to care.

---

3 Physicians who specialize in the care of critically ill patients.
4 The Organization for Economic Cooperation and Development is a forum of more than 30 countries.

Spending on R&D drives innovation, which results in the development of new technology. Once technology has been developed, its use is almost ensured. In 2012, the United States spent $119.3 billion on biomedical R&D, of which 59% was spent by the private sector, such as the pharmaceutical and biotechnology industry; the remaining 41% came from the government (Chakma et al., 2014). Apart from private funding, the federal government, through the National Institutes of Health (NIH), is the largest source of funding biomedical research. The NIH invests nearly $32.3 billion annually in medical research (NIH, 2017).

The United States leads the world in biomedical research spending. For example, U.S. R&D spending in 2014 exceeded by 46% the amount spent by all European countries on such efforts. However, some concerns have been expressed that the share of U.S. spending has declined from 50% of global spending on medical R&D in 2007 to 44.4% in 2012 (Chakma et al., 2014). Of course, if the spending, even at reduced levels, is used more efficiently and productively than in the past, there should be little reason for concern about this trend.

The major reasons that the United States leads all other nations in the development and use of technology are (1) cultural beliefs and values, (2) medical training and practice, (3) insurance coverage, and (4) competition among providers. These factors are discussed in subsequent sections of this chapter. **EXHIBIT 5.2** lists some steps that the United States could undertake to curtail the growth of technology. Implementing these measures, however, would go against the fundamental beliefs and values of Americans and would generate much controversy.

Cultural Beliefs and Values

American beliefs and values have been instrumental in determining the nature of health care delivery in the United States. Capitalism and limitations on government intervention promote innovation. An economic and political environment in which innovation thrives creates opportunities

---

EXHIBIT 5.2 Mechanisms to Control the Growth of Technology

- Implement central planning to determine how much technology will be made available and where
- Withdraw federal funding for R&D
- Change the patterns of medical training, placing greater emphasis on primary care practice
- Reduce the number of specialty residency slots for medical graduates
- Curtail insurance payments for expensive medical treatments
- Impose controls on pharmaceutical prices, which in turn will make less money available for R&D and development of new drugs

for scientists and manufacturers to develop new technology. Americans have high expectations of finding cures through science and technology, and they equate use of advanced medical technology with high-quality care. Consequently, Americans indicate overwhelmingly that advanced tests, drugs, medical equipment, and procedures are critical for improving the quality of health care (Schur & Berk, 2008). The desire to have state-of-the-art technology available, accompanied by the desire to use it despite its cost, is called the *technological imperative*.

Medical Training and Practice

The emphasis on specialty care over primary care and preventive services predominates in U.S. medical culture. This preference is reflected in the training of physicians. American medical graduates consistently choose to specialize rather than go into primary care practice. For example, it was estimated that only 20% of all 22,934 U.S. medical school students who graduated in 2012 would choose to practice primary care in 2015 (Schwartz, 2012). An oversupply of specialists has had important consequences for the development and use of new technology, because primary care physicians use less technology than specialists, even for similar medical conditions.

Insurance Coverage

Both theory and empirical research have suggested that the generosity of insurance coverage stimulates technological change (Smith et al., 2009). In general, financing of health care through insurance, either private or public, largely insulates both patients and providers from personal accountability for the utilization of medical services. Because out-of-pocket costs are of limited concern, patients expect their physicians to provide all that medical technology has to offer. Knowing that the services demanded by their patients are largely covered by insurance, providers generally show little hesitation in delivering or referring to specialty services. Other developed countries offer universal health insurance, but they use supply-side rationing to limit the overutilization of technology.

Competition Among Providers

Technology-based specialization has been used by the medical establishment as an enticement to attract insured patients. Many openly advertise the availability of the latest technology in their practices, which creates a perception of quality in the minds of consumers. State-of-the-art technology also plays a role in the ability of a hospital or clinic to recruit specialists. When hospitals develop new services and invest heavily in modernization programs, other hospitals in the area are generally forced to do the same, for competitive reasons. These trends have resulted in a tremendous amount of duplication of services and equipment and have further contributed to medical specialization.

▶ The Government's Role in Technology Diffusion

Technology diffusion has raised questions about cost, safety, benefit, and risk, among other issues. Federal legislation, in turn, has attempted to address these concerns. The government also plays a significant role in carrying out research and providing funding for research, as mentioned earlier.

Regulation of Drugs, Devices, and Biologics

The Food and Drug Administration (FDA) is an agency of the U.S. Department of Health and Human Services (DHHS) that is responsible for ensuring that drugs and medical devices are safe and effective for their intended use. The FDA also controls access to drugs by deciding whether a certain drug will be available by prescription only or as an over-the-counter purchase.

Legislation to Regulate Drugs

EXHIBIT 5.3 summarizes the main pieces of legislation that regulate drugs and medical devices in the United States. In response to legislation, the regulatory functions of the FDA have evolved over time. Under the Food and Drugs Act of 1906, the Bureau of Chemistry (predecessor of the FDA) was authorized to take action only after drugs had been marketed to consumers. It was assumed that the manufacturer would conduct safety tests before marketing the product. If innocent consumers were harmed, only then could the FDA take action (Bronzino et al., 1990, p. 198). This drug law was subsequently strengthened by the passage of the Federal Food, Drug, and Cosmetic Act of 1938 in response to the infamous Elixir Sulfanilamide disaster, which caused more than 100 deaths because of poisoning from a toxic solvent used in the liquid's preparation (Flannery, 1986). Under the revised law, drug manufacturers were required to provide scientific evidence about the safety of new products before putting them on the market.

The drug approval system was further transformed by the 1962 drug amendments (Kefauver-Harris Amendments) to the Federal Food, Drug, and Cosmetic Act. The law was tightened after thalidomide was distributed as an experimental drug to prevent morning sickness among pregnant women. In Europe, thousands of deformed infants were born

EXHIBIT 5.3 Summary of FDA Legislation

1906 *Food and Drugs Act*: FDA is authorized to take action only after drugs sold to consumers cause harm.

1938 *Federal Food, Drug, and Cosmetic Act*: Evidence of safety is required before new drugs or devices can be marketed.

1962 *Drug Amendments*: FDA takes charge of reviewing efficacy and safety of new drugs, which can be marketed only once approval is granted.

1976 *Medical Devices Amendments*: Premarket review of medical devices is authorized; devices are grouped into three classes.

1983 *Orphan Drug Act*: Drug manufacturers are given incentives to produce new drugs for rare diseases.

1990 *Safe Medical Devices Act*: Health care facilities must report device-related injuries or illness of patients or employees to the manufacturer of the device and, if death is involved, the incident must also be reported to the FDA.

1992 *Prescription Drug User Fee Act*: FDA receives the authority to collect application fees from drug companies to provide additional resources to shorten the drug approval process.

1997 *Food and Drug Administration Modernization Act*: Fast-track approvals for life-saving drugs are permitted when their expected benefits exceed those of existing therapies.

2013 *Drug Supply Chain Security Act*: Electronic systems are mandated to help protect consumers from exposure to drugs that may be counterfeit, stolen, contaminated, or otherwise harmful.

2016 *21st Century Cures Act*: Steps are designed to help accelerate medical product development and bring new innovations and advances to patients who need them.

to mothers who had used this new drug, though thalidomide was never approved for use in the United States. The 1962 drug amendments established a premarket approval system, giving the FDA authority to review the safety as well as the effectiveness of a new drug before it could be marketed. This consumer protection role for the FDA was intended to ensure that the agency could prevent harm before it occurred. The new rule, however, was criticized for slowing down the introduction of new drugs and, consequently, denying patients the early benefit of the latest treatments.

In the 1980s, pressure on the FDA from those wanting rapid access to new drugs for the treatment of human immunodeficiency virus (HIV) infection called for a reconsideration of the drug review process (Rakich et al., 1992, p. 186). The Orphan Drug Act of 1983 and subsequent amendments were passed to provide incentives, such as grant funding, for pharmaceutical firms to develop new drugs for rare diseases and conditions. As a result, many such drug therapies, called *orphan drugs*, have become available for conditions that affect fewer than 200,000 people in the United States.

In 1992, Congress passed the Prescription Drug User Fee Act, which authorized the FDA to collect fees from pharmaceutical companies to review their drug applications. According to the U.S. General Accounting Office, these fees have allowed the FDA to make new drugs available more quickly by shortening the time it takes for approvals to be issued. On the flip side, there has been an increasing trend in the number of prescription and over-the-counter drug recalls (Nagaich & Sadhna, 2015). There is clearly a trade-off between accelerating the review process and overlooking some potential safety risks.

In 1997, Congress passed the Food and Drug Administration Modernization Act. This law provides for increased patient access to experimental drugs and medical devices. It also permits fast-track approvals when the potential benefits of new drugs for serious or life-threatening conditions are considered significantly greater than those for currently available therapies.

The FDA's drug approval process remains far from perfect, however. The agency does not carry out its own testing of new drugs, but instead evaluates the drug studies conducted by pharmaceutical companies. Many times drug recalls are issued by the manufacturer or the FDA several years after a drug has been on the market and further research or use has shown the drug to be ineffective and/or unsafe. The FDA often engages in a balancing act between the demand for faster approval of new drugs on the one hand and the potential for safety recalls on the other hand. Nevertheless, the 21st Century Cures Act of 2016 provides for faster approval of new drugs and devices for life-threatening conditions.

Legislation to Regulate Devices

Medical devices include a wide range of products—from those as simple as tongue depressors and bedpans to those as complex as pacemakers and laser surgical equipment. Medical devices include general-purpose lab equipment, reagents, and test kits. Other examples include diagnostic ultrasound equipment, x-ray machines, and other imaging technology.

The FDA was first given jurisdiction over medical devices under the Federal Food, Drug, and Cosmetic Act of 1938. Initially, its jurisdiction was confined to the sale of products that were believed to be unsafe or that made misleading claims of effectiveness (Merrill, 1994). In the 1970s, however, several deaths and miscarriages were attributed to the Dalkon Shield, which had been marketed as a safe and effective contraceptive device (Flannery, 1986). The Medical Devices Amendments of 1976 extended the FDA's authority to include premarket review of medical devices divided into three classes:

- *Class I*: Devices that pose the lowest risk and are generally simple in design. These devices are subject to general controls regarding misbranding—that is, fraudulent claims regarding their therapeutic effects. Examples of Class I devices include enema kits and elastic bandages.

■   *Class II*: Devices subject to requirements for labeling, performance standards, and postmarket surveillance. Examples include powered wheelchairs and some pregnancy test kits.

■   *Class III*: Devices that come under the most stringent requirements of premarket approval regarding safety and effectiveness. Devices in this class support life, prevent health impairment, or present a potential risk of illness or injury (Rakich et al., 1992). Examples include implantable pacemakers and breast implants.

The Safe Medical Devices Act of 1990 has particular relevance for health care providers, who are required by law to report to the manufacturer, and in some cases to the FDA as well, all injuries and deaths caused by medical devices. Requirements under this act serve as an early warning system for any serious device-related problems that could potentially become widespread.

Legislation to Regulate Biologics

Biologics are derived from living organisms and include a wide range of products such as vaccines, blood and blood components, allergenics, somatic cells, gene therapy, tissues, and therapeutic proteins that are indicated for the prevention or treatment of a disease or health condition. Biologics are isolated from a variety of natural sources—human, animal, or microorganism. In contrast to most drugs that are chemically synthesized and have a known chemical structure, most biologics are complex mixtures that are not easily identified or characterized (FDA, 2009). The FDA regulates the licensing of biologics under the Public Health Service Act of 1944. Similar to drugs, the safety and effectiveness of biologics are regulated according to the Food, Drug, and Cosmetic Act of 1938, discussed previously.

The FDA in a Global Environment

A substantial quantity of drugs and devices are manufactured overseas and brought into the United States. To protect the American public against ineffective and/or harmful products, the FDA has been increasingly working in collaboration with its counterpart regulatory authorities in other countries. The FDA's involvement in developing countries to ensure the quality of drugs and devices manufactured in these countries strengthens their industries and protects the American public. Going forward, understanding the new requirements of a globalized world will become increasingly more important given the ongoing interdependencies between countries. To address global challenges, the FDA operates offices in many regions of the world. It also sends inspectors and experts from the United States to different parts of the world to conduct inspections and to participate in meetings and training sessions (Steinbach, 2016).

The Affordable Care Act and Medical Technology

In the area of medical technology, the Affordable Care Act (ACA) mainly affects devices and biologics. A 2.3% excise tax on the sale of certain medical devices by manufacturers and importers of these devices became effective in 2013. The higher costs associated with such taxes are passed on to the purchasers, mainly hospitals and physicians, and eventually filter down to consumers through higher health insurance premiums. This tax was suspended for 2016 and 2017, but a permanent repeal was still in the future at the time of this writing.

The Biologics Price Competition and Innovation Act of 2009 (incorporated into the ACA) authorized the FDA to approve biosimilars under a process similar to the approval of generic drugs. Because of their complexity, the term *generic* cannot apply to biologics; hence, the term *biosimilar* was created to apply to products that are highly similar to, or are interchangeable with, an already approved biological product. The Biosimilar User Fee Act of 2012, passed subsequently to the ACA, authorized the FDA to charge biopharmaceutical firms a user fee to pay for the review of applications for biosimilar products. It is believed that the introduction of biosimilars will create competition and drive down the cost of biologics. The first biosimilar product to be approved in the United States in March 2015 was Zarxio—biosimilar to Neupogen—which can be prescribed for the treatment of certain cancers.

Research on Technology

The Agency for Healthcare Research and Quality (AHRQ), a division of the DHHS, is the lead federal agency charged with supporting research to improve the quality of health care, reduce health care costs, and improve access to essential services. The agency's reports on technology assessment are made available to medical practitioners, consumers, and other health care purchasers.

As previously discussed, the federal government is also a major provider of financial support to private and public institutions for biomedical research. The AHRQ and the NIH support both basic and applied biomedical research in the United States.

▶ Impact of Medical Technology

The effects of advances in scientific knowledge and medical technology have been far-reaching and pervasive. These effects often overlap, making it difficult to pinpoint the precise impact of technology on the delivery of health care.

Impact on Quality of Care

Americans generally equate high-technology medicine to high-quality care, but such an association is not always accurate. Quality is enhanced only when new procedures can prevent or delay the onset of serious disease, provide better diagnosis, make quicker and more complete cures possible, increase the safety of medical treatment, minimize undesirable side effects, promote faster recovery from surgery, increase life expectancy, and add to quality of life (**EXHIBIT 5.4**). Improvements in diagnostic capabilities increase the likelihood that timely and more appropriate treatments will be provided. Technology can provide new remedies where none existed before, and can offer improved remedies that are more effective, less invasive, or safer than existing treatments. The outcomes in such cases can include increased longevity and decreased morbidity, both of which are indicators of better quality of health care.

Numerous examples can be cited that illustrate the role of technology in enhancing the quality of care. Tiny cardiac pacemakers and implantable cardioverter defibrillators can be placed in the human body to prevent sudden cardiac death. Angioplasty has reduced the need for open-heart bypass surgery. New imaging technologies such as positron emission tomography and single-photon emission computed tomography are available as advanced diagnostic tools to study brain function and identify the sources of both physical and mental disorders. Laser technology permits surgery to be performed with less trauma, better precision, and quicker postsurgical recovery; advanced lasers are used for high-precision eye surgery. Molecular and cell biology are being employed to screen for genetic disorders and provide gene therapy. New specialty drugs offer therapeutic advances for a number of conditions, such as cancer, hepatitis C, rheumatoid arthritis, and multiple sclerosis (Chambers et al., 2014).

EXHIBIT 5.4 Criteria for Quality of Care

- Prevent or delay disease onset
- Provide a more accurate diagnosis than is possible with currently available options
- Provide a quicker cure
- Provide a more complete cure
- Increase safety of treatment
- Minimize side effects
- Provide for faster recovery from surgery or illness
- Increase life expectancy
- Add to quality of life

Amid all the enthusiasm that emerging technologies might inspire, some degree of caution must prevail. Past experience shows that greater proliferation of technology does not necessarily lead to higher quality of care. Unless the effect of each individual technology is appropriately assessed, some innovations may actually be wasteful, and others may possibly be harmful.

Impact on Quality of Life

Quality of life indicates a patient's overall satisfaction with life during and after medical treatment. For example, quality of life is enhanced when technology enables people to live normal lives despite disabling conditions affecting speech, hearing, vision, and movement. Major technological advances have furnished the clinical ability to help patients cope with diabetes, heart disease, end-stage renal disease, and HIV/AIDS. Thanks to modern treatments, HIV/AIDS has become a chronic disease, not a death sentence (Komaroff, 2005). New categories of drugs are also instrumental in relieving pain and suffering. For example, for cancer pain management, new opioids have been developed for transdermal, nasal, and nebulized administration that allow needleless means of controlling pain (Davis, 2006). Finally, minimally invasive surgical procedures, such as lithotripsy, which crushes kidney and bile stones by using shock waves, have improved quality of life by reducing pain and suffering and allowing a quicker return to normal life. Similarly, procedures such as coronary artery bypass graft (CABG) surgery—an open-heart surgical procedure to correct blockage of coronary arteries—have made it possible for people with severe heart disease to return to normal activity within a few weeks after surgery. Previously, such patients would have required lifelong medication and suffered prolonged disability (Nitzkin, 1996).

Impact on Health Care Costs

Technological innovations have been the single most important factor in medical cost inflation (Institute of Medicine, 2002). In fact, they may have accounted for as much as half of the total rise in health care spending in recent years (Congressional Budget Office [CBO], 2008). Unlike other industries, in which new technology often reduces labor force and production costs, the addition of new technology in health care usually increases both labor and capital costs (Iglehart, 1982). **EXHIBIT 5.5** summarizes the main factors underlying this technology-driven cost escalation. First, there is the cost of acquiring the new technology and equipment. Second, special training for physicians and technicians to operate the equipment and to analyze the results often leads to increases in labor costs. Third, new technology may require special space and facilities (McGregor, 1989). Finally, the utilization of new technology is assured when it is covered by insurance. From a systems perspective, the costs associated with utilization of technology after it becomes available are more important than the initial purchase price.

Although it is true that many new technologies increase costs, others actually reduce costs when they replace treatments that are more expensive. For example, breakthroughs in antidepressant and antipsychotic drugs have saved money by reducing admissions for inpatient psychiatric care. **EXHIBIT 5.6** shows the main areas in which use of technology has saved health care costs.

The cost-effectiveness of individual technologies is also being evaluated. For example, in comparing the costs of open partial nephrectomy and robotic partial nephrectomy, Mano and colleagues (2015) discovered that the robotic procedure resulted in shorter hospital stays.

On other fronts, hospitals are gaining leverage on price negotiations and are clamping down on physician-preference items, such as expensive joint implants and cardiac devices (Lee, 2014; Sandier, 2015). Manufacturers from emerging economies are also increasing competitive pressures in developed nations by producing and selling their medical products at lower cost. For example, General Electric has established a major research center in India to develop diagnostic and therapeutic radiology equipment that is less costly and does not require the services of highly skilled staff (Robinson, 2015).

EXHIBIT 5.5 Cost Increases Associated with New Medical Technology

- Acquisition costs are often high because of R&D and precision manufacturing
- Training or hiring of technicians with special skills
- Facilities may require refurbishing or expansion to accommodate the new technology
- Utilization when covered by insurance (moral hazard and provider-induced demand)

EXHIBIT 5.6 Cost-Saving Medical Technology

- Replacement of earlier, more expensive procedures
- Minimally invasive procedures that eliminate the need for overnight hospital stays
- Technologies that shorten hospital stays
- Drugs that reduce inpatient psychiatric care
- Technologies that enable services to be rendered in outpatient and home care settings instead of hospitals

Impact on Access

Geographic access to health care can be improved for many people by providing mobile equipment or by using new communications technologies that allow remote access to centralized equipment and specialized personnel. Mobile equipment can be transported to rural and remote sites, making it accessible to those populations. Mobile cardiac catheterization laboratories, for example, can make the benefits of high technology available in rural settings.

Impact on the Structure and Processes of Health Care Delivery

Medical technology has transformed large urban hospitals in the United States into medical centers where the latest diagnostic and therapeutic remedies are offered, but technology also takes modern medicine to outpatient services and patients' own homes. This trend has led to reduced costs where similar technology was previously available only in hospitals. Without technological innovations, extensive adaptations of modern treatments in outpatient and home care would not have been possible. For example, monitoring devices can permit cardiac implants to transmit vital information over telephone lines, portable respirators can maintain breathing in the home, and even kidney dialyzers are being used for some patients at home. Surgical procedures now commonly performed on an outpatient basis include hernia repair, surgery for kidney and gallbladder stones, cataract removal, tonsillectomy, carpal tunnel release, left heart catheterization, knee arthroscopy, and much gynecologic surgery. Numerous diagnostic procedures, including some of the latest imaging procedures, are also performed in outpatient settings.

Impact on Global Medical Practice

As mentioned earlier, the United States leads the world in R&D spending and development of new medical technology. Many nations wait for the United States to develop new technologies that can then be introduced into their own health care systems in a more controlled and manageable fashion. As a result of this practice, European and other economies get a free ride on U.S. biomedical R&D and obtain nearly all of the benefits of U.S. medical technology at much lower health care costs (Hay, 2006).

At the same time, research partnerships overseas are extending the boundaries of knowledge about disease and strategies for diagnosis, treatment, and prevention. Such collaborations will take on added significance as global health will increasingly have repercussions for the health of Americans (Glass, 2013). In the future, the U.S. home turf will no longer be the sole domain for biomedical research and technological innovation.

Impact on Bioethics

Increasingly, technological change is raising serious ethical and moral issues. Gene mapping of humans, genetic cloning, stem cell research, genetic engineering, genetic testing, and so forth may hold potential benefits, but they also present serious ethical dilemmas. For example, research on embryonic stem cells may lead one day to the discovery of treatments and cures for diseases and other long-term degenerative illnesses such as cardiac failure, Parkinson's disease, spinal cord injury, and diabetes. However, the use of human embryos for research is highly controversial. Life support technology also raises serious ethical issues in medical decisions, including whether life support should continue when a patient may simply exist in a permanent vegetative state or whether life support should be discontinued, and if so, at what point.

▶ Assessment of Medical Technology

Health technology assessment (HTA) refers to the evaluation of medical technology to determine its efficacy, safety, and cost-effectiveness. HTA also informs various stakeholders about the ethical, legal, and social implications of medical technologies (Lehoux et al., 2009). The objective of HTA is to establish the appropriateness of medical technology for wide-spread use. Such assessment becomes essential because many technologies have not produced health benefits; some may even be harmful. Hence, HTA should govern decisions to adopt and disseminate new technology.

Efficacy and safety are the basic starting points in evaluating the over-all usefulness of medical technology. Cost-effectiveness goes a step further by evaluating the safety and efficacy of a technology in relation to its cost. Efficacy and safety are evaluated through clinical trials. A *clinical trial* is a carefully designed research study in which human subjects participate under controlled observations. Cost-effectiveness is determined by using economic models that compare the benefits of a treatment to its costs.

In the United States, it is primarily the private sector that conducts HTA; in contrast, European countries and Canada have centralized technology assessment agencies that perform this task. Since 2009, European nations have been attempting to coordinate their HTA efforts. The European Network for Health Technology Assessment was estab-lished as a facilitating organization for HTA collaboration and joint assessments in Europe.

Efficacy

Efficacy may be defined simply as the health benefit to be derived from the use of technology, or how effective a given technology is in diagnosing or treating a condition. If a product or service actually produces some health benefits, it can be considered efficacious or effective. Decisions about efficacy, however, require that the right questions be asked. For example, is the current diagnosis satisfactory? What is the likelihood that a different procedure would result in a better diagnosis? If the problem is more accurately diagnosed, what is the likelihood of a better cure? Apart from evaluating the effects on mortality and morbidity, issues related to quality of life are important when determining efficacy.

Safety

Safety refers to protection against unnecessary harm from the use of technology. As a primary benchmark, the benefits of any intervention must outweigh any negative consequences. After safety has been experimentally determined, the outcomes from the wider use of a certain technology are closely monitored over time to identify any problems.

Cost-Effectiveness

Cost-effectiveness, or cost-efficiency, goes a step beyond the determination of efficacy and safety by weighing benefits against costs. When a medical treatment is first introduced in caring for a patient, the benefits generally exceed the costs, and the use of technology is regarded as cost-effective. Over time, additional treatments then begin to lower these benefits in relation to rising costs. At some point along the timeline, continued medical interventions yield benefits that are roughly equal to the additional costs associated with their use. Optimal cost-effectiveness is achieved when additional benefits equal the additional cost of treatment. Beyond the optimal point, either additional interventions deliver no further benefits or the cost of providing additional care begins to exceed the benefits. In these cases, additional care becomes wasteful. In cost-effectiveness analysis, the potential risk from medical treatment can also be incorporated as a type of cost, recognizing that most medical procedures are associated with varying degrees of risk or potential harm.

Experts believe that much of the medical care delivered in the United States is wasteful because, after a certain point, additional care adds little or no health benefits while the costs continue to accumulate. One of the problems is that little is known about the cost-effectiveness of even well-established medical technologies. As the overall health care cost burden continues to mount, HTA will play a considerable role in future health care planning, policy, financing, and delivery. Evidence that compares the benefits and harms of various treatments (called comparative effectiveness research [CER]) can be helpful to consumers, clinicians, payers, and policymakers in making informed decisions toward improving the delivery of health care (Witt et al., 2017). It can also help prevent controversies and legal battles over medical decisions made by physicians and insurers.

▶ Benefits of Technology Assessment

From the previous section, some of the main benefits of HTA should be obvious. For example, establishing the safety and efficacy of new technology is essential to prevent potential harm to patients. Other beneficial effects discussed earlier, such as improved quality of care, better quality of life, better access, and control of costs, are all based on the use of technologies that pass rigorous examinations of their safety, efficacy, and cost-effectiveness.

Delivering Value

Possibilities regarding what technology can achieve are limitless. However, health services decision making is increasingly being governed by the answer to the question "What is appropriate?" rather than "What is possible?" (Abele, 1995). The concept of *value*—improved benefits at lower costs and health risks—is becoming important to those who finance health care, including private employers, the government, and managed care organizations. Value can be increased by improving quality, reducing cost, or doing both. The problem is that insured patients often want to use all available medical resources, regardless of how little health benefit is received in relation to their cost. Physicians often find themselves in a precarious situation when they are required to withhold treatment because of its cost-inefficiency. Payers generally get blamed as uncaring profit mongers when they intervene in the delivery of medical care based on costs. Eventually the government may find itself in a central position of issuing practice guidelines based on cost-efficiency.

Cost Containment

Simply pointing to technology as the culprit for cost escalations and putting arbitrary restraints on technology development and dissemination would be a misdirected strategy. As stated earlier, technology has the potential to not only enhance health benefits but also reduce costs. Demands for reducing costs without sacrificing quality must influence technological change. Also, a greater emphasis should be placed on developing technology specifically as a means of reducing costs.

Standardized Practice Protocols

Medical practice guidelines (or clinical practice guidelines) are systematically developed protocols to assist practitioners in delivering appropriate health care for specific clinical circumstances (Field & Lohr, 1990). HTA plays a significant role in the development of clinical protocols. Unlike in some other countries, however, cost-effectiveness has not taken central stage in health care delivery in the United States. Rising health care costs and excessive spending remain a top concern.

▶ Conclusion

Medical technology includes drugs, devices, procedures, facilities, information systems, and organizational systems. Several factors have engendered the mind-set among Americans that all available medical technology must be used regardless of its cost. The United States has the world's foremost position in both the production and the utilization of medical technology. Other countries may then adopt the technology developed in the United States, thereby avoiding the high R&D costs necessary to create the technology in the first place. In addition, these nations use supply-side rationing to contain the diffusion and use of technology. Such an approach has been deemed unacceptable by most Americans. Consequently, medical technology has been one of the primary factors in the growth of health care expenditures in the United States.

In the United States, the FDA regulates the introduction of new drugs, devices, and biologics based on their efficacy and safety, but without evaluating their cost-effectiveness. Under the Affordable Care Act, the FDA has also been given the authority to assess biosimilars and issue licenses for their adoption in medical practice. Experts believe that much of the medical care delivered in the United States is actually wasteful, but at this point, no one is quite sure how to contain Americans' insatiable demand for the almost indiscriminate use of technology.

References

1. Abele J. 1995. Health reform and technology: What does it mean for us? *Biomed Instrument Tech.* 29(6):476–478.
2. Barak A, et al. 2008. A comprehensive review and a meta-analysis of the effectiveness of Internet-based psychotherapeutic interventions. *J Technol Hum Serv.* 26(2/4):109–160.
3. Barua B. 2017. *Waiting your turn: Wait times for health care in Canada, 2017 report.* Vancouver, British Columbia: Fraser Institute.
4. Bronzino JD, et al. 1990. *Medical technology and society: An interdisciplinary perspective.* Cambridge, MA: MIT Press.
5. Chakma J, et al. 2014. Asia's ascent: Global trends in biomedical R&D expenditures. *N Engl J Med.* 370(1):3–6.
6. Chambers JD, et al. 2014. Despite high costs, specialty drugs may offer value for money comparable to that of traditional drugs. *Health Aff.* 33(10):1751–1760.
7. Clayton PD. 2001. Confidentiality and medical information. *Ann Emerg Med.* 38(3):312–316.

8. Congressional Budget Office (CBO). 2008. *Technological change and the growth of health care spending.* Washington, DC: Congressional Budget Office.

9. Davis MP. 2006. Management of cancer pain: Focus on new opioid analgesic formulations. *Am J Cancer.* 5(3):171–182.

10. Field MJ, Grigsby J. 2002. Telemedicine and remote patient monitoring. *JAMA.* 288:423–425.

11. Field MJ, Lohr KN, eds. 1990. *Clinical practice guidelines: Directions for a new agency.* Washington, DC: National Academy Press.

12. Flannery EJ. 1986. Should it be easier or harder to use unapproved drugs and devices? *Hastings Center Rep.* 16(1):17–23.

13. Food and Drug Administration (FDA). 2009. What are "biologics" questions and answers. http://www.fda.gov/AboutFDA/CentersOffices/OfficeofMedicalProductsandTobacco /CBER/ucm133077.htm. Accessed April 2015.

14. Gelijns A, Rosenberg N. 1994. The dynamics of technological change in medicine. *Health Aff.* 13(3):28–46.

15. Glass RI. 2013. What the United States has to gain from global health research. *JAMA.* 310(9):903–904.

16. Goran SF. 2012. Measuring tele-ICU impact: Does it optimize quality outcomes for the critically ill patient? *J Nurs Manag.* 20(3):414–428.

17. Haselkorn A, et al. 2007. The future of remote health services: Summary of an expert panel discussion. *Telemed J E-Health.* 13(3):341–348.

18. Hay JW. 2006. Where's the value in health care? *Value Health.* 9(3):141–143.

19. Hsiao CJ, et al. 2015. The role of health information technology in care coordination in the United States. *Med Care.* 53(2):184–190.

20. Iglehart JK. 1982. The cost and regulation of medical technology: Future policy directions. In: McKinlay JB, ed. *Technology and the future of health care.* Cambridge, MA: MIT Press; 69–103.

21. Institute of Medicine. 2002. *Medical innovation in the changing healthcare marketplace.* Washington, DC: National Academy Press.

22. Institute of Medicine. 2003. *Key capabilities of an electronic health records system.* Washington, DC: National Academy Press.

23. King J, et al. 2014. Clinical benefits of electronic health record use: national findings. *Health Serv Res.* 49(1 pt 2):392–404.

24. Komaroff AL. December 12, 2005. Beyond the horizon. *Newsweek.* 146:82–84.

25. Lee J. 2014. Supply chain: Pressure to spend less ... price transparency ... economies of scale. *Mod Healthcare.* 44(1):20–21.

26. Lehoux P, et al. 2009. What medical specialists like or dislike about health technology assessment reports. *J Health Serv Res Policy.* 14(4):197–203.

27. Lilly CM, et al. 2014. Critical care telemedicine: Evolution and state of the art. *Crit Care Med.* 42(11):2429–2436.

28. Maheu MM, et al. 2001. *E-health, telehealth, and telemedicine: A guide to start-up and success.* San Francisco, CA: Jossey-Bass.

29. Mano R, et al. 2015. Cost comparison of open and robotic partial nephrectomy using a short postoperative pathway. *Urology.* 85(3):596–603.

30. McGregor M. 1989. Technology and the allocation of resources. *N Engl J Med.* 320(2):118–120.

31. Merrill RA. 1994. Regulation of drugs and devices: An evolution. *Health Aff.* 13(3):47–69.

32. Milewa T. 2006. Health technology adoption and the politics of governance in the UK. *Soc Sci Med.* 63(12):3102–3112.

33. Morichelli L, et al. 2014. Implantable cardioverter defibrillator remote monitoring is well accepted and easy to use during long-term follow-up. *J Interv Card Electrophysiol.* 41(3):203–209.
34. Morrissey J. 2002. Hospitals offer remote control. *Mod Healthcare.* 32(51):32–35.
35. Nagaich U, Sadhna D. 2015. Drug recall: An incubus for pharmaceutical companies and most serious drug recall of history. *Int J Pharm Investig.* 5(1):13–19.
36. National Institutes of Health (NIH). 2017. Budget. https://www.nih.gov/about-nih/what-we-do/budget. Accessed January 13, 2018.
37. Nitzkin JL. 1996. Technology and health care: Driving costs up, not down. *IEEE Tech Soc Mag.* 15(3):40–45.
38. Organization for Economic Cooperation and Development (OECD). 2017. Health at a glance 2017: OECD indicators. http://dx.doi.org/10.1787/health_glance-2017-en. Accessed January 13, 2018.
39. O'Sullivan D, et al. 2014. Professional issues: decision time for clinical decision support systems. *Clin Med.* 14(4):338–341.
40. Palmer PM. 2014. Electronic health records: the unintended consequences. *AAOS Now.* 8(12):34–35.
41. Rakich JS, et al. 1992. *Managing health services organizations.* Baltimore, MD: Health Professions Press.
42. Ricciardi L, et al. 2013. A national action plan to support consumer engagement via e-health. *Health Aff.* 32(2):376–384.
43. Robinson JC. 2015. Biomedical innovation in the era of health care spending constraints. *Health Aff.* 34(2):203–209.
44. Sandier M. 2015. Device prices fall as hospitals' leverage grows. *Mod Healthcare.* 45(9):35.
45. Schur CL, Berk ML. 2008. Views on health care technology: Americans consider the risks and sources of information. *Health Aff.* 27(6):1654–1664.
46. Schwartz MD. 2012. The US primary care workforce and graduate medical education policy. *JAMA.* 308(21):2252–2253.
47. Skinner AEG, Latchford G. 2006. Attitudes to counseling via the Internet: A comparison between in-person counselling client and Internet support group users. *Counseling Psychother Res.* 6(3): 92–97.
48. Smith S, et al. 2009. Income, insurance, and technology: Why does health spending outpace economic growth? *Health Aff.* 28(5):1276–1284.
49. Steinbach, A. 2016. The US Food and Drug Administration in a globalized world: An interview with Dr. Margaret Hamburg. *Harvard Int Rev.* 37(3):59–64.
50. Tan JKH. 1995. *Health management information systems: Theories, methods, and applications.* Gaithersburg, MD: Aspen.
51. White-Williams C, et al. 2015. Hospital utilization after a telemonitoring program: A pilot study. *Home Health Care Serv Q.* 34(1):1–13.
52. Witt CM, et al. 2017. Comparative effectiveness research in integrative oncology. *J Natl Cancer Inst Monogr.* 52:43–45.

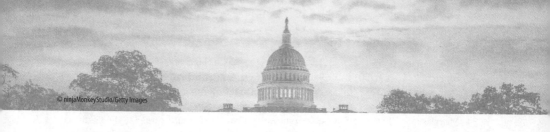

CHAPTER 6

Financing and Reimbursement Methods

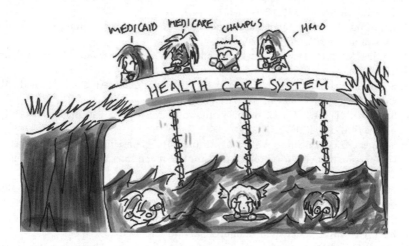

▶ Introduction

F inancing refers to any mechanism that gives people the ability to pay for health care services. For most people, health insurance provides the financing to access health care. Some uncompensated or charity care—mainly provided through free clinics, community health centers, and hospital emergency departments—is delivered to those who have little or no means to finance their health care. Such services, however, are not available in all geographic locations. In 2013, before the main insurance clauses of the Affordable Care Act (ACA) went into effect, 13.4% of Americans (42 million people) did not have health insurance for the entire calendar year (Smith & Medalia, 2015). The number of Americans who gained health insurance through ACA was estimated to be 20 million (Jost & Pollack, 2016), or 7.3% of the nonelderly U.S. population.

The complexity of financing is one of the primary characteristics of medical care delivery in the United States. Most health insurance is privately financed. Certain categories of people, however, can become eligible for tax-supported public health insurance. Almost all Americans age 65 and older qualify for Medicare, which also covers some younger adults with disabilities. Medicaid is another major public insurance program that covers many of the poor, including children in low-income households. Other public programs, such as the Department of Veterans Affairs (VA) and the military health system, cover a relatively small number of people. Under the ACA, the public sector's role in health insurance has expanded significantly.

According to data compiled by the Office of the Actuary, Centers for Medicare and Medicaid Services (CMS)—an agency under the U.S. Department of Health and Human Services (DHHS)—in 2016, government financing accounted for 45% of total U.S. health care expenditures. The most notable shift from private share of national health expenditures (NHE) to the government's share of NHE occurred soon after the Medicare and Medicaid programs were created in 1965. Since then, the government has continued to liberalize benefits and has added new programs in a piecemeal fashion. As expected, under the ACA, there was an uptick in government financing compared to private financing.

Financing also includes the various methods of paying providers for the health care they deliver. Hence, the two functions encompassed in financing are purchase of health insurance and payment for the services delivered to insured patients.

The actual payments to providers of care are handled in numerous ways. In most cases, patients directly pay a relatively small portion of the total cost of the services they receive, although cost sharing by patients has increased significantly in recent years. Various private and public insurance plans pay the bulk of the costs of health care, and they use several different types of payment mechanisms. The financing of health care through the various private and public sources ultimately aggregates into NHE, which comprise the total amount of money a nation spends on health care delivery and other health-related activities. **FIGURE 6.1** illustrates the relationships among financing, insurance, access, payment, and total expenditures.

Private employers and the government are the primary financiers of health care in the United States. From an economic perspective, one

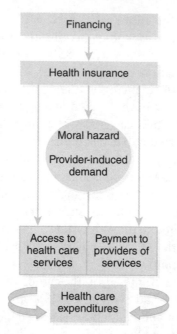

FIGURE 6.1 Relationships Among Health Care Financing, Insurance, Access, Payment, and Expenditures

could argue that Americans, through employment and taxes, finance their own health care and subsidize health care for those who cannot afford it. For instance, employer-paid health insurance actually represents an exchange for salary. Working Americans also have a Medicare tax deducted from their paychecks, which amounts to prepayment of certain Medicare benefits they can expect to start receiving at age 65. General taxes collected from working Americans subsidize health care delivered to Medicaid recipients. Certain Medicare benefits are also subsidized by taxpayers.

▶ Effects of Health Care Financing and Insurance

Health care financing produces effects that go beyond merely providing access and paying the providers of care (**EXHIBIT 6.1**). Notably, it also produces some undesirable effects.

Taken together, financing and insurance are instrumental in creating the demand for health care services. Health insurance enables people to pay for health care, but it also desensitizes both consumers and providers to the price of those services. First, it creates excessive demand from consumers who want to use their health insurance benefits. Consumers are

EXHIBIT 6.1 Health Care Financing and Its Effects

- Financing of private and public health insurance enables access to health care
- Payment to providers
- Moral hazard
- Provider-induced demand—that is, providers deliver covered services more liberally
- Technology and services with liberal reimbursement proliferate
- Total health care expenditures are greater than if the same services were to be paid by the patients

driven to utilize more health care services than they would if they had to pay the entire price out of their own pockets. Consumer behavior that leads to a higher utilization of health care services when the services are covered by insurance is referred to as *moral hazard* (Feldstein, 1993, p. 125).

Second, financing exerts powerful influences on supply-side factors, such as how much health care is delivered. Financing also indirectly affects the growth of medical technology, in that technology and services that are subject to more liberal reimbursement tend to proliferate rapidly. Conversely, when reimbursement is constrained, the supply of services is curtailed accordingly. Moreover, health insurance desensitizes providers against the price of services, with the result that providers deliver additional and more expensive services. Again, if consumers had to pay for these services out of their own pockets, many of them would not be used. The providers' ability to create demand is referred to as *provider-induced demand*. These additional services often confer little or no additional health benefits, however.

Financing eventually affects the NHE (also referred to as total health care costs or national health care spending) incurred by a health care delivery system. Both moral hazard and provider-induced demand waste health care resources and add to the rising costs of health care. To counter these effects, countries with national health insurance implement *supply-side rationing*, which focuses on restricting the availability of expensive medical technology and specialty care. Otherwise, the health care expenditures in these countries would be astronomical. Without a centrally managed health care system, the United States cannot ration health care directly. However, utilization of services is curtailed to some extent because not all Americans have health insurance coverage, despite the ACA. This indirect type of rationing is called *demand-side rationing*. When they lack insurance, people face barriers to obtaining health care unless they can either pay for the services out of pocket or receive charity care. If health insurance is extended to everyone, without other restrictions, total health care expenditures will rise at a much faster rate than they now do.

▶ Insurance: Its Nature and Purpose

Basic Insurance Concepts

Insurance is a mechanism for protecting people and organizations against risk. In the context of insurance, *risk* refers to the possibility of a substantial financial loss from some event. In health care, illnesses requiring expensive treatments and hospitalization pose substantial financial risk to most people. Similarly, the cost of most surgeries and subsequent treatment would be beyond the means of many people to pay out of pocket. Insurance, in a general sense, is primarily designed to protect people against such eventualities. Health care providers are also subject to substantial risk when they are required to treat the sick and injured people who cannot pay for their services.

An individual who is protected by insurance against the possible risk of financial loss is called the *insured*. The insured may also be referred to as the *enrollee* or *member* (in a private health insurance plan) or the *beneficiary* (in a public health insurance plan). The insuring agency that assumes risk is called the insurer or underwriter. *Underwriting* is a systematic technique for evaluating, selecting (or rejecting), classifying, and rating risks. Four fundamental principles underlie the concept of insurance (Health Insurance Institute, 1969, p. 9; Vaughn & Elliott, 1987, p. 17):

- Risk is unpredictable for the individual insured.
- Risk can be predicted with a reasonable degree of accuracy for a group or a population.
- Insurance provides a mechanism for transferring or shifting risk from the individual to the group through the pooling of resources.
- Actual losses are shared on some equitable basis by all members of the insured group.

Through the underwriting process, the insurer determines a fair price to insure the member against specified risks. The amount charged for insurance coverage is called a *premium*, which is usually paid every month. Including both the employer's and the employee's share, the average monthly cost of health insurance premiums in 2017 was $557 for an individual plan and $1,564 for a family plan (Claxton et al., 2017).

Cost Sharing

Insurance requires some type of *cost sharing* so that the insured assumes at least part of the risk. The purpose of cost sharing is to reduce the misuse of insurance benefits. Three main types of cost sharing are utilized in private health insurance: premium cost sharing, deductibles, and copayments.

In employer-sponsored health insurance, the employee is generally required to share in the total cost of the premium. Of the premium costs given previously for 2017, insured workers, on average, paid 18% of the cost for individual plans and 30.5% of the cost for family plans (up from 28% in 2011) (Claxton et al., 2011, 2017). In addition to paying a share of the costs of premiums through payroll deductions, insured individuals pay a portion of the actual costs of medical services out of their own pockets. These out-of-pocket expenses take the form of deductibles and copayments and are incurred only if and when medical care is used.

A *deductible* is the amount the insured must first pay before any benefits by the plan are payable. In most cases, the deductible must be paid annually. For example, in 2017, the average annual deductible for an individual plan was $1,505 (Claxton et al., 2017). In this case, when the insured receives medical care, the plan starts paying for benefits only after the cost of medical services received by the insured has exceeded $1,505. Deductible amounts vary considerably by the type of plan. A plan may also have separate deductibles for hospitalization and outpatient surgery. With few exceptions, all health insurance plans must provide certain recommended preventive services and immunizations without cost sharing, as mandated by the ACA.

Another type of shared cost is the *copayment*—the amount that the insured has to pay out of pocket each time health services are received after the deductible amount has been paid. For example, a plan may require a copayment of $35 for a primary care visit and $50 for a visit to a specialist. Copayment is cost sharing in the form of a dollar amount; cost sharing in the form of a percent amount is called *coinsurance*. A plan with an 80:20 coinsurance, for example, pays 80% of all covered medical expenses after the deductible requirement has been met; the insured pays the remaining 20%. Most plans include a *stop-loss* provision, which is the maximum out-of-pocket liability an insured would incur in a given year. In case of a catastrophic illness or injury, the copayment amount can add up to a substantial sum. The purpose of the stop-loss provision is to limit the total out-of-pocket costs for the insured. Once the stop-loss limit has been reached, the plan pays 100% of any additional expenses. With some exceptions, the ACA placed limits on total out-of-pocket costs per year.

Previously, $1 to $2 million lifetime limits on benefits were common. Under the ACA, lifetime limits have been prohibited.

The rationale for cost sharing is to control the utilization of health care services. Because insurance creates moral hazard by insulating the insured from the cost of health care, making the insured pay part of the cost promotes more responsible behavior in health care utilization. A comprehensive study employing a controlled experimental design conducted in the 1970s, known as the Rand Health Insurance Experiment, demonstrated that cost sharing had a material impact on lowering utilization without any significant negative health consequences.

▶ Private Insurance

The modern health insurance industry is pluralistic; that is, private insurance includes many different types of health plan providers, such as commercial insurance companies (e.g., Aetna, Cigna, Metropolitan Life, Prudential), Blue Cross/Blue Shield, self-insured employers, and managed care organizations (MCOs). The nonprofit Blue Cross and Blue Shield Associations function much like private health insurance companies.

Private insurance is generally available in the form of individual or family plans. A family plan covers the spouse and children of the subscriber in addition to the subscriber. In contrast, government programs such as Medicare and Medicaid do not offer family plans; each individual is an independent beneficiary. Five main types of private insurance are available: group insurance, self-insurance, individual private insurance, managed care plans, and high-deductible health plans (HDHPs). The distribution of health plan enrollments in 2006 (when HDHPs became available) and 2017 is illustrated in **FIGURE 6.2**.

Employment-based health insurance offer rates—that is, the percentages of employers that offer insurance—vary quite significantly according to employer characteristics (**EXHIBIT 6.2**). In 2014, 55% of all employers in the United States offered health insurance benefits, though this was before the ACA mandate for employers to provide health insurance (which was pushed back to 2015). Despite the mandate, health insurance offer rates dropped under the ACA. Whereas 98% to 99% of large employers (200 or more workers) offered health insurance even before

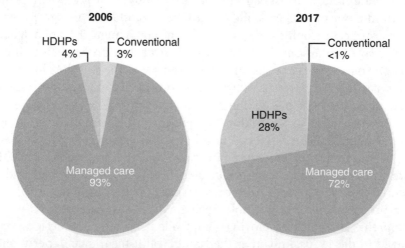

FIGURE 6.2 Distribution of Health Plan Enrollments

EXHIBIT 6.2 Employer Characteristics That Influence Health Insurance Offer Rates

- Large employers versus small employers
- Number of high-wage earners versus low-wage earners
- Full-time workers versus part-time workers
- Percentage of young workers versus older workers

the ACA, the offer rates among small employers (3 to 199 workers) actually dropped from 61% in 2012 to 53% in 2017 (Claxton et al., 2017). For many employers, the cost of health insurance became prohibitive under the ACA. In addition, the ACA incentivized employers to shift employees from full-time to part-time status, so that those employees would not necessarily qualify for health insurance benefits. Only 13% of employers offered health insurance to part-time workers in 2017 (Claxton et al., 2017). Offer rates were also lower among employers that employ a large percentage of low-wage earners, and those that employ a large percentage of young workers age 26 years and younger. Some firms provide funds to their workers so they can buy health insurance on their own.

Group Insurance

Group insurance can be obtained through an organization such as an employer, a union, or a professional organization. A group insurance program anticipates that a substantial number of people in the group will participate in purchasing insurance through its sponsor. Risk and often the cost of insurance are shared by the members of the group.

Earlier health insurance plans were designed to protect the insured against financial hardships that could occur because of the high cost of hospitalization, extended illness, and expensive surgery. These plans were referred to as major medical plans. Since the 1970s, health insurance plans have commonly combined major medical coverage with all-inclusive comprehensive coverage that includes basic and routine physician office visits and diagnostic services. More recently, preventive care services have been added to the benefits.

Self-Insurance

A large employer often has a workforce that is big enough and sufficiently well diversified in terms of risk to warrant offering its own insurance. Rather than pay insurers a dividend to bear the risk, large employers can simply assume the risk by budgeting funds to pay medical claims incurred by their employees. This practice, which is referred to as *self-insurance*, gives employers better control over the health plan.

Self-insured employers can protect themselves against any potential risk of high losses by purchasing *reinsurance* from a private insurance company. In 2017, 60% of workers were in self-insured employer plans (Claxton et al., 2017).

Direct-Purchase Private Insurance

Although most Americans obtain health insurance coverage through employer-sponsored group plans or government programs, directly purchased (nongroup) private health insurance is an important source of coverage for many Americans. The family farmer, the early retiree, the employee of a business that does not offer health insurance, and the self-employed make up the bulk of the people who rely on private non-employer-related health insurance. In 2016, an estimated 52 million people were covered under direct-purchase plans, compared to 178.5 million who were covered under employer-based plans (Barnett & Berchick, 2017).

Managed Care Plans

Managed care plans are offered mainly by health maintenance organizations (HMOs) and preferred provider organizations (PPOs). Such plans are a type of health insurance because they assume risk in exchange for an insurance premium. Unlike traditional insurance, however, MCOs assume the responsibility for obtaining health care services for their enrollees by contracting with a network of providers. MCOs also use a variety of mechanisms to monitor utilization of services, and use a variety of methods to reimburse providers for the services rendered. Managed care plans are typically sold by the same insurers that sell traditional plans. The majority of employer-sponsored plans are managed care plans.

High-Deductible Health Plans

HDHPs have grown in popularity because of their low premium costs. In 2017, 28% of employment-based health coverage was through an HDHP, up from 4% in 2006 (Figure 6.2). Generally, health plans that carry at least $1,000 deductible for individual coverage or $2,000 for family coverage are considered HDHPs.

Two types of HDHP arrangements are available, both of which link a savings account to high-deductible insurance. The savings accounts give consumers greater control over how to use the funds. Savings are also used for relatively small and routine health care expenses. Hence, these plans are also referred to as *consumer-driven health plans*. HDHPs minimize moral hazard and make consumers responsible users of health care resources. Research by the RAND Corporation (2012) unearthed strong evidence that consumer-directed health plans reduce health care spending and can lead to significant cost savings for the health care system.

The first type of HDHP includes a health reimbursement arrangement (HRA—hence HDHP/HRA for the combination). The HRA is funded by the employer; employees are prohibited from contributing to it. The funds are used to reimburse the insured for qualified medical expenses, which include payment of HDHP premiums and premiums for long-term care insurance. Employees do not pay taxes on the payments made to them from HRAs. Although participants in an HRA are not required to have an HDHP, the arrangement commonly includes both. When the HRA is coupled with an HDHP, the employee first pays for health care from the HRA and then pays for care on an out-of-pocket basis until the health plan deductible is met. Subsequently, HDHP kicks in. Unused HRA funds can generally be carried forward to the next year.

The second type of arrangement combines a health savings account (HSA) with an HDHP (HDHP/HSA) that meets federal standards. Federal regulations require caps on the yearly amounts contributed to an HSA ($3,450 for individual coverage and $6,900 for family coverage in 2018; those 55 and older can contribute an additional $1,000). Employers may contribute to the account but are not required to do so. The funds belong to the account holder and can accumulate without limit. The minimum annual deductible in 2018 was $1,350 and $2,700 for individual and family plans, respectively. Out-of-pocket expenses are capped at a maximum; in 2018, annual out-of-pocket expenses for deductibles and copayments were capped at $6,650 and $13,300 for individual and family plans, respectively. HSAs have significant tax advantages—namely, contributions are tax deductible, withdrawals used to pay for medical expenses are exempt from federal income taxes, and account earnings are exempt from taxes.

▶ The Affordable Care Act and Private Insurance

Private health insurance was envisioned as being the major way of obtaining coverage under the ACA. In reality, it did not work out that way. The majority of those persons who were newly covered under the Act gained coverage under Medicaid.

Insurance expansion is addressed through the following main mandates under the ACA:

1. Legal residents of the United States were mandated to have what is referred to as minimum essential coverage. Failing to comply resulted in an income tax penalty (called shared responsibility payment) when the person filed his or her tax

return. The Tax Cuts and Jobs Act of 2017, passed and signed into law by President Donald Trump in December 2017, effectively repealed this mandate.

2. To purchase private health insurance through government-run exchanges, subsidies were still made available in 2018 to people with incomes between 100% and 400% of the federal poverty level (FPL).[1]

3. The exchanges offer four types of standardized plans—bronze, silver, gold, and platinum—tiered according to premium cost and cost sharing. The least expensive of the four, the bronze plan, covers approximately 60% of a person's health care costs.

4. Employers with 50 or more full-time-equivalent workers must cover at least 95% of their full-time workers ("full-time" refers to an employee who works 30 hours or more per week). The insurance offered must comply with ACA requirements on coverage and cost. If they fail to meet this mandate, employers must pay heavy fines. Employers with fewer than 50 workers are exempt from this mandate.

5. As early as 2010, the ACA made it illegal to deny health insurance to people with preexisting medical conditions and required children and young adults younger than the age of 26 to be covered under their parents' health insurance plans.

▶ Public Insurance

This section discusses the financing, eligibility requirements, and covered services for the major public health insurance programs. In 2016, 40.8% of Americans who had health insurance were covered by a public insurance program, such as Medicaid, Medicare, or military health care (Barnett & Berchick, 2017).

Public financing supports *categorical programs*, each of which is designed to provide benefits to a certain category of people who meet the eligibility criteria to become beneficiaries. The United States does not have publicly financed health insurance specifically for the unemployed. Even though public insurance is financed by the government, services are purchased from providers in the private sector, for the most part. One notable exception is the Department of Veterans Affairs (VA), which runs its own health care system that provides most of the needed services to its beneficiaries.

---

1 In 2018, the FPL was an annual income of $12,060 for a single person and $24,600 for a family of four ($28,290 in Hawaii and $30,750 in Alaska).

Medicare

The Medicare program, also referred to as Title 18 of the Social Security Act, finances medical care for three categories of people:

- Persons 65 years and older
- Disabled individuals of any age who are entitled to Social Security benefits
- People of any age who have permanent kidney failure (end-stage renal disease)

Medicare is a federal program administered by the CMS. In 1966, shortly after Medicare was created, it had 19.1 million beneficiaries. By 2016, the program had grown to 56.8 million beneficiaries (CMS, 2017), or 17% of the U.S. population. Although the program was initially created for the elderly population, 16% of the beneficiaries are now persons younger than 65 years of age who qualify on the basis of their disability. With the aging of the U.S. population, this program will continue to grow. By 2024, Medicare is expected to deliver health care to one-fifth of the U.S. population (Schoen et al., 2017). Of all government programs, Medicare poses the single greatest future challenge to taxpayers, as Medicare expenditures are projected to grow faster than either workers' earnings or the nation's economy (CMS, 2017).

Deductibles, copayments, premiums, and noncovered services can leave Medicare beneficiaries with substantial out-of-pocket costs. Non-covered services include vision care, eyeglasses, dental care, hearing aids, and many long-term care services. Even for covered services, Medicare has relatively high cost-sharing requirements. In 2016, the average out-of-pocket spending on services per beneficiary was $3,024, not counting the cost of premiums. More than one-fourth of beneficiaries spent 20% or more of their incomes to pay the premiums and out-of-pocket expenses under Medicare (Schoen et al., 2017). To cover the high out-of-pocket costs, most beneficiaries have some source of supplemental coverage, such as an employer-sponsored plan for retirees (35% of beneficiaries), Medicaid for low-income individuals (19% of beneficiaries), or a privately purchased supplemental insurance plan, known as *Medigap* (23% of beneficiaries) (Jacobson et al., 2015).

For almost 30 years after its inception, Medicare had a dual structure comprising two separate insurance programs, referred to as Part A and Part B. Today, however, Medicare has a four-part structure.

Hospital Insurance (Part A)

Part A, the hospital insurance (HI) portion of Medicare, is financed by special payroll taxes paid equally by employers and employees. These taxes are paid by all working individuals, including those who are self-employed. All earnings are subject to the Medicare tax.

Part A is designed to cover hospitalization, short-term convalescence and rehabilitation in a skilled nursing facility (SNF), and home health care. For terminally ill patients, Medicare pays for care provided by a Medicare-certified hospice. **FIGURE 6.3** shows the distribution of Part A payments for various services (the managed care expenditures are for Medicare Advantage, which is discussed later). Under the ACA, the share of payments to hospitals decreased, while payments to managed care and administrative expenses increased. Payments to managed care plans were actually cut under the ACA, but the increasing enrollments in Medicare shifted the share of expenditures toward managed care plans. Consequently, the managed care share of Medicare HI spending rose from 24.5% in 2010 to 28.2% in 2015 (National Center for Health Statistics, 2017).

The structure of Part A benefits is rather complex. For hospital and nursing home stays, the timing of benefits is determined by what is referred to as a *benefit period*. It begins on the day a beneficiary is hospitalized and ends when the beneficiary has not been in a hospital or an SNF for 60 consecutive days. If after 60 days the beneficiary is hospitalized again, a new benefit period begins. The number of benefit periods a beneficiary can have over his or her lifetime is unlimited.

Services received during a hospital stay are fully paid for the first 60 days in a benefit period after a deductible ($1,340 in 2018) has been met. The Part A deductible applies to each benefit period. If ongoing hospitalization beyond 60 days is necessary, a copayment ($335 per day in 2018) must be paid from days 61 through 90. A benefit period has 90 days of maximum coverage. Beyond the 90 days, there is a lifetime reserve

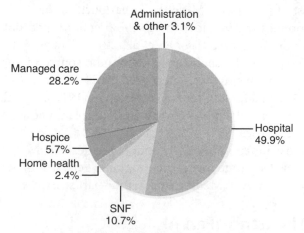

Total Part A expenditures = $278.9 billion

FIGURE 6.3 Medicare Part A Expenditures, 2015

Data from National Center for Health Statistics. Health, United States, 2016. Hyattsville, MD: U.S. Department of Health and Human Services; 2017:348

of 60 additional hospital inpatient days to which a higher copayment applies ($670 per day in 2018). Benefits for medical care in a psychiatric hospital are limited to 190 days in the beneficiary's lifetime.

For postacute care, Medicare pays for up to 100 days in a Medicare-certified SNF subsequent to inpatient hospitalization for at least 3 consecutive days, not including the day of discharge. Admission to the SNF must occur within 30 days of hospital discharge, and it must be related to the same condition for which the beneficiary was hospitalized. All covered services are fully paid for the first 20 days in the SNF. Beyond that, a copayment ($167.50 per day in 2018) must be paid from days 21 through 100.

Medicare pays for home health care when a person is homebound and requires intermittent or part-time skilled nursing care or rehabilitation therapy determined to be necessary by a physician. Services must be obtained from a Medicare-certified home health agency. Durable medical equipment (DME), such as wheelchairs, hospital beds, walkers, and medical supplies, is also covered. Home health visits do not have a deductible, but a 20% coinsurance applies to DME.

For terminally ill patients, Medicare pays for care provided by a Medicare-certified hospice. A small copayment applies for prescription drugs for these patients.

Supplementary Medical Insurance (Part B)

Part B, the supplementary medical insurance (SMI) portion of Medicare, is a voluntary program, financed partly by general tax revenues and partly by required premium contributions from the beneficiaries. Almost all persons entitled to hospital insurance also choose to enroll in SMI because they cannot get similar coverage at that price from private insurers. Coverage includes physician, ambulance, outpatient rehabilitation, an annual wellness exam, and medically needed preventive services; hospital outpatient services such as outpatient surgery, diagnostic tests, radiology, and pathology; emergency department visits; renal dialysis; prostheses; and medical equipment and supplies. Part B also covers limited home health services that are not associated with a hospital or SNF stay.

Part B premiums are income based. The standard premium for 2018 was $134 per month. For beneficiaries earning more than $85,000 and filing individual tax returns (or earning more than $170,000 and filing joint tax returns), 2018 premiums ranged between $187.50 and $428.60 depending on income. Part B also carries an annual deductible ($183 in 2018), and an 80:20 coinsurance applies to most services.

Medicare Advantage (Part C)

Part C is, in reality, not a program that offers specifically defined medical services. Part C was formerly called Medicare+Choice; this program took effect on January 1, 1998, and was mandated by the Balanced Budget Act of 1997. That law expanded the role of private managed care health plans such as HMO and PPO plans. To participate in Part C, a beneficiary must first be enrolled in both Part A and Part B. The beneficiary must pay Part B premiums to Medicare and an additional premium to the MCO (a few plans have no premiums). Beneficiaries, however, have the choice to remain in the original Medicare fee-for-service program instead of enrolling in Medicare Advantage.

By enrolling in Medicare Advantage, the beneficiary receives all Part A, Part B, and Part D services through an MCO. Medicare pays a set capitated amount of money each month to the participating managed care plans on behalf of each beneficiary. In turn, the plan manages Medicare benefits for its members. To attract Medicare enrollees, MCOs may offer extra benefits, such as basic dental and vision benefits and gym membership, which may lower the beneficiaries' out-of-pocket costs. All Part C plans include a limit on out-of-pocket costs for covered services. Part C also eliminates the need for Medigap coverage. Enrollment in Part C has steadily increased, reaching 19 million (33% of the beneficiaries) in 2017 (Jacobson et al., 2017).

Prescription Drug Coverage (Part D)

Part D was added to the existing Medicare program under the Medicare Prescription Drug, Improvement, and Modernization Act of 2003 and was fully implemented in January 2006. The program is available to anyone, regardless of income, who has coverage under Part A or Part B. Coverage is offered through two types of private plans approved by Medicare. Stand-alone prescription drug plans that offer only drug coverage are available to those who want to stay in the original Medicare fee-for-service program. Alternatively, Medicare Advantage prescription drug plans are available to those who want to obtain all health care services through the MCOs participating in Part C.

Like Part B, the Part D program is voluntary because it requires payment of a monthly premium that varies by the beneficiary's income and the type of plan selected by the beneficiary. The average basic monthly premium for 2018 was estimated to be $33.50 (National Council on Aging, 2017). The deductibles and copayments also vary by the plan selected. The maximum deductible for 2018 was $405.

Part D has complex rules to which there are exceptions. After the beneficiary and the health plan have spent a total of $3,750 on prescription drugs, the beneficiary enters a coverage gap (also called a "doughnut hole"). During this period the beneficiary must pay for drugs out of pocket. After spending $5,000 (in 2018) out of pocket, the beneficiary gets out of the coverage gap, and pays a small copayment/coinsurance for the rest of the year.

Medicaid

Also referred to as Title 19 of the Social Security Act, Medicaid is the United States' public health insurance program for the indigent; it is a federal/state collaborative effort. Each state, however, administers its own Medicaid program. Hence, eligibility criteria, covered services, and payments to providers vary considerably from state to state. Eligibility depends on income and other resources such as bank accounts, real property, and other assets. Hence, Medicaid is a *means-tested program.* Federal law specifies coverage for low-income elderly, the blind, the disabled receiving Supplemental Security Income (SSI), and some pregnant women. Medicaid is also instrumental in providing health insurance to children in low-income families (**FIGURE 6.4**; note that the data in the figure predate implementation of the ACA, which had a major impact on Medicaid enrollments). In addition, most states, at their discretion, have defined other medically needy categories. Most important among these are individuals who are institutionalized in nursing or psychiatric facilities and individuals who are receiving community-based services but would otherwise be eligible for Medicaid if institutionalized.

The Medicaid program is jointly financed by the federal and state governments. The federal government provides matching funds to the states based on the per capita income in each state. Thus, wealthier states have a smaller share of their costs reimbursed by the federal government. However, for a state to receive federal matching funds, the state must provide some specific health services (**EXHIBIT 6.3**).

Children's Health Insurance Program

The Children's Health Insurance Program (CHIP), codified as Title 21 of the Social Security Act, was enacted under the Balanced Budget Act of

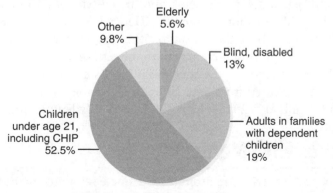

Total beneficiaries = 73.3 million

FIGURE 6.4 Medicaid Recipient Categories, 2013

Data from National Center for Health Statistics. Health, United States, 2016. Hyattsville, MD: U.S. Department of Health and Human Services; 2017:352.

EXHIBIT 6.3   Federally Mandated Services for State Medicaid Programs

- Inpatient hospital services
- Hospital outpatient services
- Physician, nurse-midwife, and nurse practitioner services
- Federally qualified health center and rural health clinic services
- Outpatient laboratory and x-ray services
- Freestanding birth center services
- Nursing facility services for beneficiaries age 21 and older
- Home health services for those eligible for nursing facility services, including medical supplies and equipment
- Medical and surgical services of a dentist
- Preventive, diagnostic, and treatment services (including vaccinations) for children up to age 21
- Family planning services and supplies
- Pregnancy-related services; tobacco cessation counseling and pharmacotherapy for pregnant women

Adapted from Paradise J. March 9, 2015. Medicaid moving forward. http://kff.org/health-reform/issue-brief/medicaid-moving-forward/. Accessed July 5, 2015.

1997. When the program was created, nearly one-fourth of the children in low-income families were uninsured. CHIP offers additional federal matching funds to states to expand Medicaid eligibility to enroll children up to 19 years of age who otherwise would not qualify for coverage because their families' incomes exceed the Medicaid threshold levels. Certain adults, such as pregnant women, parents, and caretaker relatives, may also be covered under CHIP.

In 2017, most states provided CHIP coverage to children with family incomes at or below 200% of the FPL, or about $49,200 (higher in Alaska and Hawaii) for a family of four, and if they are not covered under a private insurance plan. Nineteen states and the District of Columbia had a threshold of 300% or more of the FPL (Henry J. Kaiser Family Foundation, 2017a). States have the option to either operate CHIP as a separate program or run it in conjunction with the state's Medicaid program.

CHIP was strengthened under the ACA. As a result, enrollment in the program increased from 5.8 million in December 2013 (Smith et al., 2014) to 8.9 million in 2016 (Henry J. Kaiser Family Foundation, 2017b).

▶ Issues with Medicaid

The main problem with Medicaid is inadequate reimbursement for providers, which has prompted many physicians and some other providers to not serve Medicaid-covered patients. Medicaid reimbursement is a fraction of what is paid by Medicare and private insurers. Under the

ACA, payments were brought up to Medicare levels only temporarily. Hence, the issue of physician participation in the Medicaid program is an ongoing one.

Expansion of Medicaid under the penalty of losing matching funds if a state would not expand its Medicaid program was a significant component of the ACA. The law had also envisioned a minimum income eligibility standard of 138% of the FPL to qualify for Medicaid in any state nationwide. In a 2012 ruling, however, the U.S. Supreme Court struck down the Medicaid provision of the law, which left each state free to decide whether it would expand its existing Medicaid program. As of 2016, 31 states and the District of Columbia had expanded their Medicaid programs, thereby helping a significant number of low-income people gain health coverage.

Some evidence indicates that the ACA-linked Medicaid expansion resulted in better access to care and utilization (Antonisse et al., 2016). Better access reportedly occurred despite higher use of hospital emergency departments for routine care by Medicaid recipients (Pines et al., 2016). A shortage of primary care physicians had existed even before the ACA's passage; under the Medicaid expansion provisions of the ACA, an additional 2,000 primary care physicians would have been necessary (Roberts & Gaskin, 2015).

▶ Reimbursement Methods

Insurance companies, MCOs, Blue Cross/Blue Shield, and the government (for Medicare and Medicaid) are referred to as *third-party payers*, with the other two parties in the arrangement being the patient and the provider (Wilson & Neuhauser, 1985, p. 118). Payment made by third-party payers to the providers of services is called *reimbursement*.

Fee for Service

Fee-for-service reimbursement is based on the assumption that services are provided as sets of identifiable and individually distinct units of services. For example, physician services may include units such as an examination, x-ray, urinalysis, and a tetanus shot. For surgery, individual services may include an admission kit, numerous medical supplies (each accounted for separately), surgeon's fees, anesthesia, anesthesiologist's fees, recovery room charges, and so forth. Each of these services is separately billed.

Initially, fee-for-service charges were set by providers, and insurers passively paid the claims. Later, insurers started to limit reimbursement to a usual, customary, and reasonable amount that was determined by each payer. In this case, providers would *balance bill*—that is, ask the patients to pay the difference between the actual charges and the payments received from insurers.

Historically, providers preferred the fee-for-service method, which fell into disfavor with payers because of cost escalations. In response, private payers as well as the government have devised other methods aimed at limiting the amount of reimbursement. However, some modified versions of fee-for-service reimbursement are still in use.

Bundled Payments

In *bundled payments* or package pricing, a number of related services are included in one price. For example, normal vaginal delivery (i.e., childbirth) may have one set fee that includes predelivery and postdelivery care (Williams, 1995, p. 114). Optometrists sometimes advertise package prices that include the charges for eye exams, frames for eyeglasses, and corrective lenses. Research has shown that bundled payments can align incentives for providers to work closely together across specialties and health care settings. Consequently, Medicare is undertaking bundled payment initiatives that link payments for multiple services beneficiaries receive during an entire episode of care.

Resource-Based Relative Value Scale

Implemented in 1992 by Medicare, the resource-based relative value scale (RBRVS) is a modified form of fee for service that reimburses physicians according to a relative value assigned to each physician service. Relative values are based on the time, skill, and intensity it takes to provide a service, and the actual reimbursement is derived using a complex formula. Each year, Medicare publishes the Medicare Fee Schedule, which gives the reimbursement amount for each of the services and procedures identified by a current procedural terminology (CPT) code. The reimbursement amounts are adjusted for the geographic area in which the practice is located. Services provided by advanced-practice nurses and physician assistants and billed separately as such are paid at 85% of the full fee schedule.

Reimbursement Under Managed Care

Three distinct approaches are used by MCOs. PPOs use a variation of the fee-for-service method, in which the PPO establishes fee schedules based on discounts negotiated with providers participating in its network. HMOs sometimes have physicians on their staff who are paid a salary. *Capitation* is another mechanism used by HMOs. Under this reimbursement scheme, a provider is paid a set monthly fee per enrollee (sometimes referred to as the per member per month [PMPM] rate), regardless of whether an enrollee sees the provider or not, and regardless of how often an enrollee sees the provider. Capitation removes the incentive for provider-induced demand. It makes providers prudent and encourages them to provide only necessary services.

From Retrospective to Prospective Reimbursement

Traditionally, Medicare and Medicaid established *per diem* (daily) rates when reimbursing hospitals, nursing homes, and other inpatient facilities. The per diem rates were based on the actual costs the providers had incurred during the previous year. Because rates were set after evaluating the costs retrospectively, this method was referred to as *retrospective reimbursement*. Home health was also reimbursed on the basis of cost.

Because the retrospective method was based on costs that were directly related to length of stay, services rendered, and the cost of providing the services, providers had no incentive to control costs. Services were rendered indiscriminately because health care institutions could increase their profits by increasing costs. Because of the perverse financial incentives inherent in retrospective cost-based reimbursement, it has been largely replaced by prospective methods of reimbursement.

In contrast to retrospective reimbursement, in which historical costs are used to determine the amount paid to providers, *prospective reimbursement* uses certain preestablished criteria to determine in advance the amount of reimbursement. Medicare has been using the prospective payment system (PPS) to reimburse inpatient hospital acute care services under Medicare Part A since 1983. The four main prospective reimbursement methods currently in use are based on diagnosis-related groups (DRGs), ambulatory payment classifications (APCs), resource utilization groups (RUGs), and home health resource groups (HHRGs).

Diagnosis-Related Groups

The DRG method is used to pay for hospital inpatient services, based on a predetermined rate. Instead of a per diem rate, the reimbursement method based on DRGs prospectively sets a bundled price according to the principal diagnosis at the time of admission. The hospital receives the predetermined fixed rate for that particular DRG classification.

The primary factor governing the amount of reimbursement is the main clinical diagnosis, but additional factors can create differences in reimbursement for the same DRG. Such factors include differences in wage levels between geographic areas, an urban versus a rural hospital location, whether the institution is a teaching hospital (i.e., it has residency programs for medical graduates; adjustments in reimbursement are based on the intensity of teaching), and an adjustment related to treating a disproportionately large share of low-income patients. In 2007, Medicare Severity Diagnosis-Related Groups (MS-DRGs) were implemented; they include patient severity in determining the rates paid to better reflect use of hospital resources.

The DRG-based prospective reimbursement forced hospitals to control their costs. To keep the cost of services below the fixed reimbursement amount, this payment method has also forced hospitals to minimize the length of inpatient stay. If the total cost of services is less than the DRG-based reimbursement amount, a hospital gets to keep the difference as profit. Conversely, a hospital loses money when its costs exceed the prospective reimbursement rate. As an example, if the prospective reimbursement rate for a given DRG is $3,500 and the costs associated with each day of hospital stay are as shown in **TABLE 6.1**, a patient admitted under this DRG should be hospitalized for no more than 4 days, when the cumulative costs will equal $3,400. If the hospital discharges this patient after 3 days, it will make a profit of $700 ($3,500 – $2,800). If the patient is discharged after 5 days, the hospital will suffer a loss of $500 ($3,500 – $4,000).

To maximize their revenues under the DRG reimbursement model, hospitals would sometimes discharge patients too quickly, at the risk of returning to the hospital again. Hospitals now have disincentives to discharge patients too quickly. The ACA requires reduction in payments to hospitals that incur excessive Medicare readmissions within 30 days of discharge. In 2017, 80% of hospitals were penalized for excessive readmissions (Sanofi-Aventis, 2017). Penalties in reimbursement are also imposed for preventable conditions acquired in the hospitals, such as falls and certain infections.

Ambulatory Payment Classifications

The prospective payment method based on APCs, implemented in 2000, is associated with Medicare's Outpatient Prospective Payment System (OPPS) for services provided by hospital outpatient departments. The APC divides all outpatient services into more than 300 procedural

TABLE 6.1 Hospital Days of Stay and Costs for a Given DRG

Days of stay	1	2	3	4	5	6
Cost per day	$1,200	$900	$700	$600	$600	$600

groups, with specific reimbursement rates being associated with each APC group. The rates are also adjusted for geographic variations in wages. APC reimbursement includes services such as anesthesia, certain drugs, supplies, and recovery room charges in a package price established by Medicare.

In January 2008, Medicare implemented the OPPS to pay for facility services—such as nursing, recovery care, anesthetics, drugs, and other supplies—in freestanding (i.e., nonhospital) ambulatory surgery centers. The most common procedures performed in these centers are cataract removal and lens replacement, upper gastrointestinal endoscopy, colonoscopy, and nerve procedures. Physician services are reimbursed separately under the physician fee schedule based on RBRVS (MedPAC, 2016).

Resource Utilization Groups

Medicare pays SNFs on the basis of RUGs, but the method differs from the way in which DRG-based payments are used for hospitals. Whereas a fixed amount of reimbursement is associated with each DRG, RUG categories are used for determining an SNF's overall severity of health conditions requiring medical and nursing intervention. The aggregate of clinical severity in a facility is referred to as its *case mix*. It is determined by first evaluating each patient's medical and nursing care needs. Based on this evaluation, each patient is classified into one of 66 RUGs (according to RUG-IV classifications). The case-mix composite of an institution is then used to determine a fixed per diem amount—an all-inclusive bundled rate—associated with that case mix. The higher the case mix score, the higher the reimbursement. Adjustments to the PPS rate are made for differences in wages prevailing in various geographic areas and for facility location in urban as opposed to rural areas.

Home Health Resource Groups

Implemented in October 2000, the PPS for home health care pays a fixed, predetermined rate for each 60-day episode of care, regardless of the specific services delivered. Thus all services provided by a home health agency are bundled under one payment made on a per-patient basis. An assessment instrument called the Outcomes and Assessment Information Set (OASIS) is used to rate each patient's functional status and clinical severity level. The assessment measures translate into points; the points are totaled to determine the patient's HHRG, with payment then being based on the patient's specific HHRG category. The HHRG classification uses 153 distinct groups in which patients can be classified according to clinical severity, functional status, and the need for rehabilitation therapies.

▶ Payment Reform Initiatives

A pay-for-performance approach for hospital services was implemented in 2013 for Medicare-covered patients in each hospital. This approach was given legal weight under the ACA, which led to the creation of an inpatient hospital value-based purchasing program. This data-driven approach to payments takes into account the quality and efficiency of services delivered to Medicare-covered patients in each hospital. Preliminary results indicate that for-profit hospitals, large hospitals, non-teaching hospitals, and hospitals in less competitive markets have better outcome scores on performance measures (Haley et al., 2017).

Going forward, value-based and bundled approaches will also affect payments for outpatient services. This will be a big change, given that 95% of physician office visits in 2013 were paid on a fee-for-service basis (Zuvekas & Cohen, 2016). The payment reform was established in the Medicare Access and CHIP Reauthorization Act (MACRA) of 2015, which includes merit-based incentive payments for professional services delivered in various outpatient settings. The reformed payment system envisions data-driven numerical scores that take into account quality, resource use, clinical improvement, and meaningful electronic health record use (Rambur, 2017). Besides Medicare, private payers are moving in the direction of value-based payments.

The ACA authorized a Medicare Shared Savings Program (MSSP) for participating accountable care organizations (ACOs) that aim to coordinate services for a given patient population and take responsibility for quality while reducing costs. This program has shown some early successes in cost savings.

The ACA also created the Center for Medicare and Medicaid Innovation (CMMI). This agency has been given broad authority to conduct a wide range of demonstrations that focus on new methods to pay providers on the basis of value. These new payment models will include bundled payments as well as shared-savings and shared-risk arrangements. One challenge, of course, is how "value" will be measured. In addition, the new models will require changing the culture in which health care is practiced—how physicians practice medicine and what patients expect. In spite of the challenges that must be overcome, experts agree that the current reimbursement system is not sustainable (Smith & Walker, 2015).

▶ National Health Expenditures

National health expenditures are an estimate of the amount spent for all health services and supplies and health-related research and construction activities in a country during a calendar year. According to data from the

CMS, in 2015, the United States NHE exceeded $3.2 trillion. To interpret such large expenditures, it is common to compare the NHE to the total economic consumption. The gross domestic product (GDP) measures the total value of goods and services produced and consumed in a country. In 2015, the U.S. GDP was a little more than $18 trillion. Thus, 17.8% of the total economic output in the United States in 2015 was consumed by health care.

Another way to look at health care expenditures is in terms of the average per capita spending, which controls for changes in the size of the population. In 2015, the average per capita spending for health care amounted to $9,973 for each American. NHE from 1960 to 2015 are presented in **TABLE 6.2**.

FIGURE 6.5 shows the breakdown of how 2015 national health dollars were used. Almost 85% of the NHE was devoted to personal health services and products, which include services provided by hospitals, physician and clinical services, dental care, other professional services, nursing home care, home health care, prescription drugs, medical supplies, durable medical equipment (DME), and other personal health care products and services. The remaining 15% of national expenditures were accounted for by public health services, research, investment in structures and equipment, costs related to administration of government programs, and administrative costs of private insurance.

The annual growth in health care spending, or health care cost inflation, is a matter of concern for almost all developed nations because health care spending has been rising faster than people's incomes. Cost inflation

TABLE 6.2 National Health Expenditures, Selected Years

Year	Amount ($ billions)	Share of GDP (%)	Amount per Capita ($)
1960	27.4	5.2	147
1970	74.9	7.2	356
1980	255.8	9.2	1,110
1990	724.3	12.5	2,854
2000	1,378.0	13.4	4,881
2010	2,604.1	17.4	8,428
2015	3,205.6	17.8	9,973

Data from Health, United States, 2013, p. 327. Health, United States, 2016, p. 331. Hyattsville, MD: National Center for Health Statistics.

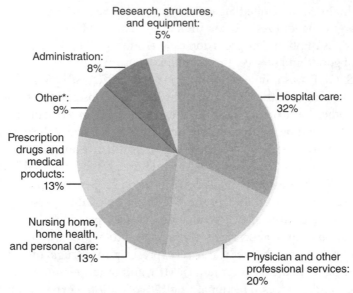

National health expenditures = $3,205.6 billion

* Dental 4%; Other professional 3%, Public health 2%

FIGURE 6.5 Breakdown of National Health Expenditures, 2015
Data from Centers for Medicare and Medicaid Services, Office of the Actuary, National Health Statistics Group

TABLE 6.3 Growth Comparisons of National Health Expenditures to the GDP and CPI, 2000–2015

	2000	2015	Average Annual Increase, 2000–2015
National health expenditures	$1,369.7 billion	$3,205.6 billion	5.8%
GDP	$10,285 billion	$18,037 billion	3.8%
Yearly average CPI	172.2	237	2.2%
GDP price deflator*	81.9	110.0	2.0%

* An alternative measure of inflation.
Data from Health, United States, 2016, pp. 314, 316. Inflationdata.com. https://inflationdata.com/Inflation/Consumer _Price_Index/CurrentCPI.asp?reloaded=true. Accessed January 30, 2018.

in health care is evaluated by comparing it to the growth of the GDP as well as to the *consumer price index* (CPI), which measures inflation in the general economy. As **TABLE 6.3** shows, in the United States, health care cost inflation has exceeded the growth in both the GDP and the CPI.

▶ Conclusion

Financing plays a critical role in health care delivery. For consumers, it pays for insurance coverage, which enables them to obtain health care services. For providers, it reimburses them for the services they deliver. The Affordable Care Act has been instrumental in expanding health insurance coverage; however, serious gaps remain.

For most services, the methods of reimbursement were changed from retrospective to prospective mechanisms after it became recognized that cost-based methods and fee-for-service reimbursement contained perverse incentives for providers to increase the cost of health care delivery. Prospective payment methods, now widely in use, and capitation, used by health maintenance organizations, contain incentives for the delivery of cost-effective health care. Comprehensive health insurance also contains perverse incentives for consumers to use more health care than needed, a phenomenon known as moral hazard. Deductibles and copayments were instituted after payers realized that these methods of cost sharing reduce the excessive use of health care. In an effort to further improve efficiencies and quality, current emphasis is on creating value-based payment models.

The financing of health care is shared between private and public sources. Contrary to what many people might think, the government incurs a sizable proportion of total health care expenditures in the United States. Hence, at least from a financing standpoint, the United States has a quasi-national health care system.

References

1. Antonisse L, et al. 2016. The effects of Medicaid expansion under the ACA: Findings from a literature review. Henry J. Kaiser Family Foundation. http://files.kff.org/attachment/Issue-brief-The-Effects-of-Medicaid-Expansion-under-the-ACA-Findings-from-a-Literature-Review. Accessed January 28, 2018.
2. Barnett JC, Berchick ER. 2017. *Health insurance coverage in the United States: 2016.* Washington, DC: U.S. Government Printing Office.
3. Centers for Medicare and Medicaid Services (CMS). 2017. 2017 annual report of the boards of trustees of the Federal Hospital Insurance and Federal Supplementary Medical Insurance Trust Funds. https://www.cms.gov/Research-Statistics-Data-and-Systems/Statistics-Trends-and-Reports/ReportsTrustFunds/Downloads/TR2017.pdf. Accessed January 25, 2018.
4. Claxton G, et al. 2011. *Employer health benefits: 2011 annual survey.* Chicago, IL: Henry J. Kaiser Family Foundation.
5. Claxton G, et al. 2017. *Employer health benefits: 2017 annual survey.* Chicago, IL: Henry J. Kaiser Family Foundation.
6. Feldstein PJ. 1993. *Health care economics.* 4th ed. New York, NY: Delmar Publishers.
7. Haley DR, et al. 2017. Hospital value-based purchasing: The association between patient experience and clinical outcome. *Health Care Manager.* 36(4):312–319.

8. Health Insurance Institute. 1969. *Modern health insurance.* New York, NY: Health Insurance Institute.

9. Henry J. Kaiser Family Foundation. 2017a. Income eligibility levels for children in Medicaid/CHIP. https://www.kff.org/medicaid/slide/income-eligibility-levels-for -children-in-medicaidchip/. Accessed January 28, 2018.

10. Henry J. Kaiser Family Foundation. 2017b. Total number of children ever enrolled in CHIP annually. https://www.kff.org/other/state-indicator/annual-chip-enrollment/?c urrentTimeframe=0&sortModel=%7B%22colId%22:%22Location%22,%22sort%22: %22asc%22%7D. Accessed January 28, 2018.

11. Jacobson G, et al. April 13, 2015. Medigap enrollment among new Medicare beneficiaries: How many 65-year olds enroll in plans with first-dollar coverage? http://kff.org/medicare/issue-brief/medigap-enrollment-among-new-medicare -beneficiaries. Accessed May 2015.

12. Jacobson G, et al. June 6, 2017. Medicare Advantage 2017 data spotlight: Enrollment market update. https://www.kff.org/medicare/issue-brief/medicare-advantage-2017 -spotlight-enrollment-market-update/. Accessed January 2018.

13. Jost TS, Pollack HA. 2016. Making health care truly affordable after health care reform. *J Law Med Ethics.* 44(4):546–554.

14. MedPAC. October 2016. *Ambulatory surgical center services payment system.* Washington, DC: Medicare Payment Advisory Commission. http://www.medpac .gov/docs/default-source/payment-basics/medpac_payment_basics_16_asc_final .pdf?sfvrsn=0. Accessed April 2018.

15. National Center for Health Statistics. 2017. *Health, United States, 2016.* Hyattsville, MD: Department of Health and Human Services.

16. National Council on Aging. August 2017. Part D in 2018: Important premium and benchmark updates. https://www.ncoa.org/wp-content/uploads/part-d -2018-premium-updates.pdf. Accessed January 28, 2018.

17. Pines JM, et al. 2016. Medicaid expansion in 2014 did not increase emergency department use but did change insurance payer mix. *Health Aff.* 35(8):1480–1486.

18. Rambur BA. 2017. What's at stake in US health reform: A guide to the Affordable Care Act and value-based care. *Policy Politics Nurs Pract.* 18(2):61–71.

19. RAND Corporation. 2012. Skin in the game: How consumer-directed plans affect the cost and use of health care. http://www.rand.org/content/dam/rand/pubs/research _briefs/2012/RAND_RB9672.pdf. Accessed May 2015.

20. Roberts ET, Gaskin DJ. 2015. Projecting primary care use in the Medicaid expansion population: Evidence for providers and policy makers. *Med Care Res Rev.* 72(5):515–561.

21. Sanofi-Aventis. 2017. *Managed care digest series: Payer digest, 2017.* Bridgewater, NJ: Sanofi-Aventis US.

22. Schoen C, et al. 2017. Medicare beneficiaries' high out-of-pocket costs: Cost burdens by income and health status. Commonwealth Fund. http://www.commonwealthfund .org/~/media/files/publications/issue-brief/2017/may/schoen_medicare_cost _burden_ib_v2.pdf. Accessed January 2018.

23. Smith JC, Medalia C. 2015. *Health insurance Coverage in the United States: 2014.* Washington, DC: U.S. Census Bureau; 2015.

24. Smith L, Walker T. 2015. Payment reform shifts to high gear. *Manag Healthcare Exec.* 25(4):6–15.

25. Smith V, et al. June 3, 2014. CHIP enrollment snapshot: December 2013. http://kff.org /medicaid/issue-brief/chip-enrollment-snapshot-december-2013. Accessed May 2015.

26. Vaughn EJ, Elliott CM. 1987. *Fundamentals of risk and insurance.* New York, NY: John Wiley & Sons.
27. Williams SJ. 1995. *Essentials of health services.* Albany, NY: Delmar Publishers.
28. Wilson FA, Neuhauser D. 1985. *Health services in the United States.* 2nd ed. Cambridge, MA: Ballinger Publishing.
29. Zuvekas S, Cohen J. 2016. Fee for service, while much maligned, remains the dominant payment method for physicians. *Health Aff.* 35(3):411–414.

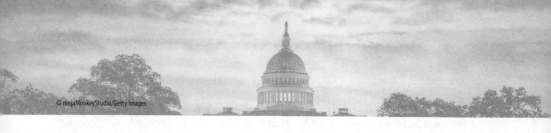
CHAPTER 7

Outpatient Services and Primary Care

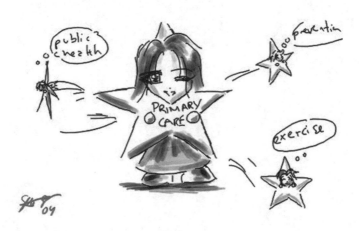

▶ Introduction

Historically, outpatient care has been independent of most other services provided in health care institutions. Previously, most physicians made home visits to treat patients, in addition to seeing patients in clinics. Outpatient care now includes more than primary care. Due to advances in medical science and for economic reasons, a variety of outpatient settings and services have become common. With technological innovation, health care delivery has shifted away from expensive stays in acute care hospitals. To capture lost revenue, hospitals gradually became the dominant players in not only inpatient care but outpatient services as well. For economic reasons, most physician practices have become group practices, and very few solo practitioners are left. Group practices generally have several providers in primary care or a single specialty.

State and local government agencies have actively sponsored limited outpatient services for underserved populations, mainly indigent patients who lack the resources to obtain health care in the private sector. Community health centers, which primarily depend on federal and state funds including grants and Medicaid, serve a number of rural and inner-city areas and provide a wide array of outpatient services.

▶ What Is Outpatient Care?

The terms *outpatient* and *ambulatory* are used interchangeably, although *outpatient* is more comprehensive. Strictly speaking, *ambulatory care* consists of diagnostic and therapeutic services and treatment for the walking (ambulatory) patient. Yet, patients do not always ambulate to health service centers to receive ambulatory care. For example, in a hospital emergency department (ED), patients may arrive by land or air ambulance. In other instances, such as with mobile diagnostic units and home health care, services are taken to the patient, rather than the patient coming to receive services. Hence, the term *outpatient service* refers to any health care services that do not require an overnight stay in a health care institution. The main settings and services for delivering outpatient care are listed in **EXHIBIT 7.1**.

▶ Scope of Outpatient Services

In 2015, according to the National Ambulatory Medical Care Survey (NAMCS), Americans made approximately 990 million visits, or 3.13

EXHIBIT 7.1 Outpatient Settings and Services

- Private practice
- Hospitals
- Outpatient clinics
- Freestanding facilities
- Mobile facilities for medical, diagnostic, and screening services
- Telephone triage
- Home care
- Hospice care
- Outpatient long-term care services
- Public health services
- Community health centers and free clinics
- Alternative medicine clinics

visits per person, to office-based physicians (National Center for Health Statistics, 2015). Physicians in general and family practice accounted for the largest share of these visits (19.5%), followed by physicians in internal medicine (14.0%), pediatrics (9.6%), and obstetrics and gynecology (8.2%), and doctors of osteopathy accounted for 5.8% of all visits.

The South led the nation in share of physician visits (35.9%), followed by the West (26.2%), Northeast (20.2%), and Midwest (17.6%) regions. Ambulatory visits per person were highest in the Northeast (3.6 visits) and lowest in the Midwest (2.6 visits).

Most physician office visits (93%) took place in metropolitan areas. Visits per person were also higher in metropolitan areas (3.3) than in rural areas (1.8), reflecting poorer access to primary care in rural areas (National Center for Health Statistics, 2015). Access to care remains a problem for certain individuals, especially the uninsured and racial/ethnic minorities (**EXHIBIT 7.2**).

Most surgeries are now performed in outpatient settings, whereas previously many of these same procedures could be performed only in hospitals. This shift toward outpatient care is expected to continue. Hospital occupancy rates have declined for more than two decades, and hospital executives have come to view outpatient care as an essential part of their health care business (Barr & Breindel, 1995; Modi et al., 2017).

The growth of non-hospital-based outpatient services has intensified competition between hospitals and community-based providers for patients using outpatient medical services. Areas of competition include home health care, ambulatory clinics for routine and urgent care, and outpatient surgery. In contrast, some other services, such as dental care and optometric services, continue to be office-based. Financing is the main reason that dental and optometric services are not integrated with other outpatient medical services: Medical insurance plans have traditionally been separate from dental and vision care plans, and there are also philosophical and technical differences. For example, chiropractic care is generally covered by most health plans, yet remains isolated from mainstream medicine. Other services, such as alternative therapies and self-care, are not covered by insurance, but patient demand continues to experience remarkable growth.

Several key changes have been instrumental in shifting the balance between inpatient and outpatient services. These factors can be broadly classified as reimbursement, technology, utilization control, and social factors.

Reimbursement

Today, both private and public payers prefer outpatient treatment because it costs less than inpatient care. Quicker discharge of patients from hospitals under prospective and capitated reimbursement methods have created a

EXHIBIT 7.2 Access to Primary Care

Did Not Get or Delayed Medical Care Due to Cost, 2015

Younger than 18 years	2.7%
18–64 years	9.8%
65 years and older	4.1%
White	9.9%
Black	11.0%
Hispanic	10.8%
Insured	7.2%
Uninsured	28.1%

Did Not Get Prescription Drugs Due to Cost, 2015

Younger than 18 years	1.6%
18–64 years	6.9%
65 years and older	3.9%
White	6.5%
Black	10.1%
Hispanic	8.3%
Insured	5.4%
Uninsured	17.3%

Did Not Get Dental Care Due to Cost, 2015

Younger than 18 years	4.1%
18–64 years	11.8%
65 years and older	7.0%
White	11.7%
Black	13.6%
Hispanic	14.5%
Insured	9.4%
Uninsured	28.2%

Data from Health, United States, 2016. National Center for Health Statistics (U.S.). Hyattsville, MD: National Center for Health Statistics (U.S.); 2017:Table 63.

substantial market for outpatient services. In response to changes in incentives for reimbursement of outpatient care, hospitals have aggressively developed outpatient services to offset declines in income from inpatients.

Technological Factors

The development of new diagnostic and treatment procedures and less invasive surgical methods has enabled services in outpatient settings that previously required inpatient hospital stays. Shorter-acting anesthetics and the proliferation of minimally invasive technologies have made many surgical procedures less traumatic and recovery times much shorter. Many office-based physicians have also acquired new technology for basic diagnostic, imaging, and surgical services.

Utilization Control Factors

Inpatient hospital stays are strongly discouraged by various payers. Prior authorization for inpatient admission and close monitoring during hospitalization have been actively pursued with the objective of minimizing length of stay.

Social Factors

Patients generally prefer receiving health care in home and community-based settings. Indeed, most people do not want to be institutionalized unless absolutely necessary. Remaining in their own homes gives individuals a sense of independence and control over their lives—elements considered important for quality of life.

▶ Outpatient Care Settings and Methods of Delivery

Certain outpatient services are now available in various settings. For example, agencies providing home health services may be freestanding, hospital-based, or nursing home-based. Many physician group practices are merging with hospitals, and hospitals and freestanding surgical clinics often compete for various types of surgical procedures. Therefore, the classifications used in this section are merely illustrative—there are many exceptions. Furthermore, in this constantly evolving system, new settings and methods are likely to emerge.

Private Practice

As office-based practitioners, physicians form the backbone of outpatient care. Most visits entail relatively limited examination and testing, and encounters with physicians are generally of a relatively short duration. The waiting time in the office (even for those with appointments) is typically longer than the actual time spent with the physician.

In the past, the solo practice of medicine and small partnership arrangements attracted the majority of practitioners. Self-employment offered a degree of independence not generally available in large organizations. Nowadays, group practices and institutional affiliations—such as employment by a hospital or managed care organization (MCO)—are the norm. Several factors account for the shift away from solo practice: uncertainties created by rapid changes in the health care delivery system, contracting by MCOs with consolidated rather than solo entities, competition from large health care delivery organizations, the high cost of operating a solo practice, the complexity of billings and collections in a multipayer system, and increased external controls over the private practice of medicine. Group practice and other organizational arrangements offer several provider benefits, including patient-referral networks, negotiating leverage with MCOs, sharing of overhead expenses, ease of obtaining coverage from colleagues for time off, and attractive starting salaries with benefits and profit-sharing plans.

Hospital Outpatient Clinics

Many hospital outpatient clinics, particularly those in inner-city areas, function as the community's safety net, providing primary care to the indigent and uninsured. Even so, outpatient services now constitute a key source of profits for many hospitals. Hospitals providing both inpatient and outpatient services have the advantage of enhancing revenues by referring postsurgical cases to their affiliated units for rehabilitation and home care follow-up. Patients also prefer a seamless transition from the hospital to its affiliated outpatient services.

Hospital-based outpatient services can be broadly classified into five main types: clinical (typically for the uninsured or those participating in research studies), surgical (patients are discharged on the day of surgery), home health care (postacute care and rehabilitation), women's health, and traditional emergency care.

Freestanding Facilities

Various types of proprietary, community-based, freestanding medical facilities are found across the United States, such as walk-in clinics, urgent care centers, and surgical centers.

Walk-in clinics provide outpatient services that range from basic primary care to urgent care and are generally used on a nonroutine, episodic basis. Primary care *retail clinics* are becoming available in stores such as Walmart, Walgreens, and CVS pharmacies. *Urgent care centers* generally offer a wide range of routine services for basic and acute conditions. The main advantages of walk-in clinics and urgent care centers are convenience of location, evening and weekend hours, and availability of services on a walk-in, no-appointment basis.

Surgicenters (short for surgical centers) are freestanding outpatient surgery centers that operate independently of hospitals. They usually provide a full range of services for surgeries that can be performed on an outpatient basis and do not require overnight hospitalization. Other types of outpatient facilities include outpatient rehabilitation centers, optometric centers, and dental clinics.

Mobile Facilities for Medical, Diagnostic, and Screening Services

Mobile health care services are transported directly to patients and constitute an efficient and convenient means for providing certain routine health services—for example, mammography, x-rays, dental care, and optometric care. They mainly benefit populations in small towns, rural communities, and nursing homes. Health screening vans, staffed by volunteers who are trained professionals, are generally operated by various nonprofit organizations and are often seen at malls and fairgrounds, where providers screen for blood pressure and cholesterol.

Telephone or Internet Triage

Telephone or Internet access, referred to as telephone or Internet triage, is a means of bringing expert opinion and advice on health care to the patient, especially during hours when physicians' offices are closed. This system is staffed by trained nurses who have access to patient medical records and provide guidance according to standardized protocols. They can consult with primary care physicians when necessary or refer patients to an urgent care facility or emergency department.

Home Care

In home health care, services are brought to patients in their own homes. Without home services, the only alternative for such patients might be institutionalization in a hospital or nursing home. Home health care is consistent with the philosophy of maintaining people in the least restrictive environment possible. Home health services typically include nursing care, such as changing dressings, monitoring medications, and help with bathing; short-term rehabilitation, such as physical therapy, occupational therapy, and speech therapy; homemaker services, such as meal preparation, shopping, transportation, and some specific household chores; and certain medical supplies and equipment, such as ostomy supplies, hospital beds and oxygen tanks, as well as walkers and wheelchairs (referred to as durable medical equipment).

Hospice Care

The term *hospice* refers to a cluster of comprehensive services for terminally ill patients with a life expectancy of 6 months or less. Hospice programs provide services that address the special needs of dying persons and their families. Hospice is a method of care, not a physical location, in which services are taken to patients and their families wherever they are located. Hospice care includes medical, psychological, and social services provided in a holistic context. The two primary areas of emphasis in hospice care are (1) pain and symptom management, referred to as *palliative care*, and (2) psychosocial and spiritual support.

Outpatient Long-Term Care Services

Long-term care (LTC) has typically been associated with care provided in nursing homes, but a number of alternative settings are now available to address a variety of needs. Two types of ambulatory LTC services are *case management* and *adult day care*. Case management provides coordination and referral among various health care services, with the objective of finding the most appropriate setting for meeting a patient's health care needs. Adult day care complements informal care provided at home by family members, with professional services available during the day.

Public Health Services

Public health services in the United States are typically provided by local health departments, and the range of services offered varies greatly by locality. Generally, public health programs are limited in scope. They include well-baby care, sexually transmitted disease clinics, family planning services, tuberculosis screening and treatment, and outpatient mental health care. States vary in the range and extent of public health services offered.

Community Health Centers

The federal government authorized the creation of Community Health Centers (CHCs) during the 1960s, primarily to extend health care services to medically underserved regions of the United States. CHCs are supported by grant funding administered by the Bureau of Primary Health Care (BPHC) within the Department of Health and Human Services (DHHS). These centers are required by law to be located in medically underserved areas and to provide services to anyone seeking care, regardless of insurance status or ability to pay (McAlearney, 2001).

CHCs provide family-oriented preventive care, primary care, and dental care, and serve as a primary care safety net. According to the BPHC, 1,367 such centers were funded through the program and provided care to approximately 25.9 million people through more than 104 million medical, dental, mental health, and substance abuse visits across the United States in 2016. Approximately 23.43% of patients were uninsured, and another 48.51% were covered under Medicaid. The vast majority (91.9%) of patients who visited CHCs had incomes less than 200% of the federal poverty level, and over 1 million were homeless.

Other health centers supported by federal funding include migrant health centers, which serve transient farm workers in agricultural communities (approximately 957,529 patients were seen in 2016), and rural health centers which are located in isolated, underserved rural areas. For example, the Community Mental Health Center Program was established to provide outpatient mental health services in underserved areas.

Free Clinics

Approximately 1,200 free clinics in the United States provide services at little or no cost to needy people. These clinics are neither operated nor supported by the government, and their services are delivered mainly by trained volunteer staff.

Alternative Medicine Clinics

Complementary and alternative medicine (CAM) refers to the broad domain of health care resources that are not intrinsic to biomedicine (CAM Research Methodology Conference, 1997). These treatment approaches aim to prevent or treat disease. Complementary interventions are used *together with* conventional medical treatments, whereas alternative interventions are used *instead of* conventional medicine.

Alternative therapies include various treatments such as homeopathy, herbal remedies, natural products used as preventive and treatment agents, acupuncture, meditation, yoga exercises, biofeedback, and spiritual guidance or prayer (Barnes et al., 2007). A significant number of adults in the U.S. exclusively use alternative medicine; one-fourth of adults with no medical practitioner visits reported using CAM therapy in 2007. Alternative medicine is not yet endorsed by most practitioners of conventional Western medicine, although interest in the efficacy of these treatments has been growing among the traditional medical establishment. Alternative treatments are generally not covered by health insurance.

▶ Primary Care

Primary care is the conceptual foundation for outpatient services, but not all outpatient care is primary care. Services beyond primary health care have become an integral part of outpatient services. As specialist services increase in supply and use, specialist physicians have become more integrated into the primary care system; however, improvement is still needed to ensure seamless coordination of care between specialists and primary care providers (Farmer et al., 2017; *United States Pharmaceuticals & Healthcare Report*, 2015). Primary care practice must evolve and adapt to recent changes in the health care system, and this transition is particularly important in light of an estimated shortage of more than 44,000 primary care physicians in the U.S. by 2035 (Petterson et al., 2015).

What Is Primary Care?

In a tri-level classification of care delivery, primary care is distinguished from secondary and tertiary care by its duration, frequency, and level of intensity. *Secondary care* is usually short-term in nature, involving sporadic consultation from a specialist for expert opinions and/or surgical or other advanced interventions that primary care physicians cannot perform. Secondary care includes hospitalization, routine surgery, specialty consultation, and rehabilitation. *Tertiary care* is the most complex level of care and is required for relatively uncommon conditions. Typically, tertiary care is institution-based, highly specialized, and technology-driven, and mostly rendered in large teaching hospitals, especially university hospitals. Examples include trauma care, burn treatment, neonatal intensive care, tissue transplants, and open-heart surgery. Some tertiary treatments may be long-term, and tertiary care physicians may assume long-term responsibility for the bulk of the patient's care.

Primary care is commonly viewed as a set of basic and routine services that include prevention, diagnostic and therapeutic services, health education and counseling, and minor surgery. More saliently, primary care should be viewed as an approach to health care rather than a set of specific services (Starfield, 1994). In this regard, the World Health Organization (WHO) and the Institute of Medicine[1] (IOM) provide useful definitions.

---

1 The Institute of Medicine was renamed the National Academy of Medicine in 2015.

WHO Definition

According to the WHO, primary health care is essential health care that is based on practical, scientifically sound, and socially acceptable methods and technology. Such care should be universally accessible to individuals and families in the community by acceptable means and at an affordable cost. Primary health care is the foundation of ambulatory services and is characterized by the first level of contact between individuals, the family, and the community on the one hand and the health care delivery system on the other hand, bringing health care as close as possible to where people live and work. It is the first element of a continuing health care process (WHO, 1978, p. 25).

IOM Definition

The IOM Committee on the Future of Primary Care defined primary care as the provision of integrated, accessible health care services by clinicians who are accountable for addressing the majority of personal health care needs, developing a sustained partnership with patients, and practicing in the context of family and community (Vanselow et al., 1995, p. 192).

Domains of Primary Care

Taken together, the WHO and IOM definitions highlight six key domains of primary care, as summarized in **EXHIBIT 7.3**.

Point of Entry

Primary care should be the point of entry into a health services system (Starfield, 1992, p. vii), that is, the first contact that a patient makes with the health care delivery system. This first-contact feature is closely associated with the gatekeeper role of the primary care practitioner. *Gatekeeping* implies that patients do not visit specialists and are not admitted to a hospital without being referred by their primary care physicians. Although gatekeeping may appear to be a controlling mechanism for

---

EXHIBIT 7.3 Domains of Primary Care

- Point of entry
- Community based
- Coordination of care
- Essential care
- Integrated care
- Accountability

denying needed care, instead primary care usually protects patients from unnecessary procedures and overtreatment (Franks et al., 1992) because specialists use medical tests and procedures to a much greater extent than do primary care providers, and such interventions carry a risk of iatrogenic (i.e., caused by the process of health care) complications (Starfield, 1994). At the same time, appropriate technology must be incorporated into primary care delivery so that costly referrals to other components of the health delivery system are made only when necessary.

Community Based

Primary care should be available in close proximity to where people live and work, and is thus characterized by convenience and accessibility. These services must also be basic, routine, and inexpensive in order to be widely available to urban, suburban, and rural communities.

Coordination of Care

One of the main functions of primary care is to coordinate the delivery of health services between the patient and the myriad components of the health care system. Therefore, primary care professionals also serve as patient advisors and advocates. Besides making referrals, they give advice regarding various diagnoses and therapies, discuss treatment options, and provide continuing care for chronic conditions (Williams, 1993). Coordination of an individual's total health care needs ensures continuity and comprehensiveness. These goals of primary care are best achieved when the patient and the provider have established a close relationship over time.

Within the overall health care delivery system, primary care can be regarded as the hub of the larger wheel. The various components of the system are located around the rim of this wheel, with the spokes of the wheel signifying the coordination of continuous, comprehensive care (**FIGURE 7.1**).

The ideal system of health care delivery is based on primary care but also closely linked with adequate and timely specialized services. Continuous, coordinated care requires that secondary and tertiary services be integrated with primary care through appropriate interaction and consultation among physicians. Coordination of care has certain advantages. Both the appropriateness and the outcomes of interventions are better when primary care physicians refer patients to specialists, rather than when patients engage in self-referral (Bakwin, 1945; Roos, 1979).

Essential Care

Primary care is regarded as essential health care. When it is made available to the vast majority of a nation's population, population health is optimized. Countries whose health systems are more oriented toward

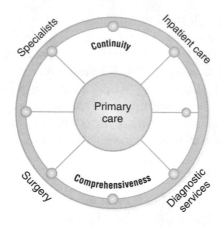

FIGURE 7.1 Coordination Role of Primary Care in Health Delivery

primary care achieve better health outcomes, higher satisfaction with services among their populations, and lower expenditures in overall health care delivery (Starfield, 1994). Even in the United States, states with higher ratios of primary care physicians to patients show better health outcomes associated with the better availability of primary care (Shi, 1992, 1994). Higher ratios of family and general practice physicians to patients are also associated with lower hospitalization rates for conditions treatable with primary care (Parchman & Culler, 1994). Adults who have primary care physicians as their regular source of care experience lower death rates and incur lower health care costs (Franks & Fiscella, 1998). However, the mixture of public and private financing for health care services in the U.S. has created a fragmented system, in which primary care is not the organizing hub for continuous, coordinated health services.

Integrated Care

Integrated care embodies the concepts of comprehensive, coordinated, and continuous services that provide a seamless process of care. Primary care is comprehensive because it addresses any health problem at any stage of a patient's life cycle. Coordination ensures that the appropriate combination of health services are provided to best meet the patient's needs. Continuity refers to care delivered over time by a single provider or a team of health care professionals.

Accountability

Within the health care system, both clinicians and patients are held accountable. On the one hand, the clinical system is accountable for quality care, patient satisfaction, the efficient use of resources, and ethical behavior. On the other hand, patients are responsible for their own health, to the extent that they are capable. Patients are also responsible for being judicious in their use of resources when they need care. An ideal patient–provider relationship is based on mutual trust, respect, and responsibility. In addition to possessing the necessary knowledge and skills, primary care clinicians must use their best judgment to involve other practitioners in diagnosis, treatment, or both when appropriate (Vanselow et al., 1995).

Community-Oriented Primary Care

Community-oriented primary care incorporates the elements of effective primary care delivery but adds a population-based approach to identifying and addressing community health problems. Current perspectives on primary care delivery have extended beyond the traditional biomedical paradigm, which focuses on medical care for the individual in an encounter-based system, to the broader biopsychosocial paradigm, which emphasizes the needs and health priorities of both the population and the individual (Gofin et al., 2015; Lee, 1994). The main challenge has been to determine the best means to bring together individual health needs in the larger context of community health needs. Workforce shortages and a lack of financial incentives to provide care beyond individual health needs have been two major obstacles to adopting the biopsychosocial paradigm.

▶ Primary Care Around the World

Primary care systems across the world face the dual challenges of a shrinking medical workforce and increasing health care demands. On the supply side, the number of medical graduates entering primary care specialties, such as general internal medicine, family medicine, or geriatrics, are decreasing in the United States and internationally (Organization for Economic Cooperation and Development [OECD], 2012; Schwartz, 2012). On the demand side, the number of patients along with their care demands are increasing substantially. In some countries, changes to health systems have also increased demand for primary care services. For example, the expansion of insurance coverage to millions of previously uninsured individuals under the Affordable Care Act (ACA) in the U.S. has further increased the demand for primary care.

Worldwide, shortages of primary care physicians along with an increased demand for primary care services have provided the impetus for delivering team-based primary care. The diversity of the primary care workforce is increasing to include a wider range of health professionals, such as nurse practitioners, registered nurses, and other clinical staff members. While transitioning to multidisciplinary teams appears necessary, approaches to implementing primary care teams differ greatly. Some approaches utilize traditional primary care health professionals but redefine or extend their roles. For example, some models refocus the roles of medical assistants on completing additional tasks such as ordering routine tests and supporting patient self-management. Other models include health care professionals not traditionally utilized in primary care, including social workers, pharmacists, or community health workers, expanding the range of expertise included in the primary care team (Freund et al., 2015).

In Canada, primary health care services have traditionally been delivered by family physicians and general medical practitioners. To solve the issues posed by a shortage of these providers, the Canadian federal government has encouraged the formation of interprofessional health care teams and greater emphasis on health promotion since 2004. All provinces and territories have designed innovative care models and multidisciplinary teams. For example, in British Columbia, interprofessional care networks care for patients with chronic health conditions. Under the aegis of the Divisions of Family Practice, groups of primary care physicians can address gaps in patient care and promote family medicine. In Ontario, the government has also developed new approaches to primary health care, such as the family health team (Ministry of Health and Long-Term Care Canada, 2012).

In Australia, primary care practices have traditionally been operated as private businesses, but the primary care landscape is changing. There is a shift away from medically qualified general practitioners working as solo practitioners and providing episodic opportunistic care, one-way referral processes, and fee-for-service financing only. More recently, general practices have included two to five primary care physicians, providing a greater focus on prevention, early intervention, and structured chronic disease management within multidisciplinary care team approaches (Naccarella et al., 2012).

▶ Effectiveness of Primary Care

Most preventive interventions are best carried out in primary care delivery, even though some believe a specialty care focus is warranted. For example, cardiac care may be concerned with cholesterol levels; testing for cholesterol levels and interventions to bring them down to desired levels are routinely performed by primary care physicians. Primary care practitioners may order further testing, such as electrocardiograms and cardiac stress tests, to assess for heart disease, and may make referrals to a cardiologist when appropriate.

U.S. states with higher ratios of primary care physicians to the total population experience lower smoking rates, less obesity, and greater use of seat belts (Shi, 1994; Shi & Starfield, 2000). Continuity of care with a single provider is also positively associated with primary preventive care, including smoking cessation and influenza immunization, in a study of 60 communities in the U.S. (Saver, 2002). An increase of one primary care physician per 10,000 population has been linked to an average reduction of 1.44 deaths per 10,000 population (127,617 deaths per year), a 2.5% reduction in infant mortality, and a 3.2% reduction in low-birthweight infants (Macinko et al., 2007).

Similarly, population subgroups with an adequate primary care source show better birthweight distributions. In 2000, among white and black populations in urban and rural areas of the United States, birthweights were higher when the source of care was a community health center designed to provide effective primary care (Politzer et al., 2001). Disadvantaged children are much more likely to have preventive care visits when their source of care is a good primary care practitioner (Gadomski et al., 1998; Kumra et al., 2017).

Early detection of breast cancer is also enhanced when primary care physicians are adequate in supply (at least relative to specialists), and a one-third increase in the supply of family physicians correlates to a 20% decrease in cervical cancer mortality rates (Barry, 2017; Ferrante et al., 2000; Macinko et al., 2007).

Hospitalizations and Use of Emergency Care

Evidence shows that lower hospitalization rates for ambulatory care–sensitive conditions (i.e., hospitalizations that can be prevented with quality primary care) are strongly associated with receiving primary care. Children receiving care from a good primary care source have lower hospitalization rates for these conditions and overall, which are associated with receiving better preventive care from primary care providers (Barry, 2017; Gadomski et al., 1998). Hospital admission rates are lower in communities where primary care physicians are more involved in caring for children both before and during hospitalization (Perrin et al., 1996). Adolescents with the same regular source of care for preventive and illness care (i.e., a source of primary care) are much more likely to receive preventive care and less likely to seek care in emergency rooms (Ryan et al., 2001). Thus strong evidence indicates that hospitalizations—especially for ambulatory care-sensitive conditions—are less frequent when primary care is available.

The geographic distribution of primary care physicians is an important factor in determining the health of the local population. Parchman and Culler (1994, p. 45) found that geographic areas with higher numbers of family and general care physicians per population experienced lower hospitalization rates for conditions that can be prevented with good primary care, including diabetes mellitus and pneumonia in children, and congestive heart failure, hypertension, pneumonia, and diabetes mellitus in adults. Women residing in primary care service areas (PCSAs) also showed increased rates of mammography recommendation and utilization (Barry, 2017). Other studies have found that poor primary care resources are independently associated with higher hospitalization rates for conditions that can be prevented by adequate primary care.

Cost of Care

Areas with higher primary care physician-to-population ratios experience lower total health care costs. This relationship has been demonstrated among elderly individuals in the U.S. who live in metropolitan areas, both for total costs (i.e., inpatient and outpatient) (Mark et al., 1996; Welch et al., 1993) and for the total population in the U.S. (Franks & Fiscella, 1998), and in international comparisons of industrialized countries (Starfield & Shi, 2002). Care for illnesses common in the population (e.g., community-acquired pneumonia) is more expensive if provided by specialists than if provided by generalists, yet no difference in outcomes is noted based on provider type (Rosser, 1996; Whittle et al., 1998).

Morbidity

A greater supply of primary care physicians has been associated with lower rates of self-reported poor health in a study of 60 representative U.S. communities, after controlling for a wide range of sociodemographic and socioeconomic characteristics (Shi & Starfield, 2000). This study also confirmed the positive impact of primary care—patients with better experiences of primary care reported better health (Shi et al., 2002).

Lower birthweight and infant mortality rates were also associated with a higher supply of primary care physicians in U.S. states, even after controlling for education, unemployment, racial/ethnic composition, income inequality, and urban–rural differences (Shi et al., 2004).

Similarly, in a recent study of the association between primary care physician supply in U.S. counties and patient health, individuals in counties with the highest numbers of primary care physician supply were found to be 20% less likely to become obese than those living in counties with the smallest numbers of primary care physician (Gaglioti, 2016).

Several studies have shown the importance of primary care as an entry point to the health care system for a majority of conditions. For example, one study demonstrated that entry-level access through primary care is associated with better outcomes for 16 common conditions in children and youth (Starfield, 1985). Another study showed that men who lack a primary care provider were at even greater risk for severe uncontrolled hypertension than men who lacked medical insurance or had alcohol-related health problems (Shea et al., 1992).

Mortality

Perhaps the most frequently cited evidence for the benefits of primary care has been mortality rates (i.e., death rates). One line of evidence comes from ecological studies of the relationship between primary care personnel-to-population ratios and various health outcomes in the U.S. Two studies found better health outcomes in states with higher primary care physician-to-population ratios after controlling for socio-demographic measures (i.e., percentage of elderly, percentage of urban residents, percentage of minority individuals, education, income, unemployment, pollution) and lifestyle factors (i.e., seat belt use, obesity, and smoking) (Shi, 1992, 1994). The supply of primary care physicians has also been shown to exert a strong and significant direct influence on life expectancy, stroke, and postnatal and total mortality (Bailey & Goodman-Bacon, 2015; Shi et al., 1999).

Studies using multiple years of data have also identified an inverse relationship between primary care physician supply and population mortality outcomes, where increases in the supply of primary care physicians are associated with decreases in overall and cause-specific population mortality rates (Shi et al., 2003; Villalbi et al., 1999). There is a strong association between life expectancy and numbers of primary care physicians—the higher the ratio of physicians per population, the longer the life expectancy of the population (Shi et al., 1999).

▶ The Medical Home Strategy

As health care delivery becomes increasingly complex, a renewed proposal for coordinating care through a *medical home* system has gained support. In 2006, the American College of Physicians (ACP) recommended the medical home care model as a fundamental change in the provision and financing of primary care. The ACP advocates patient-centered care based on a partnership between the patient and the provider combined with the incorporation of principles of the chronic care model. The chronic care model is based on the premise that chronic conditions are best managed with multidisciplinary practice-based teams, use of evidence-based guidelines, appropriate health information technology, and accountability for the quality and value of care provided (American Academy of Family Physicians et al., 2007). With one personal physician as their primary, continual medical contact, patients are wholly cared for by a directed team that is coordinated across all areas of the health system. In small-scale studies, the medical home model has been found to improve patient health outcomes and satisfaction, reduce medical errors, and add value by producing cost savings without compromising health outcomes (Rojanasarot & Carlson, 2017; Rosenthal, 2008). Studies using nationwide data have also indicated that medical home models are effective in providing comprehensive, accessible, and continuous primary care (Liang et al., 2017; Shi et al., 2017a). The medical home model offers a long-term vision of reform that can help improve and revolutionize the primary care system.

The National Committee for Quality Assurance's (NCQA's) Patient-Centered Medical Home Recognition Program is the most widely adopted patient-centered medical home (PCMH) evaluation program in the United States. More than 12,000 practices (with more than 60,000 clinicians) are recognized by the NCQA, and more than 100 payers support NCQA recognition through financial incentives or coaching. The key criteria of PCMH recognition/accreditation (displayed in **EXHIBIT 7.4**) are based on the well-known and empirically validated Wagner Chronic Care Model, which encourages the health care system to use community resources to effectively care for patients with chronic illnesses through productive interactions between activated patients and a prepared practice team. Furthermore, the NCQA recognizes practices that successfully apply systematic processes and technology in improved quality of patient care. A growing body of literature demonstrates that medical homes may improve health outcomes, reduce disparities in access and quality of care, and ultimately lower costs over time (Beal et al., 2007; Peikes et al., 2012; Shi et al., 2017a).

▶ Use of Information Technology in Primary Care

The effective use of medical information technology by primary care practices to improve quality can help practices enhance their ability to deliver both high-quality care and better patient outcomes (Higgins et al., 2015). In 2009, the federal Health Information Technology for Economic and Clinical Health (HITECH) Act, enacted under the American Recovery and Reinvestment Act, provided incentives for the meaningful use of electronic health records (EHRs). Objectives included specific requirements for using EHR data to improve health care processes and outcomes through tracking and reporting on quality measures, e-prescribing, implementing decision support, participating in health information exchanges (HIEs), and other activities. In February 2014, the Centers for Medicare and Medicaid Services reported that

EXHIBIT 7.4 Patient-Centered Medical Home Accreditation Criteria

PCMH1: Patient-Centered Access

- Appointment access
- 24/7 access to clinical advice
- Electronic access

PCMH2: Team-Based Care

- Continuity
- Medical home responsibilities
- Culturally and linguistically appropriate services
- The practice team

PCMH3: Population Health Management

- Patient information
- Clinical data
- Comprehensive health assessment
- Use data for population management
- Implement evidence-based decision support

PCMH4: Care Management and Support

- Identify patients for care management
- Care planning and self-care support
- Medication management
- Use electronic prescribing
- Support self-care and shared decision making

PCMH5: Care Coordination and Care Transitions

- Test tracking and follow-up
- Referral tracking and follow-up
- Coordinate care transitions

PCMH6: Performance Measurement and Quality Improvement

- Measure clinical quality performance
- Measure resource use and care coordination
- Measure patient/family experience
- Implement continuous quality improvement
- Demonstrate continuous quality improvement
- Report performance
- Use certified EHR technology

it had disbursed $19.2 billion in meaningful use incentives to nearly 441,000 registered providers participating in the federal EHR meaningful use program (Manos, 2014).

In addition, the ACA emphasized quality improvement and measurement in its strategic plan for health information technology (IT) and proposed the use of health IT as a tool to improve patient safety, reduce medical errors, and ensure patient-centered care (Patient Protection and Affordable Care Act of 2010). The Office of the National Coordinator (ONC) for Health Information Technology established 62 Regional Extension Centers in 2010 to provide EHR technical assistance mainly to private practices, but also to federally qualified health centers, which increase access to care for underserved communities (Heisey-Grove et al., 2013).

Even with these incentives, health IT to support quality improvement in primary care is often insufficiently or inefficiently used. Part of the reason might be that expansion of EHR use in primary care offices is relatively new. New users of health IT may not have mastered the more advanced EHR functions needed for quality improvement. Some primary care practices might find that using health IT does not automatically translate into improved quality of care. Rather, using health IT for quality improvement requires purposeful and thoughtful planning, effort, and allocation of resources—all of which require significant investments by primary care practices in capital, clinician and staff training, and time.

Despite these barriers, some primary care practices and organizations have found ways to effectively use health IT to support their quality improvement activities. Primary care practices require four interconnected factors to effectively use health IT: a practice culture with a strong commitment to using health IT for quality improvement; high-functioning health IT tools to enable data tracking and extraction; practice clinical team and staff knowledge and skills related to both health IT and quality improvement; and practice processes and workflows that incorporate the effective use of health IT for quality improvement (Higgins et al., 2015).

Regarding the use of health IT in chronic disease management, primary care facilities generally use the following types of health IT applications to address different aspects of chronic disease management:

- Clinical decision support (CDS) systems, which help providers interpret clinical results, document patients' health status, and prescribe medications
- Health information exchanges, which allow organizations to share information across organizational boundaries
- Disease registries, which capture and track key patient information to assist care team members in proactively managing patients
- Patient-centered applications, such as patient portals and integrated voice response (IVR) systems, which are designed to educate patients about their disease, medications, and self-management of chronic conditions

- EHRs with integrated decision support and chronic care management tools, which help providers manage patient information and monitor health outcomes for patients undergoing treatment for chronic diseases
- Telehealth applications that remotely connect providers and patients in co-management of chronic diseases (Agency for Healthcare Research and Quality, 2014)

▶ Assessment of Community Health Centers

In recent years, an increasing number of studies have assessed the quality, accessibility, and cost-effectiveness of CHCs.

CHCs' Quality of Care

In terms of health care quality at CHCs, it is critical that the care delivered at such centers is evidence-based, appropriate, well-coordinated, safe, and patient-centered. Through various Health Resources and Services Administration (HRSA) and other federal, private-sector, state, and community efforts and partnerships, CHCs have made major advances in adopting evidence-based practices; improving patient safety; meeting national accreditation standards, including the establishment of health centers as patient-centered medical homes; and increasing the coordination, integration, and management of health center care. To better monitor these advances, HRSA also established a core set of clinical performance measures that place a greater emphasis on health outcomes and demonstrate the value of CHC-delivered care. These measures align with those of national quality measurement organizations, and many are commonly used by Medicare, Medicaid, and private insurers to assess quality.

A number of studies have demonstrated that health centers' quality of care equals and often surpasses that provided by other primary care providers. A programmatic emphasis on quality as well as community-responsive and culturally appropriate care has also translated into impressive reductions in health disparities for patients receiving care at CHCs. These achievements are even more notable given the CHC patient population is often sicker and more at risk than the overall patient population seen nationally (HRSA, 2011).

Patients who visit CHCs report positive experiences overall, citing the centers' convenient locations and the positive interactions with providers. However, uninsured patients may be less likely to receive help from the staff in applying for government benefits and setting up appointments with other medical providers. Even though racial/ethnic and insurance coverage disparities are less prevalent at CHCs than at other primary care providers, more efforts need to be focused on assisting those without insurance in applying for benefits (Shi et al., 2013a). Results from another study showed that there was no significant difference in length of visit or number of services provided between patients seen at CHCs and those seen at office-based physician practices (Bruen et al., 2013). Across racial/ethnic groups, CHC patients were found to be more satisfied than the U.S. low-income patient population with the hours of operation and overall care received (Shi et al., 2013b).

Shin and colleagues (2013) compared CHCs' quality of care to national benchmarks of quality performance for Medicaid MCOs. Performance along three measures—diabetes control, hypertension control, and receipt of a Pap test—was evaluated. Nearly all health centers scored above the Medicaid MCO average benchmark; only 4% of CHCs ranked as low performers. In 2013, CHCs had a lower percentage of low-birthweight babies than the national estimates (HRSA, 2014). Additionally, 68% of diabetic patients had their diabetes under control, and 62% of hypertensive patients kept their blood pressure under control (HRSA, 2017).

CHCs' Access to Care

Access to preventive and primary services reduces the risk of increased disease severity, complications, and emergency medical services utilization (Laiteerapong et al., 2014). Compared to the general U.S. low-income patient population, patients served by CHCs did not experience racial/ethnic- or insurance-based disparities in access to primary care (Shi et al., 2013b). Overall, CHCs seem to be meeting the health care needs of the vulnerable populations they serve and reducing disparities in access to health care.

In comparing rates of inadequate hypertension control, poor diabetes control, and low birthweight across four racial/ethnic categories (non-Hispanic white, black/African American, Asian, and Hispanic/Latino), minimal differences and disparities for the clinical indicators were found among different races and ethnicities (Lebrun et al., 2013; Shi et al., 2017b). Thus, CHCs seem to be successful in reducing racial/ethnic health disparities, especially when compared to the disparities found nationwide. Moreover, increased federal funding for CHCs may have slowed the decline in access to care among low-income populations (McMorrow & Zuckerman, 2014).

CHCs' Cost-Effectiveness

CHC patients are found to have fewer office visits and hospitalizations, and female CHC patients are three times more likely to receive breast cancer screening compared to non-CHC patients (Laiteerapong et al., 2014). Uninsured CHC patients have fewer outpatient visits and emergency department visits and are more likely to receive dietary advice and breast cancer screening than non-CHC patients (Laiteerapong et al., 2014). The findings suggest that CHCs focus on preventive care, which results in lower rates of medical care utilization by disadvantaged groups.

CHCs and the Affordable Care Act

The ACA created the Community Health Center Fund to provide $11 billion over a 5-year period for the operation, expansion, and construction of CHCs across the country, including the District of Columbia, Puerto Rico, the U.S. Virgin Islands, and the Pacific Basin. CHCs served 19.5 million people in 2010, a number that increased to 21.7 million in 2013 (HRSA, 2014). In 2014, the ACA provided $100 million for the establishment of 150 more health centers across the United States (HRSA, 2014).

Despite the good intentions of the ACA, CHCs face significant financial challenges because Medicaid reimbursement has declined even as health centers' Medicaid patient load has increased and physicians at CHCs report overwhelming workloads and frustrations with administrative management (Cole et al., 2014). Unless these issues are resolved at a fundamental level, additional funding for the expansion of CHCs will likely accomplish little.

▶ Conclusion

Outpatient services now transcend basic and routine primary care services, as many general medical and surgical interventions are provided in ambulatory care settings. In response to changing economic incentives in the health care delivery system, numerous types of ambulatory services have emerged, and a variety of settings for the delivery of services have developed. In most settings, patients visit delivery sites to receive services. In other cases, services are brought to the patients.

The effectiveness of primary care has been demonstrated in numerous ways. However, its predominant practice can no longer be confined to the way primary care has been traditionally practiced. The broader biopsychosocial paradigm emphasizes the health of the population as well as that of the individual. A medical home model has been advocated to deliver primary care based on the principles of patient-centered care and team-based chronic disease management approaches. Community Health Centers that predominantly serve vulnerable populations have been found to deliver high-quality care cost-effectively in underserved areas; the Affordable Care Act authorized funds for the expansion of these centers. Both old and new approaches to primary care delivery face mounting challenges in the wake of workforce shortages and financial constraints.

References

1. Agency for Healthcare Research and Quality (AHRQ). 2014. Health IT for improved chronic disease management. https://healthit.ahrq.gov/ahrq-funded-projects /emerging-lessons/health-it-improved-chronic-disease-management. Accessed December 11, 2017.
2. American Academy of Family Physicians, American Academy of Pediatrics, American College of Physicians, & American Osteopathic Association. 2007. Joint principles of the patient-centered medical home, March 2007. Available at: http:// www.acponline.org/running_practice/pcmh/demonstrations/jointprinc_05_17.pdf. Accessed January 2014.
3. Bailey MJ, Goodman-Bacon A. 2015. The war on poverty's experiment in public medicine: Community Health Centers and the mortality of older Americans. *Am Econ Rev.* 105(3):1067–1104. doi: 10.1257/aer.20120070.
4. Bakwin H. 1945. Pseudodoxia pediatrica. *N Engl J Med.* 232:691–697.
5. Barnes PM, et al. 2007. Complementary and alternative medicine use among adults and children: United States. *Natl Health Stat Rep.* 12:1–23.
6. Barr KW, Breindel CL. 1995. Ambulatory care. In: Wolper LF, ed. *Health care administration: Principles, practices, structure, and delivery.* 2nd ed. Gaithersburg, MD: Aspen; 547–573.
7. Barry J. 2017. The relationship between the supply of primary care physicians and measures of breast health service use. *J Women's Health.* 26(5):511–519. doi: 10.1089 /jwh.2016.5830.
8. Beal A, et al. 2007. Closing the divide: How medical homes promote equity in health care: Results from the Commonwealth Fund 2006 Health Care Quality Survey. Washington, DC: Commonwealth Fund.
9. Bruen BK, et al. 2013. No evidence that primary care physicians offer less care to Medicaid, community health center, or uninsured patients. *Health Aff.* 32(9):1624–1630.
10. Cole AM, et al. 2014. Rewards and challenges of community health center practice. *J Prim Care Community Health.* 5(2):148–151.
11. Complementary and Alternative Medicine (CAM) Research Methodology Conference. 1997. Defining and describing complementary and alternative medicine. *Altern Ther.* 3(2):49–56.
12. Farmer SA, et al. November 22, 2017. Payment reform to enhance collaboration of primary care and cardiology: A review. *JAMA Cardiol.* doi: 10.1001 /jamacardio.2017.4308.
13. Ferrante JM, et al. 2000. Effects of physician supply on early detection of breast cancer. *J Am Board Fam Pract.* 13(6):408–414.
14. Franks P, et al. 1992. Gatekeeping revisited: protecting patients from overtreatment. *N Engl J Med.* 327(4):424–429.

15. Franks P, Fiscella K. 1998. Primary care physicians and specialists as personal physicians: Health care expenditures and mortality experience. *J Fam Pract.* 47(2):105–109.
16. Freund T, et al. 2015. Skill mix, roles and remuneration in the primary care workforce: Who are the healthcare professionals in the primary care teams across the world? *Int J Nurs Stud.* 52(3):727–743. doi: 10.1016/j.ijnurstu.2014.11.014.
17. Gadomski A, et al. 1998. Impact of a Medicaid primary care provider and preventive care on pediatric hospitalization. *Pediatrics.* 101(3):E1. http://www.pediatrics.org/cgi/content/full/101/3/e1. Accessed December 2000.
18. Gaglioti AH, Petterson S, Bazemore A, Phillips R. Access to Primary Care in US Counties Is Associated with Lower Obesity Rates. *J Am Board Fam Med.* 2016 Mar-Apr;29(2):182–190. doi: 10.3122/jabfm.2016.02.150356.
19. Gofin J, et al. 2015. Community-oriented primary care (COPC) and the Affordable Care Act: An opportunity to meet the demands of an evolving health care system. *J Primary Care Comm Health.* 6(2):128–133. doi: 10.1177/2150131914555908.
20. Health Resources and Services Administration (HRSA). 2011. Efforts to expand and accelerate health center program quality improvement. https://bphc.hrsa.gov/ftca/riskmanagement/healthcenterqualityimprovement.pdf. Accessed December 11, 2017.
21. Health Resources and Services Administration (HRSA). 2014. Health center program. http://bphc.hrsa.gov/about/healthcenterfactsheet.pdf. Accessed June 27, 2015.
22. Health Resources and Services Administration (HRSA). 2017. 2016 National Health Center Data. https://bphc.hrsa.gov/uds/datacenter.aspx. Accessed December 11, 2017.
23. Heisey-Grove D, et al. 2013. *Supporting health information technology adoption in federally qualified health centers.* ONC Data Brief, No. 8. Washington, DC: Office of the National Coordinator for Health Information Technology.
24. Higgins TC, et al. 2015. *Using health information technology to support quality improvement in primary care.* AHRQ Publication No. 15-0031-EF. Rockville, MD: Agency for Healthcare Research and Quality. March.
25. Kumra T, et al. 2017. Improving adolescent preventive care in an urban pediatric clinic: Capturing missed opportunities. *J Adolesc Health.* 60(6):734–740. pii: S1054-139X(17)30028-9.
26. Laiteerapong N, et al. 2014. Health care utilization and receipt of preventive care for patients seen at federally funded health centers compared to other sites of primary care. *Heath Serv Res.* 49(5):1498–1518.
27. Lebrun LA, et al. 2013. Racial/ethnic differences in clinical quality performance among health centers. *J Ambul Care Manage.* 36(1):24–34.
28. Lee PR. 1994. Models of excellence. *Lancet.* 344(8935):1484–1486.
29. Liang H, et al. 2017. The patient-centered care and receipt of preventive services among older adults with chronic diseases: A nationwide cross-sectional study. *Inquiry.* 54:46958017724003. doi: 10.1177/0046958017724003.
30. Macinko J, et al. 2007. Quantifying the health benefits of primary care physician supply in the United States. *Int J Health Serv.* 37(1):111–126.
31. Manos D. February 5, 2014. EHR incentives climb to $19B. *Healthcare IT News.* http://www.healthcareitnews.com/news/ehr-incentives-climb-19b. Accessed December 11, 2017.
32. Mark DH, et al. 1996. Medicare costs in urban areas and the supply of primary care physicians. *J Fam Pract.* 43(1):33–39.
33. McAlearney JS. 2001. The financial performance of community health centers, 1996–1999. *Health Aff.* 21(2):219–225.
34. McMorrow S, Zuckerman S. 2014. Expanding federal funding to community health centers slows decline in access for low-income adults. *Health Serv Res.* 49(3):992–1010.

35. Ministry of Health and Long-Term Care Canada. 2012. Family health teams. http:// www.health.gov.on.ca/en/pro/programs/fht/fht_progress.aspx. Accessed December 11, 2017.
36. Modi PK, et al. 2017. Pediatric hospitalizations for upper urinary tract calculi: Epidemiological and treatment trends in the united states, 2001–2014. *J Pediatr Urol.* pii: S1477-5131(17)30310-8.
37. Naccarella L, et al. 2012. Building the capacity of the system for team-based models of primary care: A framework for action. *Med J Aust Health Workforce Suppl.* 2(1):22–25.
38. National Center for Health Statistics. 2015. National Ambulatory Medical Care Survey: 2015 state and national summary tables. https://www.cdc.gov/nchs/data /ahcd/namcs_summary/2015_namcs_web_tables.pdf. Accessed February 14, 2018.
39. Organization for Economic Cooperation and Development (OECD). 2012. OECD health at a glance: Europe 2012. doi: 10.1787/9789264183896-en.
40. Parchman ML, Culler S. 1994. Primary care physicians and avoidable hospitalizations. *J Fam Pract.* 39(2):123–128.
41. Peikes D, et al. 2012. Early evidence on the patient-centered medical home. Prepared by Mathematica Policy Research for the Agency for Healthcare Research and Quality. https://www.pcmh.ahrq.gov/page/early-evidence-patient-centered-medical-home. Accessed March 28, 2018.
42. Perrin JM, et al. 1996. Primary care involvement among hospitalized children. *Arch Pediatr Adolesc Med.* 1996;150(5):479–486.
43. Petterson SM, et al. 2015. Estimating the residency expansion required to avoid projected primary care physician shortages by 2035. *Ann Fam Med.* 13:107–114.
44. Politzer RM, et al. 2001. Inequality in America: The contribution of health centers in reducing and eliminating disparities in access to care. *Med Care Res Rev.* 58(2):234–248.
45. Rojanasarot S, Carlson AM. 2017. The medical home model and pediatric asthma symptom severity: Evidence from a national health survey. *Population Health Manag.* doi: 10.1089/pop.2017.0066.
46. Roos N. 1979. Who should do the surgery? Tonsillectomy and adenoidectomy in one Canadian province. *Inquiry.* 16(1):73–83.
47. Rosenthal TC. 2008. The medical home: Growing evidence to support a new approach to primary care. *J Am Board Fam Med.* 21:427–440.
48. Rosser WW. 1996. Approach to diagnosis by primary care clinicians and specialists: Is there a difference? *J Fam Pract.* 42(2):139–144.
49. Ryan A, et al. 2001. The effects of regular source of care and health need on medical care use among rural adolescents. *Arch Pediatr Adolesc Med.* 155(2):184–190.
50. Saver B. 2002. Financing and organization findings brief. *Acad Res Health Care Policy.* 5(1):1–2.
51. Schwartz MD. 2012. The US primary care workforce and graduate medical education policy. *JAMA.* 308(21):2252–2253. doi: 10.1001/jama.2012.77034.
52. Shea S, et al. 1992. Predisposing factors for severe, uncontrolled hypertension in an inner-city minority population. *N Engl J Med.* 327(11):776–781.
53. Shi L. 1992. The relation between primary care and life chances. *J Health Care Poor Underserved.* 3:321–335.
54. Shi L. 1994. Primary care, specialty care, and life chances. *Int J Health Serv.* 24(3):431–458.
55. Shi L, Starfield B. 2000. Primary care, income inequality, and self-rated health in the United States: A mixed-level analysis. *Int J Health Serv.* 30:541–555.
56. Shi L, et al. 1999. Income inequality, primary care, and health indicators. *J Fam Pract.* 48:275–284.

57. Shi L, et al. 2002. Primary care, self-rated health, and reductions in social disparities in health. *Health Serv Res.* 37:529–550.
58. Shi L, et al. 2003. The relationship between primary care, income inequality, and mortality in US states, 1980–1995. *J Am Board Fam Pract.* 16(5):412–422.
59. Shi L, et al. 2004. Primary care, infant mortality, and low birthweight in US states. *J Epidemiol Community Health.* 58(5):374–380.
60. Shi L, et al. 2013a. The quality of primary care experienced by health center patients. *J Am Board Fam Med.* 26(6):768–777.
61. Shi L, et al. 2013b. Reducing disparities in access to primary care and patient satisfaction with care: the role of health centers. *J Health Care Poor Underserved.* 24(1):56–66.
62. Shi L, et al. 2017a. Patient-centered medical home recognition and clinical performance in U.S. Community Health Centers. *Health Serv Res* 52(3):984–1004 doi: 10.1111/1475-6773.12523.
63. Shi L, et al. 2017b. Access to care and satisfaction among health center patients with chronic conditions. *J Ambul Care Manag.* 40(1):69–76.
64. Shin P, et al. 2013. Quality of care in community health centers and factors associated with performance. Kaiser Commission on Medicaid and the Uninsured Report #8447. https://kaiserfamilyfoundation.files.wordpress.com/2013/06/8447 .pdf. Accessed March 28, 2018.
65. Starfield B. 1985. Motherhood and apple pie: The effectiveness of medical care for children. *Milbank Mem Fund Q: Health Soc.* 63(3):523–546.
66. Starfield B. 1992. *Primary care: Concept, evaluation, and policy.* New York, NY: Oxford University Press.
67. Starfield B. 1994. Is primary care essential? *Lancet.* 344(8930):1129–1133.
68. Starfield B, Shi L. 2002. Policy relevant determinants of health: An international perspective. *Health Policy.* 60:201–218.
69. *United States Pharmaceuticals & Healthcare Report.* 2015. (1):1–119. Ipswich, MA: Business Source Complete.
70. Vanselow NA, et al. 1995. From the Institute of Medicine. *JAMA.* 273(3):192.
71. Villalbi JR, et al. 1999. An evaluation of the impact of primary care reform on health. *Aten Primaria.* 24(8):468–474.
72. Welch WP, et al. 1993. Geographic variation in expenditures for physicians' services in the United States. *N Engl J Med.* 328(9):621–627.
73. Whittle JC, et al. 1998. Relationship of provider characteristics to outcomes, process, and costs of care for community-acquired pneumonia. *Med Care.* 36(7):977–987.
74. Williams SJ. 1993. Ambulatory health care services. In: Williams SJ, Torrens PR, eds. *Introduction to health services.* 4th ed. Albany, NY: Delmar Publishers.
75. World Health Organization (WHO). 1978. *Primary health care.* Geneva, Switzerland: WHO.

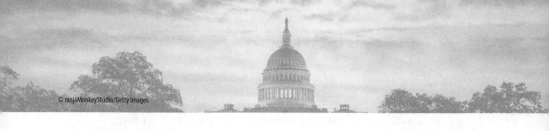

CHAPTER 8

Hospitals

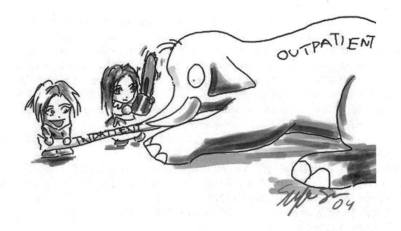

▶ Introduction

The term *inpatient* refers to an overnight stay in a health care facility, such as a hospital or a nursing home, when the patient is formally admitted with a physician's order. *Outpatient*, in contrast, refers to services provided while the patient is not lodged in the hospital or some other health care institution. This chapter describes what a hospital is, explores the hospital's evolution, and examines its current role in health care delivery.

The American Hospital Association (AHA) defines a hospital as an institution with at least six beds whose primary function is "to deliver patient services, diagnostic and therapeutic, for particular or general medical conditions" (AHA, 1994). In addition, a hospital must be licensed, it must have an organized physician staff, and it must provide continuous nursing services under the supervision of registered nurses. A hospital must appoint a governing body or board that is legally responsible for the conduct of the hospital. It must also appoint a full-time chief executive officer (CEO) to be responsible for the hospital's operations. The hospital must maintain medical records on each patient, have pharmacy services available within the institution, and provide food services to meet the nutritional and therapeutic requirements of the patients (Health Forum, 2001). The construction and operation of the modern hospital is governed by federal laws, state health regulations, city ordinances, standards of the Joint Commission (formerly the Joint Commission on Accreditation of Healthcare Organizations [JCAHO]), and national codes for building, fire protection, and sanitation.

In the past 200 years or so, hospitals have gradually evolved from basic institutions of refuge for the homeless and poor, to ultramodern facilities providing the latest medical services to the critically ill and injured. The term *medical center* is used by some hospitals, reflecting their high level of specialization and wide scope of services. Medical centers often engage in teaching and research. Since the 1980s, many hospitals have expanded their scope of services to include outpatient care.

▶ Evolution of the Hospital in the United States

The six major stages of hospital evolution in the United States are listed in **EXHIBIT 8.1**.

Stage 1

Before 1850 or so, only a few hospitals existed, all of which were found in major U.S. cities. The main health care institutions were the almshouses

---

EXHIBIT 8.1 Major Stages of Hospital Evolution

1. Almshouses as primarily institutions of social welfare
2. Community-owned private hospitals as charitable institutions supported by affluent donors
3. Institutions of medical practice and training serving the needs of all members of society and able to make a profit
4. Emergence of a relatively small number of physician-owned proprietary hospitals
5. University-based centers of medical research
6. Emergence of medical systems providing a large array of health services

(also called poorhouses) run by local governments. Pesthouses were operated to confine people with contagious diseases. Services in these institutions were more akin to social welfare than to medicine, consisting mainly of providing food and shelter to the destitute and some nursing care to the sick. Medicine and nursing as the professions we know today had not emerged. People generally stayed in these institutions for months rather than days.

Stage 2

During the latter half of the 1800s, hospitals evolved from the almshouses and pesthouses but continued to serve mainly the poor. At this time, hospitals began to transition from being primarily government-run institutions to community-owned institutions supported mainly through private charitable donations. Influential donors exercised control over the hospital through their roles as members of the board of trustees. Since this period, private (rather than government-owned) nonprofit hospitals have dominated the hospital landscape in America.

Stage 3

Medical discoveries during the latter half of the 1800s were instrumental in transforming hospitals into true institutions of medical practice. Discoveries that had a profound impact on hospital care included anesthesia, which aided significantly in advancing new surgical techniques, and the development of the germ theory of disease, which led to the subsequent discovery of antiseptic and sterilization techniques (Haglund & Dowling, 1993). From around 1850 onward, technological progress led to the development of advanced equipment, facilities, and personnel training, which became centered in the hospital. Hospitals established laboratories and x-ray units so that physicians could have convenient access to diagnostic technology. These advances made it necessary for community-based physicians to treat acute illnesses in hospitals, which also became centers where physicians received their practical training. Henceforth, hospitals came to be regarded as a necessity, because the superior medical services and surgical procedures offered there could not be obtained at home.

Stage 4

With advances in sanitation, nursing care, and medical services, hospitals began to attract well-to-do patients who could afford to pay for their care on an out-of-pocket basis. As these wealthier individuals began to use their services, hospitals found that they no longer had to depend totally on charitable contributions; indeed, they could now generate a profit. At this stage, some physicians started opening their own small hospitals, thereby laying the foundation for proprietary (for-profit) hospitals in the United States.

Stage 5

Many hospitals established formal affiliations with university-based medical schools and became centers of medical research where new discoveries were made. Even today, medical research plays a critical role in finding better cures and in disseminating research findings through publications in medical journals to advance new medical knowledge throughout the world.

During this stage, hospitals became complex organizations, and the field of hospital administration became a discipline in its own right. To manage hospitals, administrators needed expertise in financial management and good organizational and human relations skills. In addition, departments such as food service, pharmacy, x-ray imaging, and the laboratory required well-trained professional staff to manage the delivery of services.

Stage 6

Since the 1990s, local market pressures have prompted many hospitals to merge or enter into formal affiliations with other hospitals. In urban areas, *medical systems* (or health systems) have been formed. These systems are large organizations that may include more than one hospital to serve a large geographic area. They also provide a full array of health care services, including outpatient clinics, same-day surgery, outpatient imaging services, outpatient rehabilitation therapies, nursing home care, home health services, and hospice care. Many health systems have also opened special women's health centers and fitness centers. Increasingly, community services such as health education, promotion of healthy lifestyles, and prevention of disease have become an important part of a hospital's mission.

▶ Expansion and Downsizing of Hospitals in the United States

The number of hospital beds in the United States grew from 35,604 in 1872 to 907,133 in 1929 (Haglund & Dowling, 1993). This phenomenal growth started once hospitals became institutions of medical practice, serving the needs of all members of society and making a profit (stage 4 in the six-stage model). Technological advances increased the volume of surgical work, which at that time could be done only in hospitals. As new facilities with additional beds were built, they were quickly filled by patients needing acute treatment or surgery. Advances in medical science, as well as professional training of nurses and other health care professionals, played an important role in creating a demand for more beds. Additional factors contributing to the growth of hospitals from the preindustrial era to around 1980 are listed in **EXHIBIT 8.2**.

After 1930, the wider availability of private health insurance enabled more and more people to pay for hospital services, which became increasingly more costly and unaffordable. Once people had health insurance, that fact in itself generated new demand. Early insurance plans provided generous coverage for inpatient care, and few restrictions were placed on the use of hospital-based services.

In the 1940s, the U.S. government recognized that a severe shortage of hospitals existed in the country. In response, Congress passed the Hospital Survey and Construction Act of 1946, commonly known as the Hill-Burton Act. It provided federal grants to the states for the construction of new hospital beds. The objective of the Hill-Burton Act was to increase the United States' hospital capacity to 4.5 beds per 1,000 population (Teisberg et al., 1991). Indeed, the Hill-Burton program has been regarded as the greatest single factor in increasing the nation's bed supply. This building program made it possible for even small and remote communities to establish their own hospitals (Wolfson & Hopes, 1994).

The creation of Medicare and Medicaid in 1965 made public health insurance available to a large segment of the U.S. population. Hospital demand, in turn, continued to grow. Between 1965 and 1980, the number of community hospitals in the United States increased from 5,736 (741,000 beds) to 5,830 (988,000 beds) (AHA, 1990). By 1980, the United States had also reached its goal of 4.5 community hospital beds per 1,000 civilian population (National Center for Health Statistics [NCHS], 2002).

In 1983, the U.S. government decided it needed to contain the exploding cost of hospital care, mostly because of its impact on the rising

---

EXHIBIT 8.2   Factors Contributing to the Growth of Hospitals

- Broad appeal once hospitals evolved into institutions of medical practice as a result of technological advances and professional training of health care professionals
- Private health insurance
- Hill-Burton Act
- Medicare and Medicaid

cost of Medicare. **FIGURE 8.1** shows the increase in costs that occurred between 1970 and 1980. This goal of cost containment was achieved through the enactment of the Social Security amendments of 1983. The law required Medicare to stop paying hospitals per diem rates established on the basis of their costs of operation (retrospective reimbursement). Instead, a prospective payment system (PPS) was established to reimburse hospitals on the basis of diagnosis-related groups (DRGs). Under this method, hospitals received a preestablished fixed rate per admission. To ensure that they would not lose money, hospitals had to cut their costs of operation. They also had to discharge patients more quickly than had been the practice in the past, because keeping patients in the hospital longer than necessary cut into the hospital's profits. Many hospitals were forced to close when they had difficulty coping with the new method of reimbursement. Other hospitals continued to operate but had to take unused beds out of service. Thus, implementation of PPS triggered the downsizing phase in the U.S. hospital industry.

During the 1990s, the growth of managed care played a significant role in curtailing inpatient utilization even further. Managed care emphasized cost containment and efficient delivery of care through early discharge from hospitals, and, if necessary, continuity of care through home health agencies and skilled-care nursing homes. In other instances, the emphasis has been on using outpatient services whenever appropriate instead of admitting patients to hospitals.

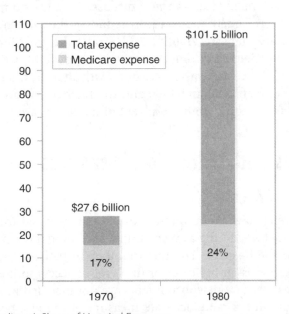

FIGURE 8.1 Medicare's Share of Hospital Expenses

Data from Department of Health and Human Services. Health, United States, 2003, p. 342; Table C-5: Selected data on community hospital expenses, 1965–95. http://aspe.hhs.gov

---

EXHIBIT 8.3   Factors Contributing to the Downsizing of Hospitals

- Change in Medicare reimbursement to hospitals from a retrospective to a prospective method, leading to shorter hospital stays
- Hospital closings
- Managed care's emphasis on cost containment and use of services such as outpatient, home health, and skilled nursing care

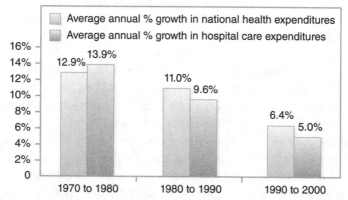

FIGURE 8.2   Comparison of Growth in Hospital and National Health Expenditures

Data from National Center for Health Statistics. Health, United States, 2002. Hyattsville, MD: Department of Health and Human Services, 2002:291.

The three main factors just discussed (and summarized in **EXHIBIT 8.3**) were largely successful in reducing the growth of national spending on hospital care. **FIGURE 8.2** illustrates the growth of spending on hospital inpatient care compared with the growth of national health expenditures. Notice the slower rates of growth after the implementation of the PPS between 1980 and 1990 and the further slowdown between 1990 and 2000 resulting from the advent of managed care.

▶ Access and Utilization Measures

Measures of Access

Discharges refer to the total number of patients released from a hospital's acute care beds during a given period, including those patients who die while in the hospital. The total number of patient discharges per 1,000 population is an indicator of the level of access to hospital inpatient services. Because newborn infants are not included in admissions, discharges provide a more accurate measure of the number of people served by a hospital. Thus, discharges measure the number of patients who received hospital inpatient services.

Measures of Utilization

An *inpatient day* (also referred to as a patient day or a hospital day) is a night spent in the hospital by a patient. The average number of days a patient spends in the hospital is called the *average length of stay* (ALOS). The total number of inpatient days incurred by a population over a given period of time is referred to as *days of care*. Mathematically,

$$Days\ of\ care = discharges \times ALOS$$

National data on days of care per 1,000 population show that elderly individuals spend more time in hospitals than do younger people. Even after adjusting for childbearing among women 18 years and older, women are admitted to hospitals more often than men, but men incur longer stays. Hospital utilization is higher among blacks than whites, and is also higher among the poor than the nonpoor. Various factors (e.g., education, socioeconomic status, behaviors, lifestyles, heredity, access to primary care) interact to produce differences in health status and onset of acute conditions for the various population groups; hence, some groups incur more frequent hospitalizations and require longer stays once admitted. From this information, it can be concluded that overall hospital utilization is higher among Medicare and Medicaid recipients compared to the rest of the population. Demand for and utilization of hospital services are also influenced by overall population growth, advances in medical technology, and health insurance.

For the past decade, the ALOS for community hospitals in the United States has ranged between 5.4 and 5.5 days. The PPS, as noted earlier, had a marked influence on the decline in the ALOS, as did the introduction of managed care during the 1990s. The sharp decline in ALOS during the 1990s became possible with the growth of alternative services, such as home health and subacute long-term care, which enabled people to be discharged earlier than was previously possible, and yet receive continuity of care in a non-hospital setting. Thanks to the development of these substitute sites of care and more advanced technology, there has been no evidence that quicker discharges of patients from hospitals under the PPS or managed care payment systems resulted in medical harm to patients.

Utilization of Hospital Capacity

Capacity refers to the number of beds set up, staffed, and made available by a hospital for inpatient use. Of all community hospitals in the United States, 84% have fewer than 300 beds. The average size of a community hospital is approximately 160 beds (NCHS, 2017).

TABLE 8.1 Relationship Between the Selected Measures of Capacity Utilization

Day Number	Census	Patient Days
1	100	100
2	104	204
3	101	305
4	99	404
5	98	502
6	102	604
7	103	707

Patient days for this week: 707. Average daily census: 707/7 = 101. If hospital capacity is 153, the occupancy rate is 66% [(101/153) × 100].

The term *census* refers to the number of patients in a hospital on a given day or the number of beds occupied on a given day. The cumulative census over a given period of time is called *patient days* or *days of care*. The average census over a period of time is called the *average daily census* (**TABLE 8.1**). Mathematically,

$$\text{Average daily census} = \frac{\text{Patient days over a given period}}{\text{Number of days in the period}}$$

The *occupancy rate* is the percentage of capacity used during a given period of time. It is calculated by dividing the average daily census for that period by the capacity (Table 8.1). The fraction is expressed as a percentage (percent beds occupied). An individual hospital's performance in capacity utilization can be meaningfully compared with local and national composite occupancy rates. In 2014, the occupancy rate for all U.S. community hospitals was 62.8% (NCHS, 2017).

▶ Hospital Employment

According to the Bureau of Labor Statistics (BLS), in November 2017, the health care and social assistance sector in the United States employed more than 19.6 million workers. Of these, more than 5 million (26%) were employed in hospitals (BLS, 2018). In terms of job growth, however, the outpatient services sector continues to lead the way. Interestingly, between 2000 and 2010, while the overall employment in the United States declined by a little more than 2%, hospital employment grew by almost 16%; overall health occupation jobs grew by 25% over the same period (Center for Health Workforce Studies, 2012). Recent job growth in hospitals has been largely focused on health occupations as opposed to non-health care positions, such as food service or janitorial staff. Between 2014 and 2024, hospitals are expected to see the lowest job growth as opposed to job growth in the other sectors of the health care industry (Martiniano et al., 2016). Nevertheless, between 2014 and 2016, hospital staffing per occupied bed increased particularly for registered nurses, and to a lesser extent for staff physicians and occupational therapists. Of particular note was a decrease in staffing for licensed practical nurses (Sanofi-Aventis, 2017).

▶ Types of Hospitals

The United States supports a variety of institutional forms, including both private and government-owned hospitals (**FIGURE 8.3**). A hospital can be classified under more than one category.

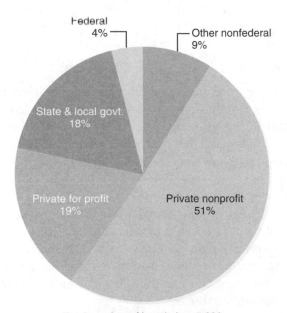

Total number of hospitals = 5,686
Note: Due to rounding, the data do not add up to 100%.

FIGURE 8.3 Types of Hospitals, 2016

Data from Health Forum LLC, an affiliate of the American Hospital Association. Fast facts on U.S. hospitals. 2018. https://www.aha.org/system/files/2018-

EXHIBIT 8.4 Characteristics of a Community Hospital

- Nonfederal: hospitals operated by local and state governments can be community hospitals
- Short stay: average length of stay must be 25 days or less
- Open to the general public
- Private for-profit or nonprofit; general or specialty

Community Hospitals

More than 87% of all U.S. hospitals are community hospitals. The identifying characteristics of these hospitals are listed in **EXHIBIT 8.4**. By definition, a *community hospital* is a nonfederal, short-stay hospital whose services are available to the general public. This definition excludes federal hospitals, such as those operated by the Department of Veterans Affairs (VA) and military systems, and the hospital units of some institutions, such as prisons and infirmaries in colleges and universities, because their services are not available to the general public. In contrast, most hospitals operated by local and state governments are community hospitals. Also excluded from the definition of a community hospital are long-stay hospitals, such as psychiatric facilities, tuberculosis hospitals, and other chronic disease hospitals. In long-stay hospitals, the average length of stay is more than 25 days.

Public Hospitals

In health care, the word *public* connotes government ownership. *Public hospitals*, therefore, are hospitals owned by agencies of federal, state, or local governments. An estimated one-fourth of the U.S. hospitals are in the public sector. A public hospital is not necessarily a hospital that is open to the general public. For example, because they are government owned, federal hospitals are classified as public hospitals, even though they do not serve the general public. Federal hospitals are maintained primarily for special groups of federal beneficiaries such as Native Americans, military personnel, and veterans.

State governments have generally limited themselves to the operation of mental and tuberculosis hospitals, reflecting the government's early role in protecting communities by isolating the mentally ill and persons with contagious diseases.

Local governments, such as counties and cities, operate hospitals that are open to the general public. Hence, these hospitals are also classified as community hospitals. Government-owned community hospitals are often located in large urban areas where they serve mainly the inner-city indigent and disadvantaged populations. Due to the generally poor health status of these populations and inner-city violence, these hospitals incur higher utilization than hospitals located in suburban areas. Most of these hospitals are of small to moderate size. Some large public hospitals are affiliated with medical schools, and they play a significant role in training physicians and other health care professionals. Medicare, Medicaid, and state and local tax dollars finance most of the services these hospitals provide. These hospitals also provide a substantial amount of charity care and often suffer financial losses that are covered by funneling tax dollars into the operations.

Because of increasing financial pressures, many public hospitals have undergone privatization or had to close in recent years. Consequently, the number of state and local government-owned community hospitals has steadily declined, from 1,444 in 1990 to 1,003 in 2014 (NCHS, 2017).

Private Nonprofit Hospitals

Private nonprofit hospitals are also called *voluntary hospitals*. A little more than half of the hospitals in the United States are under private nonprofit ownership (see Figure 8.3). These hospitals are owned by nongovernment entities such as community associations, philanthropic foundations, or religious groups. The primary mission of these hospitals is to benefit the communities in which they are located. Their operating expenses are covered from patient fees, third-party reimbursement, donations, and endowments.

Church-owned hospitals play a significant role in delivering hospital services in the United States. For example, the Catholic Church operates more than 600 hospitals (more than 116,000 beds) in all 50 states and delivers care to one-sixth of all hospital patients each year (Catholic Health Association of the United States, 2015). Some Protestant denominations and Jewish philanthropic organizations also operate numerous community hospitals. These hospitals are not discriminatory in terms of access to care, but are generally sensitive to the special spiritual or dietary norms of the sponsoring denomination (Raffel & Raffel, 1994, pp. 131–132). In one report, church-owned hospitals were found to be superior to other ownership types in delivering high value to their communities, offering reliable high quality and efficiency and having high patient perception of care at a reasonable cost (Foster et al., 2013). According to the same report, government hospitals demonstrated the weakest balanced performance.

Lay people make a common assumption that nonprofit (sometimes referred to as not-for-profit) organizations do not make a profit.

The reality is that every corporation, regardless of whether it is for profit or nonprofit, has to make a profit (a surplus of revenues over expenses) to remain operational over the long term. No business can survive for long if it continually spends more than it takes in. This statement is as true for nonprofit organizations as it is for the for-profit sector.

The Internal Revenue Code, Section 501(c)(3), grants tax-exempt status to nonprofit organizations. As such, these institutions are exempt from federal, state, and local taxes such as income, sales, and property taxes. In exchange for the tax benefit these organizations receive, they must (1) provide some defined public good, such as service, education, or community welfare, and (2) not distribute the profits to any individual. The rationale behind tax exemption is that these facilities provide an essential community benefit, principally for charitable, training, or research purposes. There are ongoing debates and court cases over what does or does not constitute a community benefit.

Research has shown considerable variation in the level of community benefits provided by nonprofit hospitals. A national study found that, on average, these hospitals spent 7.5% of their expenses on community benefits; more than 85% of these expenses were devoted to charity care and other patient care services (Young et al., 2013). Although for-profit and nonprofit hospitals engage in similar competitive behaviors, on average nonprofit hospitals do appear to spend more on charity care than their investor-owned counterparts, but the difference tends to be small (Rubin et al., 2015).

To comply with the requirements of the Affordable Care Act (ACA), nonprofit hospitals must assess community health needs and develop strategies to meet those needs, under a new section—501(r)—of the tax code. These hospitals must develop and publicize written financial assistance policies and limit billing and collection actions against patients who are eligible for assistance.

Private For-Profit Hospitals

Private for-profit hospitals, also referred to as *proprietary hospitals* or investor-owned hospitals, are owned by individuals, partnerships, or corporations. They are operated for the financial benefit of the entity that owns the institution—that is, the stockholders.

More than 260 hospitals in roughly 33 states are owned by physicians, representing approximately 5% of U.S. hospitals. These relatively small hospitals usually specialize in heart or orthopedic surgeries (Rau, 2013). According to the Physician Hospitals of America (PHA), a professional association representing this industry sector, 67% of the hospitals participating in the star-rating system developed by the Centers for Medicare and Medicaid Services (CMS) received 4 or 5 stars compared to 41% of all hospitals nationwide (PHA, 2015). The ACA put severe restrictions on the creation and expansion of physician-owned hospitals, even though with respect to efficiency, patient satisfaction, and outcomes these hospitals perform favorably compared to other hospitals (Lundgren et al., 2016).

For-profit corporations operate some of the largest multihospital chains in the United States. Among the largest are Hospital Corporation of America (156 hospitals in 2014), Community Health Systems (208 hospitals), and Tenet Health System (76 hospitals). A significant trend over the past few years has been the building or acquisition of a substantial number of hospitals by large investor-owned corporations. Even so, most multihospital health care systems today are operated by nonprofit corporations. Although a major goal for a for-profit organization is to provide a return on investment to its shareholders, it achieves this goal primarily by excelling at accomplishing its basic mission. The basic mission of any health services provider is to deliver the highest quality of care possible at the most reasonable price possible.

General Hospitals

A *general hospital* provides diagnostic, treatment, and surgical services for patients with a variety of acute medical conditions. Its services may include general and specialized medicine, general and specialized surgery, and obstetrics. Most hospitals in the United States are general hospitals, but they are not all community hospitals because most federal hospitals are general hospitals too.

The term *general hospital* does not imply that these hospitals are less specialized or that their care is inferior to that of specialty hospitals. The difference lies in the nature of services, not the quality. General hospitals provide a broader range of services for a larger variety of conditions, whereas specialty hospitals provide a narrow range of services for specific medical conditions or patient populations.

Specialty Hospitals

Specialty hospitals primarily engage in treating specific types of diseases or medical conditions—such as heart disease or cancer—or serving a specific patient population such as children. Specialty hospitals also provide services such as psychiatric care, rehabilitation, and orthopedic surgery. Specialty hospitals forge a distinct service niche in a given market. These hospitals are also considered community hospitals as long as they meet the criteria discussed previously. In some of the specialty areas, these hospitals compete with general hospitals that offer the same services.

Psychiatric Hospitals

The primary function of a psychiatric hospital is to provide diagnostic and treatment services for patients who have mental illnesses. Specifically, such an institution must have facilities to provide psychiatric, psychological, and social work services. A psychiatric hospital must also have a written agreement with a general hospital for the transfer of patients who may require medical, obstetric, or surgical care (Health Forum, 2001, p. A3). Historically, state governments took the primary responsibility for establishing facilities to care for the mentally ill, but as new pharmaceuticals have become available to treat mental illness, private psychiatric facilities and outpatient treatment centers have assumed the task of delivering most mental health services.

Substance abuse treatments are generally provided in non-hospital settings. However, a hospital may have a specialized unit to deliver substance abuse therapies, such as detoxification and medically managed withdrawal, before referring the patient to an outside agency for a comprehensive drug addiction treatment.

Rehabilitation Hospitals

Rehabilitation hospitals specialize in intensive therapeutic services to restore the maximum level of functioning in patients who have suffered recent disability due to illness or accident. Such hospitals serve patients who generally cannot be cured but whose functioning can be improved. Such patients include amputees, victims of accidents or sports injuries, stroke victims, and others. Patients often transfer to such facilities after undergoing orthopedic surgery or receiving trauma care in a general hospital. Facilities and staff are available to provide physical, occupational, and speech and language therapy.

Children's Hospitals

Children's hospitals are community hospitals that typically have special facilities and trained staff to deal with the unique medical problems of children, particularly those with complex and rare conditions. Most of the inpatients in children's hospitals are treated for chronic or congenital conditions. The remaining patients require intensive care for a variety of needs, such as cancer treatment, treatment of cystic fibrosis, and tissue transplants.

Children's hospitals have equipment and furnishings that are specially designed for children—from newborn babies requiring intensive care to teens with chronic illness. They also maintain a nurse staffing ratio that is higher than that in general hospitals because children require more nursing care compared to adults.

Rural Hospitals

A *rural hospital* is one that is located in a county that is not part of a metropolitan statistical area (MSA). The U.S. Bureau of the Census has defined an MSA as a geographic area that includes at least (1) one city with a population of 50,000 or more or (2) an urbanized area of at least 50,000 inhabitants and a total MSA population of at least 100,000. Compared with other hospitals, rural hospitals generally treat a larger percentage of poor and elderly patients. Their remote geographic location, small size, and limited workforce, along with physician shortages and typically inadequate financial resources, pose a unique set of challenges for rural hospitals (AHA, 2017).

To save some of the very small rural hospitals from having to close, the Balanced Budget Act of 1997 allowed certain rural hospitals to operate as *critical access hospitals* (CAHs). According to Medicare rules, a CAH should have no more than 25 beds and must provide 24-hour emergency medical services. An additional 10 beds may be operated for psychiatric and/or rehabilitation services. CAHs are reimbursed according to the retrospective cost-plus method, instead of the PPS method.

Teaching Hospitals

To be designated as a *teaching hospital*, a hospital must offer one or more graduate residency programs approved by the American Medical Association. Hence, one of the primary roles of a teaching hospital is to train physicians. Although these hospitals may also be actively involved in training nurses and other health professionals, such as therapists and dietitians, unless they train physicians, they cannot be called teaching hospitals.

Most major teaching hospitals are affiliated with medical schools of universities. The term *academic medical center* applies to an organization in which there is active collaboration among the university, medical school, hospital/health system, and health care professionals. An academic medical center is uniquely capable of conducting basic and applied clinical research, providing health care services, and offering medical education (Daniels & Carson, 2011). Among the largest and most prestigious teaching hospitals are the members of the Council of Teaching Hospitals and Health Systems, which has approximately 400 members in both the United States and Canada.

In addition to fulfilling a substantial teaching and research mission, teaching hospitals deliver specialized care for a variety of complex medical problems. These institutions often operate several intensive care units, possess the latest medical technologies, and attract a diverse group of physicians representing most specialties and many subspecialties.

Major teaching hospitals also offer many unique tertiary care services not generally found in other institutions, such as burn care, trauma care, and organ transplantation.

Osteopathic Hospitals

Osteopathic medicine represents an approach to medical practice that employs all the methods traditionally associated with allopathic medicine, such as pharmaceuticals, laboratory tests, x-ray diagnostics, and surgery. Osteopathic medicine, however, takes a holistic approach and goes a step further in advocating treatment that involves correction of the position of the joints or tissues and in emphasizing diet and environment as factors that prevent disease and improve health. For many years after osteopathy was established as a separate branch of medicine in 1874, osteopaths had to develop their own hospitals because of antagonism toward their profession demonstrated by the established allopathic medical practitioners. In 1970, osteopathic hospitals became eligible to apply for registration with the AHA (AHA, 1994). Since then, allopathic and osteopathic physicians have practiced side by side in the same clinics and hospitals.

For all practical purposes, osteopathic hospitals are community general hospitals. However, with the integration of medical practice, having separate hospitals has become economically unnecessary. Also, the operation of osteopathic hospitals has been found to be more costly and less productive in comparison to their counterparts (Sinay, 2005). Hence, a large number of osteopathic hospitals have closed.

▶ Licensure, Certification, and Accreditation

A hospital is legally required to have a *license* from the state in which it operates. The licensure function is usually carried out by each state's department of health. State licensure standards strongly emphasize compliance with building codes, fire safety, climate control, space allocations, and sanitation. States have also established minimum standards for equipment and personnel that health care organizations must meet to be licensed.

Certification by the federal government gives a hospital the authority to participate in the Medicare and Medicaid programs. The U.S. Department of Health and Human Services (DHHS) has developed health, safety, and quality standards referred to as *conditions of participation* and has the authority to enforce those standards. Hospitals accredited by the Joint Commission or the American Osteopathic Association have been automatically deemed to meet all the health and safety requirements for participation in Medicare and Medicaid.

The Joint Commission, a private nonprofit body, was formed in 1951 with the approval of the various medical and hospital organizations. Upon compliance with its standards, the Joint Commission accredits most of the nation's general hospitals, as well as many of the long-term care facilities, psychiatric hospitals, substance abuse programs, outpatient surgery centers, urgent care clinics, group practices, community health centers, hospices, and home health agencies. Different sets of standards apply to each category of health care organization. Over the years, the Joint Commission has refined its accreditation standards and process of verifying compliance to put greater emphasis on quality of care. Seeking accreditation is voluntary, but Medicare regulations confer *deemed status* on accredited hospitals, allowing these hospitals to participate in Medicare and Medicaid without having to be certified.

▶ Hospital Organization

Hospitals are complex organizations. A hospital is generally responsible to numerous external stakeholders, such as the community, the government, managed care organizations, and accreditation agencies. Internally, hospital governance involves three major sources of power, whose motivations are sometimes at odds. The organizational structure of a hospital also differs substantially from that of other large organizations. The CEO receives delegated authority from the governing body (board) and is responsible for managing the organization with the help of senior executives. In large hospitals, these senior executives often carry the title of senior vice president or vice president responsible for various key service areas, such as nursing services, rehabilitation services, human resources, finance, and so forth. Most physicians belong to a separate organizational structure that operates in parallel to the administrative structure (**FIGURE 8.4**). Such a dual structure is rarely seen in other types of businesses and presents numerous opportunities for conflict to arise between the CEO and the medical staff. Sometimes matters can be further complicated because most physicians are not employed by the hospital, yet they must be closely involved in its operations. Also, the nursing staff, pharmacists, diagnostic technicians, dietitians, and others are administratively accountable to the CEO but professionally accountable to the medical staff (Raffel & Raffel, 1994, p. 139).

One major exception to the medical staff organization described here occurs with employment of physicians on salary in organizations such as VA hospitals. Other hospitals employ a small number of salaried hospitalists, who manage the care of patients once they are hospitalized.

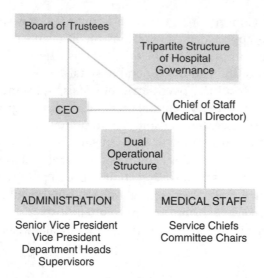

FIGURE 8.4 Hospital Governance and Operational Structure

▶ **Ethics and Public Trust**

Ethical issues arise in all types of health services organizations, but the most significant ones occur in acute care hospitals. Advanced technologies create situations requiring decision making under complex circumstances. Constraints on reimbursement often make it essential to cut costs or eliminate unprofitable services, which also can raise ethical concerns. Many physicians must deal with issues such as legalized abortion, physician-assisted suicide, artificial prolongation of life, and experimental treatments.

Ethical Challenges

Physicians and other caregivers have moral responsibilities when delivering clinical care. These professionals are guided by the principles of beneficence and nonmaleficence. *Beneficence* means that a health services organization has an ethical obligation to do all it can to alleviate suffering caused by ill health and injury. This obligation includes providing essential services, such as emergency care, to needy individuals who do not have the ability to pay. Closely related to beneficence, *nonmaleficence* means that health services personnel have a moral obligation not to harm the patients. This principle requires physicians to use their best professional judgment in choosing interventions that maximize the potential health benefits at minimum risk.

No less challenging is the ethical issue surrounding the definition of extraordinary or heroic measures to sustain a person's life. Medical and legal experts differ on the controversial issue of withdrawing nutrition and other means of life support for dying patients (Bresnohan & Drane, 1986). The questions raised in such cases do not have easy answers, and most of the time physicians must follow their own consciences, apply their personal ethical values, or follow hospital policy. Other legal and ethical standards in medical treatment require the patient's consent before treatment is rendered, a discussion of the various treatment alternatives, and the patient's participation in decision making and the selection of treatment options. Health care providers are also duty bound to hold all patient information in strict confidence. Likewise, fairness, equality, and nondiscrimination are essential in the delivery of health care.

Addressing Ethical Issues

Many health care organizations, especially large acute care hospitals, have ethics committees. The *ethics committee* is charged with the responsibility of developing guidelines and standards for ethical decision making in the delivery of health care (Paris, 1995). In addition, ethics committees are responsible for resolving issues related to medical ethics. Such committees are interdisciplinary, involving physicians, nurses, clergy, social workers, legal experts, ethicists, and administrators.

Certain legal mechanisms are also available to help deal with difficult decisions about life and death. The Patient Self-Determination Act of 1990 applies to all health care facilities participating in Medicare or Medicaid. This law requires hospitals and other facilities to provide all patients, on admission, with information on patients' rights.

Informed consent is a basic patient right. Every patient has the right to make an informed choice regarding his or her medical treatment, including the choice to refuse treatment. For a patient who is mentally capable, physicians must provide all the information the patient asks for or should have to make a properly informed decision.

Patients also have the right to formulate *advance directives*, allowing the patient to express in advance his or her wishes regarding continuation or withdrawal of treatment in the event that he or she becomes incompetent. When advance directives are not available, the burden of ethical decision making falls squarely on the shoulders of those responsible for providing health care services. In actual practice, however, discussions between physicians and patients about the prognosis at the end of life are infrequent and limited in scope (Bradley et al., 2011). Hence, relatively few people use advance directives. Physicians can play an important role by engaging their patients in discussions about the patients' preferences regarding end-of-life decisions.

Public Trust

Communities must place a high degree of trust in their hospitals, but occasionally the behavior of some hospitals has called this trust into question. Hospital administrators have a fiduciary responsibility, meaning that they are responsible for acting prudently in managing the affairs of the organization. Because a hospital's mission is to benefit the community, the hospital should be viewed as a community asset regardless of whether it is an investor-owned or nonprofit institution. When such a viewpoint is lost, and a hospital's board and its executives start placing other priorities ahead of their main responsibility to serve the community, a breach of public trust can occur. Although hospitals must maintain their financial and operational integrity, a real danger arises when financial concerns are put above a genuine concern for the welfare of the patients and the community. Because hospitals form the institutional hub of health care delivery, their integrity within the system is crucial. Scandals with regard to delays in care and alleged deaths resulting from such delays in VA hospitals received national media attention in 2014. When the critical services promised to the nation's veterans are not delivered, and there is little accountability for the billions of taxpayer dollars spent ineffectively, faith and confidence in the system are severely jeopardized.

▶ Conclusion

Any facility that treats patients on the basis of an overnight stay is called an inpatient facility. The most common types of inpatient facilities are hospitals and nursing homes. Both of these institutions trace their beginnings to the almshouses of the 18th and 19th centuries, but as medical science advanced, hospitals emerged as institutions specializing in acute care and surgical services. In many parts of the United States, medical systems serve large geographic areas, delivering a full array of health care services.

Hospitals in the United States went through an expansion and then a contraction phase, both of which were triggered primarily by government policy. Hospital employment has steadily risen over time, and this trend is expected to continue.

Hospitals can be classified in a number of different ways. The majority of hospitals in the United States are private, nonprofit facilities. These hospitals have been required to provide community benefits; the Affordable Care Act has tightened this requirement. The ACA also placed severe restrictions on the expansion of physician-owned hospitals. Most hospitals are community hospitals, meaning that they are nonfederal, short stay, and open to the public.

Licensure of hospitals is a legal requirement. Accreditation by the Joint Commission confers deemed status that enables a hospital to admit Medicare and Medicaid patients. Hospitals confront numerous ethical challenges and must operate in a way that strengthens public trust.

References

1. American Hospital Association (AHA). 1990. *Hospital statistics 1990–1991 edition.* Chicago, IL: AHA.
2. American Hospital Association (AHA). 1994. *AHA guide to the health care field 1994 edition.* Chicago, IL: AHA.
3. American Hospital Association (AHA). 2017. Factsheet: Rural and small hospitals. https://www.aha.org/system/files/2018-02/2017-01-rural-fs_0.pdf. Accessed April 2018.
4. Bradley EH, et al. 2011. Documentation of discussions about prognosis with terminally ill patients. *Am J Med.* 111(3): 218–223.
5. Bresnohan JF, Drane JF. 1986. A challenge to examine the meaning of living and dying. *Health Prog.* 67:32–37, 98.
6. Bureau of Labor Statistics (BLS). 2018, February 8. Health care and social assistance: NAICS 62. https://www.bls.gov/iag/tgs/iag62.htm. Accessed February 9, 2018.
7. Catholic Health Association of the United States. 2015, January. Catholic health care in the United States. http://www.chausa.org/docs/default-source/general-files/cha-us-health-care-at-a-glance_january-2015.pdf?sfvrsn=0. Accessed May 2015.
8. Center for Health Workforce Studies, University at Albany, State University of New York. 2012, March. Health care employment projections: An analysis of Bureau of Labor Statistics occupational projections 2010–2020. http://www.healthit.gov/sites/default/files/chws_bls_report_2012.pdf. Accessed May 2015.
9. Daniels RJ, Carson LD. 2011. Academic medical centers: Organizational integration and discipline through contractual and firm models. *JAMA.* 306(17):1912–1913.
10. Foster D, et al. 2013, June. Hospital performance differences by ownership. Truven Health Analytics. http://www.nonprofithealthcare.org/uploads/Hospital_Performance_Differences_by_Ownership.pdf. Accessed April 2018.
11. Haglund CL, Dowling WL. 1993. The hospital. In: Williams SJ, Torrens PR, eds. *Introduction to health services.* 4th ed. Albany, NY: Delmar Publishers, 135–176.
12. Health Forum. 2001. *AHA guide to the health care field.* 2001–2002 ed. Chicago, IL: Health Forum.
13. Lundgren DK, et al. 2016. Are the Affordable Care Act restrictions warranted? A contemporary statewide analysis of physician-owned hospitals. *J Arthroplasty.* 31(9):1857–1861.
14. Martiniano R, et al. 2016, April. Health care employment projections, 2014–2024: An analysis of Bureau of Labor Statistics projections by setting and by occupation. Rensselaer, NY: Center for Health Workforce Studies, School of Public Health, SUNY Albany.
15. National Center for Health Statistics (NCHS). 2002. *Health, United States, 2002.* Hyattsville, MD: Department of Health and Human Services.
16. National Center for Health Statistics (NCHS). 2017. *Health, United States, 2016.* Hyattsville, MD: Department of Health and Human Services.
17. Paris M. 1995. The medical staff. In: Wolper LF, ed. *Health care administration: Principles, Practices, structure, and delivery.* 2nd ed. Gaithersburg, MD: Aspen Publishers, 32–46.

18. Physician Hospitals of America (PHA). 2015. Physician-owned hospitals excel in CMS star ratings. http://www.physicianhospitals.org/news/228189. Accessed May 2015.

19. Raffel MW, Raffel NK. 1994. *The U.S. health system: Origins and functions.* 4th ed. Albany, NY: Delmar Publishers.

20. Rau J. 2013, April 12. Doctor-owned hospitals prosper under health law. http://kaiserhealthnews.org/news/doctor-owned-hospitals-quality-bonuses. Accessed May 2015.

21. Rubin DB, et al. 2015. Tax-exempt hospitals and community benefit: New directions in policy and practice. *Ann Rev Public Health.* 36:545–557.

22. Sanofi-Aventis. 2017. *Managed care digest series: Provider digest, 2017.* Bridgewater, NJ: Sanofi-Aventis US.

23. Sinay T. 2005. Cost structure of osteopathic hospitals and their local counterparts in the USA: Are they any different? *Soc Sci Med.* 60(8):1805–1814.

24. Teisberg ED, et al. 1991. *The hospital sector in 1992.* Boston, MA: Harvard Business School.

25. Wolfson J, Hopes SL. 1994, July. What makes tax-exempt hospitals special? *Healthc Financ Manage.* 56–60.

26. Young GJ, et al. 2013. Provision of community benefits by tax-exempt U.S. hospitals. *N Engl J Med.* 368(16):1519–1527.

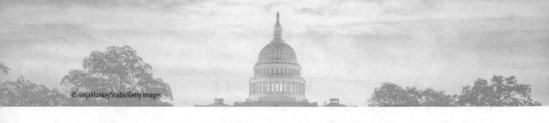

CHAPTER 9

Managed Care and Integrated Systems

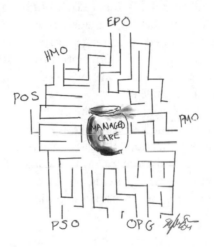

▶ Introduction

Since around 1990, managed care has been the single most dominant force that has fundamentally transformed the delivery of health care in the United States. At first, some observers viewed the managed care phenomenon as an aberration. However, as private employers began to realize cost savings and public policymakers and administrators saw the opportunity to slow down the growth of Medicare and Medicaid expenditures, they increasingly turned to managed care as a means of delivering health care. Managed care is now firmly entrenched in the U.S. health care system, and some features of managed care have also been adopted by other nations.

When employment-based private health insurance emerged as the dominant form of coverage in the United States, neither the employers nor the insurance companies had any incentive to manage the delivery of services or payments made to providers. Providers showed a strong preference to be paid on a fee-for-service basis. Over time, however, both the delivery of health care and the payments for care got out of control. For example, between 1980 and 1990, the consumer price index—a measure of price increases (inflation) in the economy—rose by 59%, but inflation in medical care was 117% during the same time period (Department of Health and Human Services [DHHS], 1996, p. 241). Managed care was designed to slow down the growth in health care spending by limiting both the quantity of health care delivered and the amount of reimbursement given to providers.

Managed care has experienced unprecedented success. For example, only 27% of all employees insured through employer-sponsored health insurance were enrolled in managed care plans in 1988. By 2002, however, 95% were enrolled in managed care. This growth occurred despite attacks on managed care from both physicians and consumers. Today, fewer than 1% of workers are enrolled in employer-sponsored conventional health insurance plans.

By enrolling a large segment of the insured U.S. population and taking responsibility to procure cost-effective health care for the enrollees, managed care organizations (MCOs) garnered enormous buying power. To a large extent, the organizational consolidation of providers represented a response to this growing power of MCOs. These changes have given rise to new organizational arrangements that are discussed in this chapter.

▶ What Is Managed Care?

Managed care is a mechanism of providing health care services in which a single organization takes on the management of financing, insurance, delivery, and payment.

- *Financing*. Premiums are negotiated between employers and the MCO. Generally, a fixed premium per enrollee includes all health care services provided for in a contract.
- *Insurance*. The MCO collects premiums for insuring groups of enrollees. It then functions like an insurance company by assuming all risk. In other words, it takes financial responsibility if the total cost of services provided exceeds the revenue from fixed premiums. Under the Affordable Care Act (ACA), an MCO is allowed to retain no more than 20% of the premium dollar (15% for some MCOs)

to manage risk and to cover its own administrative expenses. The remainder of the premium that is spent on health care services is called the *medical loss ratio*.

- *Delivery.* Unlike conventional insurance, the MCO arranges to provide health care to its enrollees. To do so, most MCOs establish contracts with physicians, clinics, hospitals, and medical systems. These providers operate independently but are linked to the MCO through legal contracts. Some very large MCOs have their own physicians on salary and operate their own clinics; in some instances, MCOs even operate their own hospitals. To keep costs under control, MCOs use various methods to manage the utilization of health care services.

- *Payment.* MCOs use three main types of payment arrangements with providers: capitation, discounted fees, and salaries. The three methods allow risk sharing in varying degrees between the MCO and the providers. Risk sharing puts the burden on the providers to be cost conscious and to curtail unnecessary utilization of services. Sometimes, a limited amount of fee-for-service is used for specialized services. Under *capitation*, the provider is paid a fixed monthly sum per enrollee, often called a per member per month (PMPM) payment. The provider receives the capitated fee per enrollee regardless of whether the enrollee uses health care services and regardless of the quantity of services used. The provider is responsible for delivering all needed health care services determined to be medically necessary. A provider can lose money if services are delivered indiscriminately. The discounted fee arrangement uses a modified form of fee for service, in which the provider can bill the MCO for each service separately but is paid according to a schedule of fees. The fee schedule is prenegotiated and is based on discounts off the regular fees the provider would otherwise charge. Providers agree to discount their regular fees in exchange for the volume of patients the MCO brings them. In the third method of payment, salaries for physicians are often coupled with bonuses for efficient delivery of services.

The main characteristics of managed care are summarized in **EXHIBIT 9.1**.

Accreditation and Quality Indicators

Since 1991, MCOs have been accredited by the National Committee for Quality Assurance (NCQA); accreditation is voluntary. The NCQA has also designed a set of standardized performance measures for MCOs. Commonly referred to as managed care report cards, the national standards and performance reports on individual MCOs are contained in the Healthcare Effectiveness Data and Information Set (HEDIS). The report

---

EXHIBIT 9.1   Main Characteristics of Managed Care

- MCOs manage financing, insurance, delivery, and payment for providing health care.
- Premiums are usually negotiated between MCOs and employers.
- MCOs function like an insurance company and assume risk.
- MCOs arrange to provide health care, mainly through contracts with providers.
- MCOs manage the utilization of health care services.
- Three main payment methods are capitation, discounted fees, and physicians on salary.

---

cards are voluntary efforts that were begun out of concerns that controlling health care utilization could adversely affect the quality of care. HEDIS measures have been used quite extensively to evaluate and compare the quality of care in health plans.

The Centers for Medicare and Medicaid Services (CMS) rates the relative quality of Medicare Advantage plans (MA; Medicare Part C) on a one- to five-star scale, with five stars representing the highest quality. The star rating, which provides an overall measure of a plan's quality, is a cumulative indicator of the quality of care, access to care, responsiveness, and beneficiary satisfaction provided by the plan. The star rating incorporates HEDIS as one of the four measures. Ratings are available on Medicare's website to help beneficiaries choose from among the various MA plans if they want to enroll in Part C of Medicare. The ACA authorized incentive payments to reward plans that scored higher on the star ratings.

▶ Evolution of Managed Care

In the early 1900s, certain railroad, mining, and lumber companies located in isolated areas employed salaried physicians to provide medical care to their workers. In other instances, such companies contracted with physicians and hospitals at a flat fee per worker. Such arrangements can be viewed as prototypes of managed care.

The first known private health insurance plan started at the Baylor University Hospital in Dallas, Texas, in 1929 was also based on capitation. For a predetermined fixed fee per month, Baylor, and subsequently other hospitals, provided inpatient services.

Later, during the 1940s, some large health plans emerged in New York, California, Washington, and St. Louis. These plans also provided comprehensive health care to enrolled populations for a capitated fee. For example, the well-known Kaiser Permanente plan started in California in 1942 when the industrialist Henry J. Kaiser was faced with the problem of providing health care to his 30,000 workers. In 1945, the Permanente Health Plan was made available to the general public; today, the Kaiser Foundation Health Plan, operated by Kaiser Permanente, is the largest health maintenance organization (HMO) in the United States. In the rest of the country, however, delivery of health care typically continued to follow the fee-for-service system. Commercial insurance companies were the dominant players in the private health insurance market.

The Health Maintenance Organization Act of 1973 was passed out of concern for escalating health care expenditures. Subsequent to the creation of Medicare and Medicaid, national health expenditures rose at more than double the rate of growth in the consumer price index during the 5-year period from 1966 to 1971 (**FIGURE 9.1**). The 1973 law was designed to provide an alternative to the traditional fee-for-service practice of medicine; it aimed to stimulate the growth of HMOs by providing federal funds to establish new HMOs (Wilson & Neuhauser, 1985, p. 206). The reasoning behind promoting HMO growth was the perception that it would encourage competition among health plans, increase efficiency, and slow the rate of growth in health care expenditures. The law's objective was to create 1,700 HMOs to serve 40 million members by 1976 (Iglehart, 1994). By the end of the 1970s, however, HMOs had enrolled fewer than 10 million members.

During the 1980s, managed care experienced relatively slow growth, but in states such as California and Minnesota, growth was faster than in most parts of the United States. As pointed out earlier, health care costs continued to rise uncontrollably over this period, and private businesses

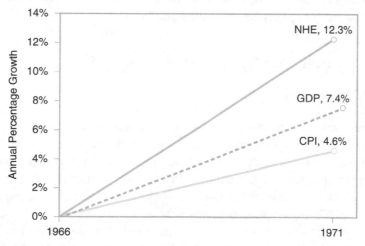

FIGURE 9.1 Average Annual Rates of Increase in National Health Expenditures (NHE), Gross Domestic Product (GDP), and Consumer Price Index (CPI), 1966–1971

Data from Bureau of Labor Statistics, National Center for Health Statistics.

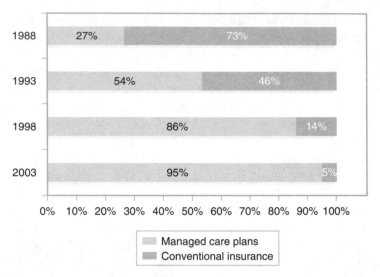

FIGURE 9.2 Enrollment of Workers in Employer-Sponsored Health Plans, Selected Years

Modified from Claxton G., et al. 2007. The Kasier Family Foundation and Health Research and Educational Trust Employer Health Benefits 2007 Annual Survey. Menlo Park, CA: Henry J. Kaiser Foundation and Chicago, IL; Health Research and Educational Trust, p. 65

were increasingly threatened by the erosion of their profits resulting from double-digit increases in the cost of health insurance premiums for their employees. Consequently, employers started switching from traditional health insurance to managed care plans during the 1980s. Even so, it was not until the early 1990s that a veritable managed care revolution got under way, after private employers experienced a total increase of 217% (12.2% average annual increase) in the cost of health insurance between 1980 and 1990. **FIGURE 9.2** illustrates the growth of enrollment in managed care plans between 1988 and 2003.

▶ Growth and Transformation of Managed Care

As the market for managed care grew, competition among MCOs gave rise to new forms of managed care plans. To differentiate among themselves, some new organizations adopted variations in payment schemes. Preferred provider organizations (PPOs), for example, differentiated themselves by using discounted fee payments instead of capitation. Other MCOs differentiated themselves according to how the medical care providers were organized. Still others offered their enrollees a choice between providers who were contractually affiliated with the organization and those who were not. MCOs also adopted various methods to control health care costs by actively monitoring utilization of services.

Private Insurance Enrollment

As pointed out previously, managed care has become the primary vehicle for delivering health care to the vast majority of Americans and is now a mature industry in the United States. In essence, private health insurance can now be equated with managed care, whether it is obtained through a small or large employer. High-deductible health plans are also commonly offered in the form of managed care plans.

Medicare Enrollment

Medicare beneficiaries have the choice of enrolling in a managed care plan under the MA program or remaining in the traditional fee-for-service program. Even though the latter option has been more popular with Medicare beneficiaries, enrollment in MA plans doubled between 2005 (14% of beneficiaries) and 2013 (28% of beneficiaries) (Sanofi-Aventis, 2014). More recently, the rate of growth in MA enrollment has slowed somewhat, reaching 31.7% in 2015 (Sanofi-Aventis, 2016a).

Medicaid Enrollment

Waivers under the Social Security Act, particularly Sections 1115 and 1915(b), allowed states to enroll their Medicaid recipients in managed care plans. Later, the Balanced Budget Act of 1997 gave states the authority to implement mandatory managed care enrollments without federal waivers (Moscovice et al., 1998). Since then, enrollment of this patient population in managed care has grown at a rapid pace, from 56% of all Medicaid beneficiaries in 2000 to almost 85% in 2015 (Sanofi-Aventis, 2013, 2016a).

Managed Care Backlash

Managed care made significant headway during the decade of the 1990s and achieved notable success in slowing down the growth of national health care expenditures. Toward the latter half of the 1990s, however, it drew a backlash from consumers, providers, and politicians. The American media also played a role in shaping public opinion against managed care by presenting, in many instances, one-sided and subjective "news" stories focusing on denial of services.

For consumers, dissatisfaction with managed care was associated mainly with the erosion of choice resulting from the limited number of providers associated with the plans and some restrictions in direct access to specialized services. Dissatisfaction on the part of physicians, hospitals, and other providers was related to the control that MCOs exerted over utilization and limits on reimbursement. Risk sharing under capitation became particularly controversial. Politicians responded by passing laws to contain some of the perceived excesses of managed care. In the process, however, all parties had to accept certain compromises.

Transformation of Managed Care

In response to the backlash, HMOs moved away from tight management of health care services, albeit without totally abandoning utilization controls. They also incorporated fee-for-service reimbursement, along with capitation for certain services, into their payment schemes. PPOs emerged, offering greater choice of access to providers. Both consumers and providers welcomed these changes. In the end, enrollees had to give up unconditional freedom over choice, providers had to accept some controls over how they would practice medicine and settle for lower rates of reimbursement than what they were getting under fee-for-service arrangements, and MCOs had to relax their tight management of health care utilization.

Even though some differences between individual plans still exist, relaxed controls and flexibility have become common features of all plans. Managed care today is quite different from what it was initially intended to be: an organizational mechanism that would tightly control the financing and delivery of health care. It is because of these compromises that managed care became enormously successful—practically replacing traditional health insurance in the United States. At the same time, these compromises have eroded managed care's full potential to reverse the rising tide of health care spending.

▶ Utilization Control Methods in Managed Care

MCOs use three main approaches to monitor and control the utilization of services:

- Expert evaluation of which services are medically necessary in a given case. Such an evaluation ensures that only medically necessary services are actually provided.
- Determination of how services can be provided most inexpensively while maintaining acceptable standards of quality. For example, often similar services can be obtained as an outpatient or as an inpatient; outpatient services cost less. Similarly, generic drugs cost less than brand-name drugs.
- Review of the process of care and changes in the patient's condition to revise the course of medical treatment if necessary.

The methods most commonly used for utilization monitoring and control are gatekeeping and utilization review. Generally, HMOs employ tighter utilization controls than other types of managed care plans, which are discussed later in this chapter.

Gatekeeping

Commonly used by HMOs, *gatekeeping* is an arrangement that requires a primary care physician to coordinate all health care services needed by an enrollee. The physicians have contracts with the HMO as in-network providers. Gatekeeping also emphasizes preventive care, routine physical examinations, and other primary care services that are delivered by the primary care gatekeeper. Secondary care services, such as diagnostic testing, consultation from specialists, and admission to a hospital, are provided only on referral from the gatekeeper. In this way, the gatekeeper controls access to costly medical services.

Utilization Review

Utilization review is the process of evaluating the appropriateness of services provided. It is sometimes misunderstood to be a mechanism for denying services, but its main objective is actually to review each case and to determine the most appropriate level of services. Three main types of utilization review are employed: prospective, concurrent, and retrospective.

Prospective Utilization Review

Under the prospective utilization review method, the medical necessity of certain treatments is determined before the care is actually delivered. An example of prospective utilization review is the decision by a primary care gatekeeper to refer or not refer a patient to a specialist. Not all managed care plans use gatekeepers; instead, some plans require the enrollee or the provider to obtain prior approval or *precertification* from the plan administrators before certain services are provided. Most plans use established clinical guidelines to determine the appropriateness of services. Preauthorization of hospital admissions and second opinions for surgical procedures are additional examples of precertification. In case of an emergency admission to an inpatient facility, plans generally require notification within 24 hours. One of the main objectives of prospective review is to prevent unnecessary or inappropriate institutionalization or other courses of treatment such as surgery.

Concurrent Utilization Review

Concurrent utilization review occurs when decisions regarding appropriateness are made during the course of health care utilization. The most common examples of this type of review involve monitoring the length of inpatient stays. When a patient is hospitalized, a certain number of inpatient days are generally preapproved. A trained nurse then monitors the patient's status and reviews the case with a physician if a longer stay is necessary. A decision is made to authorize or deny additional days.

   Discharge planning is an important component of concurrent utilization review. A patient's prognosis for recovery, expected outcomes, and anticipated day of discharge are critical elements of concurrent review. Discharge planning deals with the patient's ongoing care and evaluates any special requirements that are necessary after discharge. For example, if a patient is admitted with a fractured hip, it is important to decide whether home health care or a skilled nursing facility would be more appropriate for convalescent care. If the patient requires care in a skilled nursing facility, then discharge planning must find out whether the appropriate level of rehabilitation services would be available and for how long insurance will pay for rehabilitation therapy in a long-term care setting.

Retrospective Utilization Review

Retrospective utilization review determines the appropriateness of utilization after services have already been delivered. Such review is based on an examination of medical records to assess the appropriateness of care. It may involve an assessment of individual cases, and large claims may be reviewed for billing accuracy. Retrospective review may also involve an analysis of data to examine patterns of excessive utilization or underutilization. *Underutilization* occurs when medically necessary care is not delivered; *overutilization* occurs when medical services that are not necessary are delivered.

▶ Types of Managed Care Plans

Three main factors led to the development of different types of managed care plans. The first and most important involved the choice of providers. HMOs were the most common type of MCOs in the 1970s, but HMO plans had inherent weaknesses, especially with regard to choice of providers. Other types of MCO plans that offered greater choice were developed mainly to compete with the more restrictive HMO plans. Second, different ways of arranging the delivery of services led to different forms of MCOs because there is no single way to arrange providers into a delivery network. Payment and risk sharing make up the third major factor. The main differences between the three different types of managed care plans discussed in this section are presented in **EXHIBIT 9.2**.

EXHIBIT 9.2 Differences Among the Three Main Types of Managed Care Plans

Main Distinguishing Factors
1. Choice of providers
2. Delivery of services
3. Payment and risk sharing

HMO Plans	PPO Plans	POS Plans
Use of only in-network providers is permitted	Use of both in-network and out-of-network providers is permitted	Use of both in-network and out-of-network providers is permitted
Providers on staff and/or contracted providers	Contracted providers only	Contracted providers only
Use of gatekeeping Focus on prevention and primary care Specialty services are obtained upon referral	No gatekeeping Unrestricted access to specialty services	Unrestricted access to specialty services
Providers are paid mostly under capitation: Some fee for service Risk sharing with providers under capitation	Providers are paid according to discounted fee schedules No risk sharing	Combination of capitation and fee for service Some risk sharing

Note: There may be some variations to the above for individual plans.

HMO Plans

HMOs were the first type of managed care plans to appear on the market. An HMO is distinguished from other types of plans by its focus on wellness care. Such an organization not only provides medical care during illness, but also offers a variety of services to help people maintain their health—hence the name "health maintenance organization." HMOs emphasize preventive and screening services through routine checkups and tests. Prevention of disease and early detection and treatment save health care costs in the long run when the course of a disease is checked before it turns into a more complex case. As an incentive to the enrollees to seek wellness care, HMO plans typically do not have annual deductibles, and they have lower copayments than do other types of plans.

Initially, HMOs used only capitation to reimburse providers, but providers disliked the risk-sharing feature of capitation. HMOs, therefore, had to compromise by raising PMPM rates and, in many instances, switching to fee-for-service reimbursement. In 2015, 67% of HMOs used capitation; 57.5% used fee-for-service reimbursement to pay physicians (Sanofi-Aventis, 2016b).

The utilization of services is coordinated and managed by the HMO, mainly through primary care gatekeepers. Enrollees must obtain services from in-network hospitals, physicians, and other health care providers. Specialty services, such as mental health and substance abuse treatment, are frequently carved out. A *carve-out* is a special contract outside the regular capitation scheme, which is funded separately by the HMO. A state may also enroll its Medicaid beneficiaries into a specialized managed behavioral health organization (MBHO).

The four most widely used HMO models differ from each other according to the arrangements they make with participating physicians. These models are the staff, group, network, and independent practice association models.

Staff Model HMO

A staff model HMO employs its own salaried physicians. The physicians are typically paid fixed salaries. An HMO may also have a bonus program combined with the salary, in which case end-of-the-year bonuses are based on each physician's productivity and the HMO's profitability. Physicians work only for their employer HMO and provide services to that HMO's enrollees. Staff model HMOs must employ physicians in all of the common specialties to provide for the health care needs of their members. In addition, contracts with selected subspecialties are established for less frequently needed services. The HMO operates one or more outpatient clinics, which contain physicians' offices, support staff, and sometimes ancillary support facilities, such as laboratory and radiology departments. In most instances, the HMO contracts with area hospitals for inpatient services.

Compared with other HMO models, staff model HMOs are able to exercise a greater degree of control over the practice patterns of their physicians, which makes it easier to monitor utilization. Even so, the fixed salary expense can be high, which requires that these HMOs have a large number of members to support the operating expenses. Enrollees generally have a limited choice of physicians. Because of its disadvantages, the staff model has been the least popular type of HMO with both consumers and physicians.

Group Model HMO

A group model HMO contracts with a multispecialty group practice and separately with one or more hospitals to provide comprehensive services to its members. The group practice is an independent practice, employing its own physicians who can treat non-HMO-covered patients as well. The HMO generally pays an all-inclusive capitation fee to the group practice to provide physician services to its members. Under a different scenario, the HMO may own the group practice, which is organized as a separate corporation but one that is administratively tied to the HMO. In this case, the group practice may provide services exclusively to the HMO's members. Ownership or an exclusive contract enables the HMO to exercise better control over utilization. Even when it is not an exclusive contract, the HMO brings a block of business to the group practice, which gives the HMO a fair amount of leverage regarding financial terms and utilization controls.

Network Model HMO

Under the network model, the HMO contracts with more than one medical group practice. This model is particularly well suited for operations in large metropolitan areas and across widespread geographic regions where group practices are located. Each group practice is paid a capitation fee based on the number of enrollees. The group is responsible for providing all physician services. It can make referrals to specialists but is financially responsible for reimbursing them for any referrals it makes. The network model is generally able to offer enrollees a wider choice of physicians than the staff or group models. The main disadvantage is the dilution of utilization control.

Independent Practice Association Model HMO

Of the four HMO models, the independent practice association (IPA) model has been the most successful in terms of the largest share of enrollments. The IPA model became popular with both providers and enrollees. IPAs gave small groups and individual physicians the opportunity to participate in managed care and, therefore, were preferred by physicians. The enrollees generally have the greatest choice of providers under the IPA model.

An IPA is a legal entity separate from the HMO. The IPA, not the HMO, establishes contracts with both independent solo practitioners and group practices. The HMO, in turn, contracts with the IPA for physician services. Physicians do not have a contract with the HMO, but with the IPA. Hence, the IPA functions as an intermediary representing a large number of physicians. The IPA, which is generally paid a capitation amount by the HMO, retains administrative control over how it pays its physicians. For example, it may reimburse physicians through capitation or some other mechanism, such as modified fee for service. The IPA often shares risk with the physicians and assumes the responsibility for utilization management and quality assessment.

Under the IPA model, the HMO is still responsible for providing health care services to its enrollees, but the logistics of arranging physician services are shifted to the IPA. As a consequence, the HMO is relieved of the administrative burden of establishing contracts with numerous providers and controlling utilization. Financial risk is also shared with the IPA.

IPAs may be independently established by community physicians, or the HMO may create an IPA and invite community physicians to participate in it. An IPA may also be hospital based and structured so that only physicians from one or two hospitals are eligible to participate in it (Wagner, 1995). One major disadvantage of the IPA model is that if a contract is lost, the HMO loses a large number of participating physicians.

PPO Plans

PPO plans were created by insurance companies in response to the growth of HMOs. PPOs differentiated themselves by offering out-of-network options for enrollees. By the early 1990s, PPOs became more popular and their market share began to exceed that of HMOs.

PPO enrollees can either choose in-network preferred providers with whom the PPO has established contracts or use physicians and hospitals outside the network. Higher copayments apply for using nonpreferred providers. The additional out-of-pocket expenses largely act as a deterrent to going outside the network for care.

PPOs make discounted fee arrangements with providers. The discounts typically range between 25% and 35% off the providers' regular fees. Negotiated payment arrangements with hospitals can take a variety of forms, such as payments based on diagnosis-related groups, bundled charges for certain services, and discounts. Hence, no direct risk sharing with providers is involved. PPOs also apply fewer restrictions to the care-seeking behavior of enrollees. In most instances, they do not use gatekeeping, which allows enrollees to see specialists without being referred by a primary care physician. Precertification (prospective utilization review) is generally employed only for hospitalization and high-cost outpatient procedures (Robinson, 2002).

Point-of-Service Plans

Point-of-service (POS) plans combine features of classic HMOs with some of the characteristics of patient choice found in PPOs. Through this combination, POS plans overcome the drawback of restricted provider choice but retain the benefits of tight utilization management. Many POS plans are actually offered by HMOs to give members an optional plan that allows utilization of out-of-network providers. From the consumer's perspective, free choice of providers was a major selling point for POS plans, but after reaching a peak in popularity in 1998–1999, enrollment in POS plans gradually declined mainly because of the high out-of-pocket costs associated with them.

▶ Impact on Cost, Access, and Quality

Influence on Cost Containment

Other countries assign the task of cost containment to the government, which controls health care expenditures by budgeting system-wide expenditures (global budgets) and imposing limits on services (supply-side rationing) and payments to providers. In the United States, the primary responsibility for cost containment falls on the private sector, but the government also has pioneered various approaches, mostly aimed at controlling Medicaid and Medicare costs. The private-sector approach to cost containment has involved the expansion of managed care, which has been widely credited for slowing down the rate of growth in health care expenditures during the 1990s. Because of the backlash against managed care, however, the full cost-containment potential of managed care was never realized. Moreover, certain government regulations imposed as part of the backlash against managed care actually caused premiums to rise and reversed any gains in cost containment made by MCOs (Dugan, 2015).

From a cost-containment perspective, enrollment of Medicare and Medicaid beneficiaries in managed care has been controversial. On the one hand, some recent evidence suggests that MA plans offer care of equal or higher quality and for less cost than traditional fee-for-service Medicare, thereby delivering higher value (Newhouse & McGuire, 2014). On the other hand, the experience does not appear to be the same with Medicaid managed care. For example, a study encompassing all 50 states showed that shifting Medicaid recipients from fee-for-service models into managed care did not reduce Medicaid spending (Duggan & Hayford, 2013).

Impact on Access

Baker and colleagues (2004) found that timely breast cancer and cervical cancer screenings were twice as likely for women receiving services in geographic areas with greater HMO market share, compared to women in areas with low managed care penetration. More recent studies report similar findings on health screenings, diabetes care, and favorable ratings of physicians by the patients (Ayanian et al., 2013). In MA plans, better access to primary care may have been responsible for lowering the risk of preventable hospitalizations, particularly for ethnic/minority groups (Basu, 2012). Behavioral health carve-outs have also been instrumental in addressing long-standing challenges in access and utilization of behavioral health care (Frank & Garfield, 2007).

In contrast, in Medicaid managed care, Caswell and Long (2015) found an increased probability of emergency department use (instead of primary care) and difficulty in seeing a specialist by Medicaid enrollees. This experience has been repeated among Medicaid enrollees who benefited from the expansion of Medicaid under the ACA. In one survey, only one-fourth of the physicians participating in Medicaid managed care offered appointments within 2 weeks of the contact date (Taitsman, 2015).

Influence on Quality of Care

Despite anecdotes, individual perceptions, and isolated stories propagated by the news media, no comprehensive research to date has clearly demonstrated that the growth of managed care has come at the expense of the quality of care delivered to Americans. Actually, the available evidence points to the opposite conclusion: The quality of health care provided by MCOs has improved over time (Hofmann, 2002). The financial pressures associated with managed care do not seem to lead to significant changes in physician behavior, because under capitation a physician takes full responsibility for the patient's overall care (Eikel, 2002).

A comprehensive review of the literature by Miller and Luft (2002) concluded that HMO and non-HMO plans provided roughly equal quality of care as measured by a wide range of conditions, diseases, and interventions. At the same time, HMOs lower the use of hospital and other expensive resources. Hence, medical care delivered through managed care plans has been cost-effective. Evidence also suggests that the race, ethnicity, and socioeconomic status of managed care enrollees have little or no effect on the quality of care they receive (Balsa et al., 2007; Brown et al., 2005). Conversely, evaluation of the existing literature does point to lower access and lower enrollee satisfaction ratings for HMO plans compared with non-HMO plans (Miller & Luft, 2002). Also, quality-based star ratings by the CMS are higher for nonprofit MA plans compared to for-profit plans (Peng et al., 2015). Earlier studies (e.g., Schneider et al., 2005) reached similar conclusions regarding quality of care in for-profit versus nonprofit health plans. In recent years, the significant growth in Medicaid managed care enrollments by states across the country has become controversial, as many observers have suggested that this approach is being adopted without consistent evidence showing that Medicaid managed care plans reduce expenditures and improve access and quality of care.

▶ Integrated Systems

Organizational integration became necessary for economic reasons in a changing health care landscape. It began with hospital mergers and acquisitions during the 1990s. Subsequently, consolidation with physician group practices was viewed as beneficial for both hospitals and physicians as health care services increasingly moved from the inpatient to the outpatient sector. Diversification into services that an organization had not offered before was the next step in integration. Many of these transformations can be attributed to the growth of managed care, which came to dominate the U.S. health care landscape. For example, managed care gained enormous bargaining power over independent hospitals and physician clinics, and these organizations came under growing pressure to reduce costs and deliver services efficiently to populations spread over large geographic areas. More recently, the ACA added another twist by requiring certain integrated organizations to be held accountable for people's health. Today, the U.S. health care market includes two main types of highly integrated health care systems: integrated delivery systems (IDSs) and accountable care organizations (ACOs).

Since the passage of the ACA, consolidation through mergers and acquisitions has picked up in the health care industry; such deals tend to curtail competition. It is not clear, however, whether this consolidation has occurred in response to the ACA.

Integrated Delivery Systems

An *integrated delivery system* (IDS) includes several organizations under ownership or contractual arrangements that provide an array of health care services to large communities. There can be degrees of integration, but a highly integrated health network operates as a one-stop shopping environment that is centered on one or more hospitals and includes outpatient clinics and surgical centers, one or more long-term care facilities, home health and hospice services, and ownership of or contract with one or more MCOs. Specialized cardiac care clinics and rehabilitation facilities may be included. Other services, such as imaging centers, dialysis centers, and mental health centers, may also be incorporated.

In 2016, 81% of acute care hospitals in the United States were affiliated with an IDS. Moreover, between 2010 and 2016, the number of medical group practices affiliated with an IDS almost doubled to 5,705

(Sanofi-Aventis, 2017). Clearly, the wave of the future is toward organizational integration because of the many advantages that IDS-affiliated facilities enjoy over non-IDS-affiliated facilities. Notably, inpatient and outpatient caseloads, including outpatient surgery, are higher at IDS-affiliated hospitals. They also have lower average lengths of stay, rising revenues, and lower total costs per discharge compared with non-IDS-affiliated hospitals (Sanofi-Aventis, 2017).

IDSs help achieve cost savings through resource sharing and elimination of duplication. Research shows that IDSs have positive effects on quality of care, as well as the potential to lower health service utilization and produce costs savings (Hwang et al., 2013).

Accountable Care Organizations

In a general sense, an *accountable care organization* (ACO) is an integrated group of providers—including hospitals, physicians, and post-discharge care delivery organizations—that work together to deliver coordinated care and take responsibility for quality and efficiency of services delivered to a given population of patients. The ACA authorized formation of ACOs to serve Medicare beneficiaries enrolled in the traditional fee-for-service program. According to Medicare rules, an ACO must be a legal entity. Hence, organizations formed through contractual arrangements—such as alliances and virtual organizations, discussed later—do not qualify as ACOs to serve Medicare patients. The ACO must also have a governing body to provide oversight and be held legally accountable for its actions.

In conjunction with the formation of ACOs, the ACA authorized a Medicare Shared Savings Program (MSSP) that is designed to reward ACOs that lower the growth of health care expenditures while meeting performance standards on quality of care (CMS, 2015). ACOs are motivated to eliminate unnecessary care because their contract payments from insurers cover the entire continuum of care (Song & Fisher, 2016), from primary care to specialty services to acute care to rehabilitation. To realize the expectations of cost and quality, ACOs use mechanisms already prevalent in managed care and IDSs—disease management, care coordination, sharing of cost savings with providers, and use of information technology, among others (Burns & Pauly, 2012).

Although this model of care delivery is still in its infancy, early signs point to some successes being achieved. In terms of provider participation, 64% of medical group practices participated in ACOs in 2016. ACOs participating in the MSSP program enrolled 7.3 million Medicare beneficiaries in 2015; these ACOs generated average savings of $11.7 million on average spending of $187 million. Going forward, it seems likely that providers will continue to assume risk in arrangements that tie reimbursement to quality and cost outcomes (Sanofi-Aventis, 2017). Projecting from current trends, ACOs could potentially become the main providers of services to the majority of Medicare beneficiaries. Some states are also experimenting with ACOs to serve their Medicaid populations. Based on past history, managed care organizations are likely to follow suit.

More than 560 ACOs have formed across the United States; since 2012, provider participation in MSSP has jumped 1,678% (Sanofi-Aventis, 2017). Among these ACOs, 51% have been physician led, compared with 33% that have been jointly led by hospitals and physicians; only 3% have been led by hospitals alone (Colla et al., 2014). Clearly, physicians hold the key to the future success of ACOs. These organizations are more likely to form in geographic areas where IDSs that have experience working under capitation already exist (Auerbach et al., 2013).

ACOs have already come under criticism from providers. A survey by the National Association of ACOs indicated that two-thirds of the ACO participants were unlikely to remain in the ACO program. Yet, for the program to be successful, 800 to 900 Medicare ACOs would be needed by 2018 (Perez, 2015). Hence, it remains to be seen how ACOs might evolve in the future.

▶ Types of Integration

Integration Based on Major Participants

Physicians and hospitals have been two key participants in the formation of integrated organizations because, in almost all instances, one entity cannot function without the other. Hence, a *physician–hospital organization* (PHO) has been a common type of integrated organization. A PHO is a legal entity that represents an alliance between a hospital and local physicians and combines their services under the aegis of a single organization. It allows both entities to have greater bargaining power in contract negotiations with MCOs. PHO formation is often initiated by the hospital, but it is unlikely to succeed without the participation of the medical staff leaders. PHOs provide the benefits of integration while preserving the independence and autonomy of physicians. The ACA specified that PHOs could qualify as ACOs (Casalino et al., 2013).

Integration Based on Type of Ownership or Affiliation

The objectives of organizational integration can be accomplished in ways other than outright ownership. For example, relatively simple cooperative arrangements, sharing of resources, and joint responsibilities through contracts can be established.

Acquisitions and Mergers

Acquisition refers to the purchase of one organization by another. The acquired company ceases to exist as a separate entity and is absorbed under the name of the purchasing corporation. A *merger* involves a mutual agreement to unify two or more organizations into a single entity. The separate assets of two organizations are brought together, typically under a new name. Both former entities cease to exist, and a new corporation is formed.

Small hospitals may merge to gain efficiencies by eliminating the duplication of services. Acquisitions and mergers can also help an organization expand into new geographic markets. A large hospital may acquire smaller hospitals to serve as satellites in a large metropolitan area with sprawling suburbs. A regional health care system may be formed after a large hospital has acquired other hospitals and diversified into services such as outpatient care, long-term care, and rehabilitation.

Joint Ventures

A *joint venture* results when two or more institutions share resources to create a new organization to pursue a common purpose (Pelfrey & Theisen, 1989). Each of the participants in a joint venture continues to conduct business independently. The new company created by the participants also remains independent. Joint ventures are often used by organizations to diversify into new services when the participants can benefit by joining hands rather than competing against each other. For example, hospitals in a given region may engage in a joint venture to form a home health agency that benefits all partners. An acute care hospital, a multispecialty physician group practice, a skilled nursing facility, and an insurer may join to offer a managed care plan (Carson et al., 1995, p. 209). In this scenario, each of the participants would continue to operate its own business, and all would have a common stake in the new HMO or PPO.

Alliances

In one respect, the health care industry is unique because organizations often develop cooperative arrangements with rival providers. Cooperation instead of competition, in some situations, eliminates duplication of services while ensuring that all the health needs of the community are fulfilled (Carson et al., 1995, p. 217). An *alliance* is an agreement between two organizations to share their resources without joint ownership of assets. For example, a hospital may form an alliance with a medical group practice to conduct community health assessments, jointly create programs that minimize health risks, and work to improve the community's health.

Alliances are relatively simpler to form than mergers. An alliance may be a first step that gives both organizations the opportunity to evaluate the advantages of a potential merger. Such arrangements require little financial commitment and can be easily dissolved if the anticipated benefits do not materialize.

Virtual Organizations

When contractual arrangements between two or more organizations form a new organization, the resulting entity is referred to as a *virtual organization*, or an organization without walls. The formation of a health network based on contractual arrangements is called *virtual integration*. IPAs are a prime example of virtual organizations; a PHO may also be a virtual organization. The main advantage of virtual organizations is that they require less capital to enter new geographic or service markets (Gabel, 1997). They also help bring together scattered entities under one mutually cooperative arrangement.

Integration Based on Service Consolidation

Horizontal Integration

Horizontal integration is a growth strategy in which a health care organization extends its core product or service. For example, an acute care hospital that adds coronary bypass surgery to its existing surgical services or that builds a suburban acute care facility is integrating horizontally (Rakich et al., 1992, p. 326). Multihospital chains, nursing facility chains, and a chain of drugstores, all under the same management with member facilities offering the same core services or products, are other examples of horizontal integration. The main objective of horizontal integration is to achieve geographic expansion. Diversification into new products or services is not achieved through horizontal integration.

Vertical Integration

Vertical integration links services that are at different stages in the production process of health care—for example, organization of preventive services, primary care, acute care, and postacute service delivery around a hospital. The intended purpose of vertical integration is to increase the comprehensiveness and continuity of care; in essence, it is a diversification strategy. This type of integration may be achieved through acquisitions, mergers, joint ventures, or alliances. To add just one or two new services, internal development strategies may be used. For example, CVS Health operates walk-in retail clinics inside its pharmacy stores in many locations. IDSs are also formed through vertical integration.

▶ Conclusion

Most insured Americans today—either through private or government sources—receive health care through a managed care organization. MCOs have been credited with helping contain the costs of health care, and enrollment in managed care plans has continued to grow. Yet, the full potential of managed care was never realized because of widespread opposition.

Integrated delivery systems emerged as hospitals and physicians, in particular, faced growing pressures from managed care to deliver services at reduced costs. Integration has enabled large health care organizations to win sizable managed care contracts and, in some instances, to offer their own health insurance plans. However, the delivery of health care has become complex from the standpoint of providers and consumers. Through the Affordable Care Act, the U.S. government is now experimenting with accountable care organizations in the hope that they may be able to reduce costs and improve quality. Some early results are promising. If the successes in providing value are consistently achieved, ACOs could well become the providers of choice to contract with Medicare, Medicaid, and managed care organizations for the delivery of most services to enrolled populations.

References

1. Auerbach DI, et al. 2013. Accountable care organization formation is associated with integrated systems but not high medical spending. *Health Aff.* 32(10):1781–1788.
2. Ayanian JZ, et al. 2013. Medicare beneficiaries more likely to receive appropriate ambulatory services in HMOs than in traditional Medicare. *Health Aff.* 32(7):1228–1235.
3. Baker L, et al. 2004. The effect of area HMO market share on cancer screening. *Health Serv Res.* 39(6):1751–1772.
4. Balsa A, et al. 2007. Does managed health care reduce health care disparities between minorities and whites? *J Health Econ.* 26(1):101–121.
5. Basu J. 2012. Medicare managed care and primary care quality: Examining racial/ethnic effects across states. *Health Care Manag Sci.* 15(1):15–28.
6. Brown AF, et al. 2005. Race, ethnicity, socioeconomic position, and quality of care for adults with diabetes enrolled in managed care. *Diab Care.* 28(12):2864–2870.
7. Burns LR, Pauly MV. 2012. Accountable care organization may have difficulty avoiding the failures of integrated delivery networks of the 1990s. *Health Aff.* 31(11):2407–2416.
8. Carson KD, et al. 1995. *Management of healthcare organizations.* Cincinnati, OH: South-Western College Publishing.
9. Casalino LP, et al. 2013. Independent practice associations and physician–hospital organizations can improve care management for smaller practices. *Health Aff.* 32(8):1376–1382.
10. Caswell KJ, Long SK. 2015, April 16. The expanding role of managed care in the Medicaid program: Implications for health care access, use, and expenditures for nonelderly adults. *Inquiry.* [Epub ahead of print].

11. Centers for Medicare and Medicaid Services (CMS). 2015. Shared savings program. http://www.cms.gov/Medicare/Medicare-Fee-for-Service-Payment/sharedsavingsprogram/index.html. Accessed August 16, 2015.

12. Colla CH, et al. 2014. First national survey of ACOs finds that physicians are playing strong leadership and ownership roles. *Health Aff.* 33:964–971.

13. Department of Health and Human Services (DHHS). 1996. *Health, United States, 1995.* Hyattsville, MD: DHHS.

14. Dugan J. 2015. Trends in managed care cost containment: An analysis of the managed care backlash. *Health Econ.* 24(12):1604–1618.

15. Duggan M, Hayford T. 2013. Has the shift to managed care reduced Medicaid expenditures? Evidence from state and local level mandates. *J Policy Anal Manage.* 32(3):505–535.

16. Eikel CV. 2002. Fewer patient visits under capitation offset by improved quality of care: Study brings evidence to debate over physician payment methods. *Findings Brief: Health Care Financ Org.* 5(3):1–2.

17. Frank RG, Garfield RL. 2007. Managed behavioral health care carve-outs: Past performance and future prospects. *Ann Rev Public Health.* 28(1):303–320.

18. Gabel J. 1997. Ten ways HMOs have changed during the 1990s. *Health Aff.* 16(3):134–145.

19. Hofmann MA. 2002. Quality of health care improving. *Bus Insurance.* 36(38):1–2.

20. Hwang W, et al. 2013. Effects of integrated delivery system on cost and quality. *Am J Manag Care.* 19(5):e175–e184.

21. Iglehart JK. 1994. The American health care system: Managed care. In: Lee PR, Estes CL, eds. *The nation's health.* 4th ed. Boston, MA: Jones and Bartlett, 231–237.

22. Miller RH, Luft HS. 2002. HMO plan performance update: An analysis of the literature, 1997–2001. *Health Aff.* 21(4):63–86.

23. Moscovice I, et al. 1998. Expanding rural managed care: Enrollment patterns and perspectives. *Health Aff.* 17(1):172–179.

24. Newhouse JP, McGuire TG. 2014. How successful is Medicare Advantage? *Milbank Q.* 92(2):351–394.

25. Pelfrey S, Theisen BA. 1989. Joint venture in health care. *J Nurs Admin.* 19(4):39–42.

26. Peng X, et al. 2015. Relationship between Medicare Advantage contract characteristics and quality-of-care ratings: An observational analysis of Medicare Advantage star ratings. *Ann Intern Med.* 162(5):353–358.

27. Perez K. 2015. ACOs: From unicorns to pacesetters in four years. *Healthc Financ Manag.* 69(5):108–109.

28. Rakich JS, et al. 1992. *Managing health services organizations.* 3rd ed. Baltimore, MD: Health Professions Press.

29. Robinson JC. 2002. Renewed emphasis on consumer cost sharing in health insurance benefit design. *Health Aff Web Exclusives.* W139–W154.

30. Sanofi-Aventis. 2013. *Managed care digest series, 2013: Public payer digest.* Bridgewater, NJ: Sanofi-Aventis US.

31. Sanofi-Aventis. 2014. *Managed care digest series: Public payer digest, 2014.* Bridgewater, NJ: Sanofi-Aventis US.

32. Sanofi-Aventis. 2016a. *Managed care digest series, 2016: Public payer digest.* Bridgewater, NJ: Sanofi-Aventis US.

33. Sanofi-Aventis. 2016b. *Managed care digest series, 2016: HMO-PPO digest.* Bridgewater, NJ: Sanofi-Aventis US.

34. Sanofi-Aventis. 2017. *Managed care digest series: Provider digest, 2017.* Bridgewater, NJ: Sanofi-Aventis US.

35. Schneider EC, et al. 2005. Quality of care in for-profit and not-for-profit health plans enrolling Medicare beneficiaries. *Am J Med*. 118(12):1392–1400.

36. Song Z, Fisher ES. 2016. The ACO experiment in infancy: Looking back and looking forward. *JAMA*. 316(7):705–706.

37. Taitsman J. 2015. Medicaid managed-care patients face hurdles in getting care. *Mod Healthc*. 45(1):27.

38. Wagner ER. (1995). Types of managed care organizations. In: Kongstvedt PR, ed. *Essentials of managed health care*. Gaithersburg, MD: Aspen Publishers, 24–34.

39. Wilson FA, Neuhauser D. 1985. *Health services in the United States*. 2nd ed. Cambridge, MA: Ballinger Publishing.

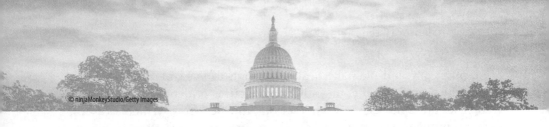

CHAPTER 10

Long-Term Care Services

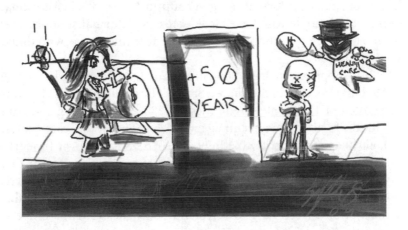

▶ Introduction

Long-term care (LTC) services are needed under three main circumstances: (1) physical or mental deficits that limit a person's ability to do regular daily tasks, creating the need for support and assistance; (2) need for continuity of care after hospitalization because of a severe illness, injury, or surgical episode; or (3) need for care in specialized environments. For example, elderly patients with Alzheimer's disease and children and adolescents with birth-related disorders may need specialized environments of care delivery. On the one hand, the elderly—people 65 years of age or older—are the primary clients of LTC, though most older adults do not need LTC services. In fact, most elderly persons are physically and mentally healthy enough to live independently. On the other hand, many young adults are victims of debilitating diseases, such as multiple sclerosis, and serious injuries from vehicle crashes, sports mishaps, and industrial accidents. In many cases, these individuals require LTC services.

LTC is delivered in a variety of community-based settings as well as in nursing homes (skilled nursing facilities, subacute care facilities, and specialized care facilities). Hence, the LTC delivery system has two major sectors: community-based care and institutional care. In the United States, most LTC is actually provided informally by family, friends, and surrogates who receive no payment for their time and effort. Current estimates of the extent of informal caregiving are hard to come by. Previous estimates suggested that 80% of those persons receiving LTC at home receive that care exclusively from unpaid caregivers; an additional 14% receive both unpaid and paid help (Thompson, 2004). Informal caregiver support forestalls institutionalization. Older people who have close access to informal support often continue to live in the community much longer than those who do not have such support.

In 2014, approximately 67,000 paid, regulated LTC providers served about 9 million people in the United States. The multifaceted LTC industry consisted of 15,600 nursing homes, 30,200 assisted living and similar facilities, 12,400 home health agencies, 4,800 adult day care centers, and 4,000 hospices (Harris-Kojetin et al., 2016). Surveys over time have shown that the vast majority of older Americans wish to stay in their own home indefinitely. Hence, community-based services are preferred by most older people, and these services have grown more rapidly than LTC institutions. According to Kaye and colleagues (2010), compared to noninstitutional LTC populations, those receiving institutional care are older (median age = 82 years), are single or widowed, and are more likely to have *cognitive impairment*—that is, a mental disorder associated with memory and learning issues, ability to concentrate, and making decisions.

Even though most elderly people are in good health, the aging process leads to chronic, degenerative conditions that resist cure. As a consequence, as people grow older, the odds increase that they will require LTC. Moreover, LTC cannot be an isolated component of the health care delivery system, but rather non-LTC services must be closely integrated with those of LTC. To address the total health care needs of patients requiring LTC, the delivery system must allow ease of transition among various types of health care settings and services.

Chronic conditions are the leading cause of illness, disability, and death in the United States today. *Chronic conditions* are characterized by

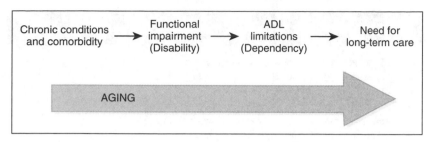

FIGURE 10.1 Progressive Steps Toward the Need for Long-Term Care Among the Elderly

persistent and recurring health consequences lasting over a long period, which are generally irreversible. Arthritis, diabetes, asthma, heart disease, and dementia are some examples of chronic conditions. A person's age or the mere presence of a chronic condition does not predict the need for LTC, but as a person ages, chronic ailments, *comorbidity* (multiple health problems), disability, and dependency tend to follow each other, depending on the individual's lifestyle and compliance with medical directives. This progression increases the probability that a person will need LTC (**FIGURE 10.1**). Approximately one-third of the elderly have functional impairments of one kind or another. Among those age 85 and older, two-thirds have functional impairments (Congressional Budget Office [CBO], 2013).

By 2050, 20% of the U.S. population will be elderly, up from 12% in 2000. The number of people age 85 and older will grow the fastest (CBO, 2013). Growth of the elderly population will bring a corresponding surge in the number of elderly people with functional and cognitive limitations. Thus, the need for LTC will increase sharply in coming decades.

The rest of the developed world also faces aging-related problems and challenges in providing adequate LTC services, very similar to those noted in the United States. Indeed, the elderly population as a proportion of the total population in other developed countries, such as Japan, Germany, France, and Great Britain, is already higher than it is in the United States.

▶ What Is Long-Term Care?

LTC can be defined as a variety of individualized, well-coordinated services that promote the maximum possible independence for people with functional limitations and that are provided over an extended period of time in accordance with a holistic approach, while maximizing the person's quality of life. The seven essential characteristics of LTC are summarized in **EXHIBIT 10.1** and are explained in this section.

EXHIBIT 10.1 Seven Essential Characteristics of Long-Term Care

- LTC includes a variety of health care services.
- Services are individualized.
- Services must be well coordinated.
- The goal is to promote maximum possible functional independence.
- Services are needed over an extended period of time.
- Patients' physical, mental, social, and spiritual needs must be met.
- Patients' quality of life must be maximized.

A Variety of Health Care Services

Clients receiving LTC need a variety of services for two main reasons:

- The need for services varies greatly from individual to individual. Even the elderly, who are the predominant users of LTC services, are not a homogeneous group. For example, some people just require supportive housing, whereas others require intensive treatments. Hence, LTC includes services such as housing programs, transportation, case management, recreation, nutrition, nursing, medical care, and social services.
- Even for the same individual, the need for the various types of services generally changes over time. Such change is not necessarily progressive, developing from lighter to more intensive levels of care. Depending on the change in condition and functioning, the individual may shift back and forth between the various levels and types of LTC services. For example, after hip surgery, a patient may require extensive rehabilitation therapy in a nursing facility for 2 or 3 weeks before returning home, where he or she receives continuing care from a home health agency. After that, the individual may continue to live independently but require a daily meal from Meals on Wheels. Later, this same person may suffer a stroke and after hospitalization have to stay indefinitely in an LTC facility.

Clients often require both LTC and non-LTC services, such as primary care and acute care. Hence, LTC is not a self-contained system of comprehensive health care services, nor can it function independently of primary, acute, mental health, and ancillary services such as pharmaceuticals and diagnostics.

LTC must also include both therapeutic and preventive services. The primary goal of preventive services is to prevent or delay the need for institutionalization in LTC facilities. Preventive measures include ensuring that the elderly receive good nutrition and have access to preventive medical care. For example, older adults must have access to services such as vaccination against pneumonia, annual flu shots, glaucoma screening, diabetes screening, and cancer screening.

For those elderly persons who live independently, certain social support programs also serve a preventive function. Programs such as homemaker, chore, and handyman services can assist with a variety of tasks that older adults may no longer be able to perform. Examples include shopping, light cleaning, general errands, lawn maintenance, and minor home repairs.

Individualized Services

An assessment of the patient's physical, mental, and emotional condition and past medical and social history, former occupation, leisure activities, and cultural factors is used to determine which services would be most suitable for the individual. An individualized plan of care is developed, and services are rendered according to that plan.

Coordination of Services

The mere availability of a spectrum of services may not be sufficient to meet the varied and changing needs of LTC clients unless those services are well coordinated. As it is, many people find the health care delivery system difficult to navigate. Such difficulties are often compounded in the case of elderly and disabled individuals. For example, acute episodes, such as pneumonia, bone fracture, or stroke, require admission to a general hospital. Many acute care services are now delivered in a variety of outpatient settings instead of hospitals. After acute care delivery, a patient may be transferred to a hospital-based transitional care unit for intensive rehabilitation. The patient may subsequently have to be moved to an LTC facility for ongoing care. Depression may create a need to visit an outpatient mental health clinic. The same individual may also require dental or optometric care.

Maximum Possible Functional Independence

Two standard measures are used to determine a person's level of dependency. First, the activities of daily living (ADLs) scale is used to assess a person's ability to perform certain common tasks referred to as *activities of daily living* (**EXHIBIT 10.2**). Severe ADL limitations often indicate the need for institutional care. For example, functional deficits in three or more ADLs dramatically increase the probability that an individual will need institutional care. Second, the *instrumental activities of daily living* (IADLs) scale incorporates activities that are necessary for living independently in the community, such as using the telephone, driving a car

---

EXHIBIT 10.2   Activities of Daily Living

The classic ADL scale includes six basic activities:

- Eating
- Bathing
- Dressing
- Using a toilet
- Maintaining bowel and bladder control
- Transferring, such as getting out of bed and moving into a chair

   Sometimes grooming and walking a distance of 8 feet are also included in the scale.

EXHIBIT 10.3   Age-Related Progression of Long-Term Care Intensity

- Independent living
- Decline in IADLs
  - Informal care for those who have adequate social support
  - Informal care supplemented by paid community-based services
- Decline in ADLs
  - For light ADLs (eating, dressing, using a toilet), informal care with supplemental services may continue
  - Institutionalization

---

or traveling alone by bus or taxi, shopping, preparing meals, doing light housework, taking medicine, and handling money. IADLs are not generally used as a criterion for care in institutional settings because institutionalized persons are not required to perform many IADLs (Ostir et al., 1999). The probability of having limitations in ADLs and IADLs increases significantly with age; **EXHIBIT 10.3** illustrates the age-related progression of LTC intensity.

The main goal of LTC is to enable the individual to maintain functional independence to the maximum level that is practicable. In many instances, a person's functional status can be improved by the use of adaptive devices, such as walkers, wheelchairs, special utensils, and many other types of equipment, and by modification of the living environment with safety features such as grab bars. However, as dependency increases, the need for LTC services also increases (see Figure 10.1).

Restoration of function may be possible to some extent through appropriate rehabilitation therapy, but in most cases a full restoration of normal functioning is an unrealistic expectation. Caregivers must render care and assistance wherever the patient is either unable to do things for himself or herself or absolutely refuses to do so. The focus should be on maintaining whatever functional ability the patient still has and on preventing further decline of that ability. Caregivers should motivate and help patients do as much as possible for themselves.

Extended Period of Time

Compared to acute care, LTC is sustained over a longer period of time. The period of care and institutional stays, when needed, generally extend to weeks, months, and years instead of days. Even when institutional LTC is indicated for a short period (90 or fewer days), LTC services may continue in the patient's own home after the patient has been discharged from a long-term care facility. At other times, long-range confinement to a nursing home may be necessary.

Holistic Approach

The holistic model of health not only focuses on a person's physical and mental needs, but also emphasizes well-being in every aspect of what makes a person whole and complete. A patient's physical, mental, social, and spiritual needs and preferences are incorporated into medical care delivery and the living environment. The following are brief descriptions of the four aspects of holistic caregiving:

1. *Physical.* The physical aspect refers to the technical aspects of care, such as medical examination, nursing care, medications, diet, and rehabilitation treatments. It also includes comfort factors such as appropriate temperature and cozy furnishings, cleanliness, and safety in home and institutional environments.

2. *Mental.* The emphasis with mental care is on the total mental and emotional well-being of each individual. Such care may include treatment of mental and behavioral problems, if necessary. Maintaining mental health goes beyond diagnosis and treatment of mental conditions, however. In an institutional setting, it includes appropriate layout, décor, and engagement techniques that help overcome disorientation and confusion; mental stimulation to help overcome boredom and depression; and an environment that promotes positive feelings. For example, the living atmosphere can be enhanced through live plants, flowers, moving water, pleasant aromas, and soothing music. Pet animals, fish in aquariums, and birds create a vibrant living environment.

3. *Social.* Almost everyone enjoys warm friendships and social relationships. Visits from family, friends, or volunteers provide numerous opportunities for socializing. Many nursing homes have created indoor and outdoor spaces such as game

rooms, alcoves, balconies, and patios where people can sit and enjoy one another's company.

4. *Spiritual.* The spiritual dimension operates at an individual level. It includes personal beliefs, values, and commitments in a religious and faith context. Spirituality and spiritual pursuits are very personal matters, but for most people, they also require continuing interaction with members of their faith community.

Quality of Life

Quality of life refers to the total living experience that results in overall satisfaction with one's life. It is particularly relevant to LTC facilities because people typically reside there for an extended period. Quality of life factors include lifestyle pursuits, living environment, clinical palliation, human factors, and personal choices, as discussed here:

- Lifestyle factors are associated with personal enrichment and making one's life meaningful through enjoyable activities. For example, many older people still enjoy pursuing their former leisure activities, such as woodworking, crocheting, knitting, gardening, and fishing.
- The living environment must be comfortable, safe, and appealing to the senses. Cleanliness, décor, furnishings, and other aesthetic features are important.
- Clinical *palliation* should be available to provide relief from unpleasant symptoms such as pain or nausea—for instance, when a patient is undergoing chemotherapy.
- Human factors refer to caregiver attitudes and practices that emphasize caring, compassion, and the preservation of human dignity for the patient.
- Institutionalized patients generally find it disconcerting to have lost their autonomy and independence. Quality of life is enhanced when residents have some latitude to govern their own lives and make personal choices regarding food and daily routines. Residents in LTC facilities also desire an environment that gives them adequate privacy.

▶ Community-Based Long-Term Care Services

Community-based LTC services have four objectives: (1) to deliver LTC in the most economical and least restrictive setting whenever appropriate for the patient's health care needs; (2) to supplement informal caregiving when more advanced skills are needed to address the patient's needs; (3) to provide temporary respite to family members from caregiving stress; and (4) to delay or prevent institutionalization. These goals are accomplished through an administrative network that includes the Federal Administration on Aging, State Units on Aging, and Area Agencies on Aging. Nationally, more than 600 Area Agencies on Aging administer funds appropriated by the U.S. federal government under the Older Americans Act of 1965.

For the financially needy, Title III of the Older Americans Act may finance such community-based services as adult day care (ADC), home maintenance, health promotion and disease prevention (e.g., medication management, nutrition, and health screening), telephone reassurance, and transportation services. States may also have some federal funds available under Title XX Social Services Block Grants. In addition, community-based LTC services have grown under the Home and Community Based Services waiver program that was enacted under Section 1915(c) of the Social Security Act. Medicare and Medicaid may partially cover certain LTC services; the remainder must be covered by individual savings and private donations.

Home Health Care

Home health care refers to health care provided in the home of the patient by health care professionals. The organizational setup commonly requires a hospital-based or freestanding home health agency that sends health care professionals and paraprofessionals (such as home care aides) to patients' homes to deliver services approved by a physician.

Home health services typically include nursing care, such as changing dressings, monitoring medications, and providing help with bathing; short-term rehabilitation, such as physical, occupational, and speech therapy; homemaker services, such as meal preparation, shopping, transportation, and some specific household chores; and certain medical supplies and equipment, such as ostomy supplies, hospital beds, oxygen tanks, walkers, and wheelchairs. Not all home health agencies provide all of these services, however.

As the largest single payer for home health services, Medicare covered 40% of home health expenditures in the United States in 2015 (National Center for Health Statistics [NCHS], 2017). To qualify for home care under the Medicare program, patients must (1) be homebound, (2) have a plan of treatment that is periodically reviewed by a physician, and (3) require intermittent or part-time skilled nursing and/or rehabilitation therapies.

Under Medicaid, states have several different options available to deliver home health services. In essence, states can develop community programs to deliver services to Medicaid beneficiaries if these people would otherwise end up in an institution. In 2015, Medicaid paid for 36% of home health expenditures (NCHS, 2017).

Adult Day Care

Adult day care is a daytime, community-based, group program that is designed to meet the needs of functionally and/or cognitively impaired adults and to provide a partial respite to family caregivers. Such care is designed for people who live with their families but because of physical or mental conditions cannot remain alone during the day when the family members are working.

Most ADC services are highly focused on prevention and health maintenance, with the objective of preventing or delaying institutionalization, but they also incorporate nursing care, psychosocial therapies, and rehabilitation. As such, ADC services, in many instances, have become alternatives to home health care and assisted living and function as a transitional step before placement in a long-term care institution. Nearly half of the participants have dementia, and 50% of ADC centers offer specialized programs for these patients (MetLife Mature Market Institute, 2010).

Adult Foster Care

Adult foster care is defined as a service characterized by small, family-run homes providing room, board, oversight, and personal care to non-related adults who are unable to care for themselves ("AARP Studies Adult Foster Care," 1996). Foster care generally provides services in a community-based dwelling in an environment that promotes the feeling of being part of a family unit (Stahl, 1997). Participants in these programs are elderly or disabled individuals who require assistance with one or two ADLs, and many of the residents have a psychiatric diagnosis.

Typically, the caregiving family resides in part of the home. To maintain the family environment, most states license fewer than 10 beds per family unit. Each state has established its own standards for licensing foster care homes. As states have continued to shift Medicaid funds from institutional to community-based services, use of adult foster care has grown. Medicare does not pay for services provided by the adult foster care home but may cover rehabilitation services.

Senior Centers

Senior centers are local community centers for older adults where seniors can congregate and socialize. Many centers serve a noon meal daily. Others sponsor wellness programs, health education, counseling services, recreational activities, information and referral, and some limited health care services. Health care services typically offered at senior centers include health screening, especially for glaucoma and hypertension.

Approximately 11,000 senior centers have been established across the United States, serving 1 million older adults every day. To maintain operations, senior centers rely on a variety of public and private sources of funding from various branches of government, businesses, donations, and volunteer hours (National Council on Aging, 2015).

Home-Delivered and Congregate Meals

The Elderly Nutrition Program operates under the U.S. Administration on Aging and serves congregate meals in senior centers and home-delivered meals, referred to as Meals on Wheels, to homebound elderly persons 60 years of age and older. The main goal of this program is to improve the nutritional intake of older Americans. The program generally provides one hot noon meal for 5 days a week.

In the Meals on Wheels program, meals are prepared by local institutions and delivered by volunteers. The volunteers also perform an important service by checking on the welfare of homebound elderly and are encouraged to report any health or other problems that they may notice during their visits.

Homemaker and Handyman Services

Some older adults are relatively healthy but cannot carry out a few simple tasks necessary for independent living. These tasks may be as urgent as repairing a burst plumbing pipe or as mundane as cleaning the house. Some tasks, such as grocery shopping, must be performed often, whereas others, such as replacing storm windows, require attention just once or twice a year. Homemaker, household chore, and handyman services can assist older adults with a variety of such tasks, including shopping, light cleaning, general errands, and minor home repairs. Homemaker programs may be staffed largely or entirely by volunteers.

Emergency Response Systems

A personal emergency response system, also called a medical emergency response system, consists of an electronic device that enables people to summon help in an emergency. This kind of system is specifically designed for disabled or elderly people who live alone and may not otherwise need ongoing medical or supportive care. Other patients, after returning home from hospitals and nursing homes, are plagued by anxiety about relapses or accidents because they are often unprepared for self-management after returning home. Usually they either wear or carry a transmitter unit that enables them to send a medical alert to a 24-hour monitoring and response center. Such a system is available for a reasonable fee.

Case Management

In the LTC context, *case management* refers to a method of linking, managing, and coordinating services to meet the varied and changing health care needs of elderly clients (Zawadski & Eng, 1988). Case management services assess the special needs of older adults, formulate a care plan to address those needs, identify which services are most appropriate, determine eligibility for services, make referrals and coordinate delivery of care, arrange for financing, and ensure that clients are receiving services in accordance with the plan of care. Case managers often assist the adult children of disabled elderly persons who may be living far from each other.

▶ Institutional Long-Term Care

Generally, institutional LTC is more appropriate for patients whose needs cannot be adequately met in a less clinical, community-based setting. However, a variety of institutional options are available to meet the varying needs of the elderly who no longer can live alone safely. Available options today include retirement centers, residential or personal care facilities, assisted living facilities, and nursing homes. These facilities provide varying levels of assistance.

An evaluation of the extent of functional impairment often determines which services are best suited to the individual, but personal preferences, and often the availability of financing, also play a significant role. Because people generally prefer to receive care in their own home, when institutionalization becomes necessary, they prefer a homelike, nonclinical setting. Nevertheless, medical needs must often override personal preferences, especially when severe physical or mental problems develop.

FIGURE 10.2 illustrates, on a continuum, six types of elder care institutions that can be classified under three general categories: retirement homes, personal care homes, and nursing homes. Continuing-care retirement communities (CCRCs) offer all three options within one campus-like setting. Based on the concept of aging-in-place, CCRCs can address people's changing needs over time.

Retirement Facilities

Retirement facilities do not deliver nursing care services, but rather emphasize privacy, security, independence, and active lifestyles. Some

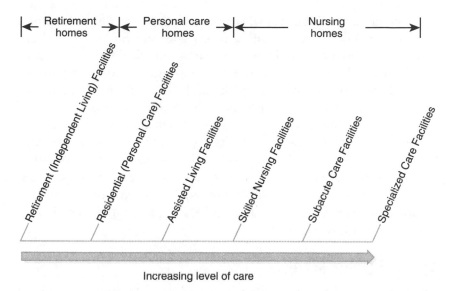

FIGURE 10.2 Long-Term Care Institutions for the Elderly

basic personal care such as assistance with bathing may be available in some retirement facilities, but in most instances, when additional nursing or rehabilitation services are needed, arrangements are made for a local home health agency to provide them.

The special features and amenities in retirement facilities are designed to create a physically supportive environment that promotes independence. For example, the living quarters are equipped with emergency call systems. Many facilities provide monthly blood pressure and vision screenings. Most organize programs for socializing, physical fitness, recreation, and local outings for shopping and entertainment. Some basic hotel services, such as one meal a day and periodic housekeeping, are generally provided. Apartment units or detached cottages equipped with kitchenettes and private baths are the most common types of retirement facilities. Common laundry rooms are often shared with other residents. Many upscale retirement centers abound, in which one can expect to pay a fairly substantial entrance fee plus a monthly rental or maintenance fee. At the other end of the income scale, many communities have government-subsidized housing units for the low-income elderly and disabled individuals.

Personal Care Facilities

Personal care can be defined as nonmedical custodial care. *Custodial care* comprises basic assistance provided in a protected environment; it does not include active medical or rehabilitative treatments.

Facilities providing personal care may be called by different names, such as domiciliary care facilities, board-and-care homes, foster care homes, residential care facilities, or personal care facilities. These facilities provide physically supportive dwelling units, monitoring and/or assistance with medications, oversight, and light assistance with certain ADLs such as bathing and grooming. To maintain a residential rather than an institutional environment, many such facilities limit the admission of residents who use wheelchairs. Most of these facilities are relatively small and can be viewed as community-based alternatives rather than institutions. Staff members are mostly nursing paraprofessionals, such as personal care aides, who do not require a license or professional certification to deliver care. Similar workers employed in nursing homes must be certified by the state.

Assisted Living Facilities

An assisted living facility provides personal care, 24-hour supervision, social activities, recreational activities, and some nursing and rehabilitation services. The most common areas of assistance with ADLs are bathing, dressing, and toileting. These facilities maintain a skeleton staff of licensed nurses—generally licensed practical nurses (referred to as licensed vocational nurses in some states)—to do admission assessments and deliver basic nursing care and medication management. Hence, these facilities can be classified on the LTC continuum somewhere between personal care homes and nursing homes. Advanced nursing care and rehabilitation therapies can be arranged through a home health agency. Approximately 59% of the residents eventually move into a skilled nursing facility and one-third die while residing in the assisted living facility (National Center for Assisted Living, 2013).

Skilled Nursing Facilities

A skilled nursing facility is a typical nursing home that provides a full range of clinical LTC services, from skilled nursing care to rehabilitation to assistance with all ADLs. *Skilled nursing care* is medically oriented care provided by a licensed nurse. The plan of treatment is authorized by a physician. The majority of direct care with ADLs is delivered by paraprofessionals, such as certified nursing assistants and therapy assistants, but under the supervision of licensed nurses and therapists.

A variety of disabilities, including problems with ambulation, incontinence, and behavior, often coexist among a relatively large number of patients in need of skilled care. Compared to other types of facilities, these nursing homes have a significant number of patients who are cognitively impaired because of confusion, delirium, or dementia. The social functioning of many of the patients in such facilities is also in severe decline.

Licensed professionals who work in skilled care facilities include registered nurses (RNs), licensed practical/vocational nurses, and registered therapists (physical therapists, occupational therapists, respiratory therapists, and speech/language pathologists). Rehabilitation is often an important component of skilled care, as are therapeutic diets and nutritional supplements. The patient's assessment requires multidisciplinary input from various health care professionals, and the plan of care is highly individualized.

Subacute Care Facilities

Subacute care is a blend of intensive medical, nursing, and other services that are technically complex and provided in an LTC setting. Examples include complex wound care, intravenous therapy, blood transfusion, ventilator support, and AIDS care. Subacute care is a substitute for services that were previously provided in acute care hospitals; its popularity has grown because it is a cheaper alternative to a hospital stay.

Subacute care generally follows hospitalization and is required for a relatively short period of time, such as between 20 and 90 days. Services are available in three main settings:

1. Long-term care hospitals (LTCHs), according to federal regulations, must be certified as acute care hospitals and must have an average length of stay greater than 25 days.
2. Many skilled nursing facilities have opened subacute care units by raising the staff skill mix through hiring additional RNs and having therapists on staff.
3. Some subacute-type services are rendered by community-based home health agencies. Thanks to new technology, certain subacute services can be provided in a patient's own home.

Specialized Care Facilities

By their very nature, both subacute care and specialized care place high emphasis on medical and nursing services. Some skilled nursing facilities have opened specialized care units for patients requiring ventilator care, wound care, services for Alzheimer's disease, intensive rehabilitation, or closed head trauma care. Other freestanding facilities have chosen a niche, specializing only in Alzheimer's care, rehabilitation, or AIDS care.

▶ Licensing and Certification of Nursing Homes

Nursing homes are heavily regulated through licensure and certification requirements. In the United States, it is illegal to operate a nursing facility without a license. To serve Medicare and/or Medicaid beneficiaries, a facility must be certified by the federal government.

Licensing

Every state requires nursing homes to be licensed by the state. Annual renewal of a license is required for existing nursing homes. To keep their licenses in good standing, it is essential that facilities comply with the state's standards for nursing homes. These standards vary from state to state, except for national fire safety regulations. The Life Safety Code, published by the National Fire Protection Association, encompasses national building and fire safety rules that have become a part of licensure standards. In addition, each state has crafted basic standards for nursing care and other services. Compliance with standards is verified through periodic inspections, generally once a year. A state's department (board or division) of health or department of human services generally has nursing home licensing and oversight responsibilities.

Certification

The Centers for Medicare and Medicaid Services (CMS), an agency of the U.S. Department of Health and Human Services, is responsible for certifying a nursing home that wants to serve Medicaid and/or Medicare clients. To be certified, a nursing home must first be licensed by the state. Thus, licensure and certification serve different purposes. A license allows a facility to operate and do business, whereas certification allows a nursing home to admit patients who are on public assistance. It is possible for a facility to have only a license, but in that case, it cannot receive payments from Medicaid or Medicare.

Three distinct federal certification categories exist, and facilities in all three categories are generically referred to as nursing homes:

1. SNF certification allows a facility to admit patients whose care is financed by Medicare; Medicare pays for postacute skilled care only after a patient has stayed in a hospital for a minimum of 3 days, not counting the day of discharge. The maximum coverage in an SNF-certified facility is 100 days, but in actual

practice the average length of stay is much shorter due to the complex Medicare rules that the facility must follow to determine the length of stay. Medicare pays the full cost of skilled nursing care only for the first 20 days; the beneficiary must pay a substantial copayment ($167.50 per day in 2018) for days 21 through 100.

2. NF certification allows a facility to admit patients whose care is financed by Medicaid. Unlike Medicare, Medicaid allows patients to stay in an NF-certified nursing home indefinitely as long as the patient's physician authorizes the need for nursing care and the patient qualifies for Medicaid assistance. The beneficiary is required to turn over most of his or her monthly income to the facility; Medicaid pays the remaining costs. Many patients are initially admitted to a facility with a private-pay source of funding. When their private funds are exhausted, these patients generally become eligible for Medicaid assistance.

3. Intermediate care facility for individuals with intellectual disabilities (ICF/IID)—previously called intermediate care facility for the mentally retarded (ICF/MR)—certification allows a nursing facility to serve patients who are intellectually/developmentally disabled, also referred to as mentally retarded/developmentally disabled. A *developmental disability* is a physical incapacity that generally accompanies below-average intellectual functioning and often arises at birth or in early childhood. ICF/IIDs provide specialized programming and care modules for patients with mental retardation and associated disabilities. The reimbursement is derived mostly from Medicaid.

Certification is granted on the basis of compliance with federal standards. The same standards apply to both SNF and NF certifications, but different standards apply to ICF/IID certification. A facility may be dually certified as both an SNF and an NF. Facilities having dual certification can admit Medicare and/or Medicaid patients to any part of the facility.

The small number of facilities that have elected not to be certified can admit only those patients who have a private source of funding for nursing home care. Such private-pay patients—those not covered by either Medicare or Medicaid for long-term nursing home care—are not restricted to noncertified facilities, however. In most certified nursing homes, private-pay patients are placed alongside those who depend on Medicare and Medicaid.

▶ Other Long-Term Care Services

Respite Care

Family caregivers often experience physical and emotional problems. Caregiving responsibilities can ignite family conflicts and encroach on caregivers' employment and leisure activities. Under these circumstances, many caregivers experience stress and burnout. *Respite care* enables family caregivers to take some time off to deal with their feelings of stress and frustration. Virtually any kind of LTC service—adult day care, home health care, and temporary institutionalization—can be viewed as respite care, as long as the focus is on giving informal caregivers some time off while meeting the disabled person's needs for assistance (Doty et al., 1996).

Restorative Care

Restorative care refers to therapeutic interventions designed to help patients regain or improve function. Restorative rehabilitation involves intensive short-term treatments rendered by physical therapists, occupational therapists, and speech–language pathologists. Examples of persons requiring rehabilitation therapy include individuals who have experienced orthopedic surgery, stroke, limb amputation, and prolonged illness.

Maintenance rehabilitation has the goal of preserving the present level of function and preventing further decline. Assistance with ambulation and range-of-motion exercises are examples of maintenance rehabilitation.

Adaptive rehabilitation improves function despite deficits that remain. Examples include adaptive equipment and training in its proper use, splints that can help a person use his or her arms to perform certain ADLs, and braces or orthotics to support the knee or foot so a person can ambulate safely.

Hospice Care

Approaches to terminal illness and death with the objective of maintaining the patient's dignity and comfort have received increased attention in the delivery of health care. Almost three-fourths of all deaths occur among those persons age 65 and older. The common causes of death among the elderly are heart disease, cancer, chronic respiratory disease, stroke, and Alzheimer's disease (Murphy et al., 2013). Hence, dealing with death and dying is very much a part of LTC.

End-of-life care is commonly associated with *hospice*, a cluster of comprehensive services for terminally ill persons who have a life expectancy of 6 months or less. Hospice is a method of care, not a location, although some freestanding hospice facilities have been established. Hospice can be a part of home health care when the services are provided in the patient's home. In other instances, hospice services are taken to patients in nursing homes, retirement centers, or hospitals.

▶ The Affordable Care Act and Long-Term Care

The main implications of the Affordable Care Act (ACA) for long-term care services are as follows:

- States have the option to provide home- and community-based attendant services under a program called Community First Choice through an increase in Medicaid federal matching payments.
- The Elder Justice Act of 2010 was incorporated into the ACA to counter elder abuse, neglect, and exploitation. Nursing facilities that receive federal payments must comply with certain reporting and notification requirements.
- All certified nursing facilities must comply with a Quality Assurance Performance Improvement (QAPI) requirement with the objective of preventing or decreasing the likelihood of quality problems.

▶ Nursing Home Industry and Expenditures

During the past several years, the number of nursing homes, bed capacity, number of residents in U.S. nursing homes, and occupancy rates have continued to decline (**TABLE 10.1**). This downward trend largely reflects the growth of community-based LTC alternatives and other institutional options and government policies that incentivize the use of community-based care. The need for various types of LTC services will continue to increase given a growing population with chronic conditions, comorbidities, and subsequent disability, but with increased life span.

The nursing home industry in the United States is dominated by private, for-profit nursing home chains. In 2014, 70% of all U.S. nursing homes had for-profit ownership; 24% were operated by private nonprofit entities. Only 6% were government owned, and most of these are owned and operated by local counties. Of all nursing homes, 97% were certified for Medicare; of this group, 95% were also certified for Medicaid. Among nursing home residents, 85% were elderly, 67% were female, and half had a diagnosis of Alzheimer's disease or some other dementia (Harris-Kojetin et al., 2016).

Nursing home expenditures are shown in **TABLE 10.2**. In recent years, the share of U.S. nursing home expenditures has been shifting from the

TABLE 10.1 Nursing Home Trends (Selected Years)			
	2000	**2010**	**2015**
Number of nursing homes	16,886	15,690	15,656
Number of beds	1,795,388	1,703,398	1,694,777
Average beds per nursing home	106.3	108.6	108.3
Number of residents	1,480,076	1,396,473	1,360,970
Occupancy rate*	82.4%	82.0%	80.3%

* Percentage of beds occupied (number of residents per 100 beds). These data do not include long-term care facilities that are not classified as nursing homes (Figure 10.2).
Data from National Center for Health Statistics. Health, United States, 2007 (pp. 370–371); Health, United States, 2012 (pp. 317–318); Health, United States, 2016 (pp. 312–313).

TABLE 10.2 Sources of National Health Expenditures for Nursing Care Facilities and Continuing Care Retirement Centers, 2016		
	Billions of Dollars	**Percent**
Total expenditures	**162.7**	
Medicare	37.5	23.0
Medicaid	50.0	30.7
Veterans Administration	5.0	3.1
Other public	3.3	2.0
Total public sources		**58.8%**
Private out of pocket	43.8	26.9
Private health insurance	14.8	9.1
Other private	8.3	5.1
Total private sources		**41.1%**

Data from CMS, Office of Actuary. National Health Expenditures by Type of Service and Source of Funds, CY 1960-2016. https://www.cms.gov/Research-Statistics-Data-and-Systems/Statistics-Trends-and-Reports/NationalHealthExpendData /NationalHealthAccountsHistorical.html. Accessed February 13, 2018.

government to private sources. In 2011, for example, expenditures from private sources amounted to 37.5% of the total expenditures for nursing home and continuing care retirement centers. In 2016, the private share of expenditures increased to 41.1%. Although out-of-pocket payments constitute a substantial source of financing for nursing home care, for many years Medicaid has remained the largest single source of financing. Medicare pays for eligible beneficiaries under Part A, but the coverage is for a short duration, representing mostly postacute care after discharge from a hospital. Just 9% of nursing home services are paid through private insurance. In 2014, only 11% of adults age 65 and older had private LTC insurance coverage (Johnson, 2016). Insurance premiums are generally expensive; hence, few people purchase LTC insurance.

▶ Conclusion

LTC should be viewed not as an isolated component of the health care delivery system, but rather as a continuum of both community-based and institution-based services that are rationally linked to the rest of the health care delivery system. LTC includes medical care, social services, and housing alternatives. Hence, it involves a range of services that can vary according to individual needs. Chronic conditions and comorbidities can lead to physical and/or mental disability, which in turn may impair the performance of ADLs and IADLs. LTC services often complement what people with impaired functioning can do for themselves. Informal caregivers provide the bulk of these services, and respite care can provide these family members with temporary relief from the burden of caregiving.

When the required intensity of care exceeds the capabilities of informal caregivers, available alternatives include professional community-based services to supplement informal care or admission to a long-term care facility. Services offered at these facilities range from basic personal assistance to more complex skilled nursing care and subacute care. Specialized facilities caring for patients with Alzheimer's disease, AIDS, intellectual/developmental disabilities, or head trauma have also proliferated. Some LTC patients require long-range custodial care without the prognosis of a cure; others may require short-term postacute convalescence and therapy. Still others may need end-of-life care through a hospice program.

With the aging of the baby boomer population, both demand and supply for LTC services are expected to grow at a rapid rate in the future. With rising costs, however, a greater emphasis is being placed on community-based services compared to nursing home care. Overall, public sources of financing pay for the bulk of LTC services in the United States.

References

1. AARP studies adult foster care for the elderly. 1996. *Public Health Rep.* 111(4):295.
2. Congressional Budget Office (CBO). 2013. *Rising demand for long-term services and supports for elderly people.* Washington, DC: Congressional Budget Office.
3. Doty P, et al. 1996. Informal caregiving. In: Evashwick CJ, ed. *The continuum of long-term care: An integrated systems approach.* Albany, NY: Delmar Publishers, 125–141.
4. Harris-Kojetin L, et al. 2016. *Long-term care providers and services users in the United States: Data from the National Study of Long-Term Care Providers, 2013–2014.* Hyattsville, MD: National Center for Health Statistics.
5. Johnson RW. 2016, August. Who is covered by private long-term care insurance? Urban Institute. https://www.urban.org/sites/default/files/publication/83146/2000881-Who-Is-Covered-by-Private-Long-Term-Care-Insurance.pdf. Accessed February 12, 2018.
6. Kaye HS, et al. 2010. Long-term care: who gets it, who provides it, who pays, and how much? *Health Aff.* 29(1):11–21.
7. MetLife Mature Market Institute. 2010. *The MetLife national study of adult day services.* Westport, CT: Metropolitan Life Insurance Company.
8. Murphy SL, et al. 2013. Deaths: Final data for 2010. *Natl Vital Stat Rep.* 61(4). Hyattsville, MD: National Center for Health Statistics.
9. National Center for Assisted Living. 2013. Resident profile. https://www.ahcancal.org/ncal/facts/Pages/Residents.aspx. Accessed April 2018.
10. National Center for Health Statistics (NCHS). 2017. *Health, United States, 2016.* Hyattsville, MD: U.S. Department of Health and Human Services.
11. National Council on Aging. 2015. Fact sheet: Senior centers. http://www.ncoa.org/assets/files/pdf/FactSheet_SeniorCenters.pdf. Accessed June 2015.
12. Ostir GV, et al. 1999. Disability in older adults 1: Prevalence, causes, and consequences. *Behav Med.* 24(4):147–156.
13. Stahl C. 1997, September 29. Adult foster care: An alternative to SNFs? *ADV Occup Ther.*
14. Thompson L. 2004. *Long-term care: Support for family caregivers.* Washington, DC: Health Policy Institute, Georgetown University.
15. Zawadski RT, Eng C. 1988, December. Case management in capitated long-term care. *Health Care Financing Rev Ann Suppl.* 75–81.

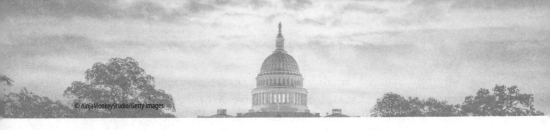
© ninjaMonkeyStudio/Getty Images

CHAPTER 11

Populations with Special Health Needs

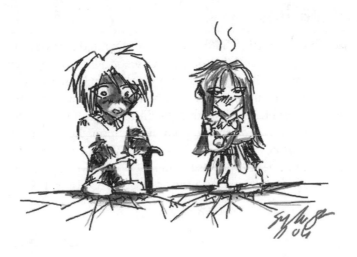

▶ Introduction

Differences in health that are avoidable and unjust—referred to as health disparities or health inequities—are greater in the United States than in other developed countries, such as Canada or high-income European countries (Avendano et al., 2009; Lasser et al., 2006; Siddiqi et al., 2015; van Hedel et al., 2014). Certain population groups in the United States either face greater barriers than the general population in accessing timely and needed health care services or have special health-related issues that may go unaddressed. Members of these groups, who face a greater risk of poor physical, psychological, and social health (Aday, 1994), may be referred to as underserved populations, medically underserved, medically disadvantaged, underprivileged, or vulnerable populations; marginalized groups; or American underclasses. The causes of their vulnerability are largely attributable to inequalities in social, economic, health, and geographic conditions. Special population groups encompass racial and ethnic minorities, uninsured women and children, persons living in rural areas, the homeless, the mentally ill, the chronically ill and disabled, and individuals with human immunodeficiency virus/acquired immunodeficiency syndrome (HIV/AIDS). This chapter defines these population groups, describes their health needs, and summarizes the major challenges that they typically experience in the United States.

▶ Framework to Study Vulnerable Populations

The vulnerability model (**FIGURE 11.1**) is an integrated approach to studying vulnerability. *Vulnerability* denotes susceptibility to negative events that result in poor health or illness. Poor health can be manifested physically, psychologically, and socially. Health needs are greater for individuals who experience problems along multiple dimensions, because poor health along one dimension is often compounded by poor health along others. Vulnerability does not represent a personal deficiency inherent to certain populations, but rather the effects of interactions between multiple factors over which individuals may have little or no control (Aday, 1999).

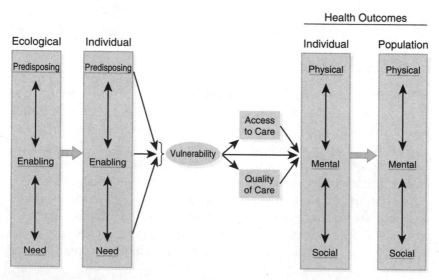

FIGURE 11.1 General Framework to Study Vulnerable Populations

EXHIBIT 11.1 Predisposing, Enabling, and Need Characteristics of Vulnerability

- Predisposing characteristics
  - Racial/ethnic characteristics
  - Gender and age (women and children)
  - Geographic location (rural health)
- Enabling characteristics
  - Insurance status (uninsured)
  - Homelessness
- Need characteristics
  - Mental health
  - Chronic illness/disability
  - HIV/AIDS

Vulnerability is determined by a convergence of (1) predisposing, (2) enabling, and (3) need characteristics at both individual and ecological (contextual) levels (**EXHIBIT 11.1**). Not only do these characteristics act synergistically to determine individuals' access to health care, but they also ultimately influence individuals' risk of contracting illness or recovering from an existing illness. Individuals with multiple risks (i.e., a combination of two or more vulnerability traits) typically experience poorer access to care, lower-quality care, and inferior health status than those with fewer vulnerability traits.

Understanding vulnerability as a combination or convergence of disparate factors is preferred to studying individual factors separately, because vulnerability best captures reality when it is defined as a convergence of risks. Furthermore, this approach reflects the concurrence of risk factors and underscores the belief that it is difficult to address disparities in one risk factor without also addressing disparities in others.

The vulnerability model presented here has a number of distinctive characteristics. First, it is a comprehensive model, including both individual and ecological attributes of risk. Second, it is a general model, focusing on the attributes of vulnerability for the total population rather than for subpopulations. Although there are individual differences in exposure to risks, a number of common, cross-cutting traits affect all vulnerable populations. Third, the model emphasizes the effects of experiencing multiple vulnerability traits, which lead to cumulative consequences.

▶ Predisposing Characteristics

Attributes that predispose individuals to vulnerability include demographic characteristics, belief systems, and social structure variables.

These attributes are associated with social position, access to resources, health behaviors, and variations in health status, which individuals have relatively little control over. Unfortunately, these attributes may lead to discrimination on account of race, gender, financial status, sexual preference, or other traits. The following subsections discuss some of these predisposing characteristics, including race and ethnicity, gender, age, and geographic distribution.

Racial/Ethnic Minorities

The main categories for race recognized by the U.S. Census Bureau are white, black or African American, Hispanic or Latino, American Indian or Alaska Native, Asian, Native Hawaiian or other Pacific Islander, and a nondescript category called "some other race." *Asian* refers to persons originating from the Far East, Southeast Asia, or the Indian subcontinent, including those from Cambodia, China, India, Japan, Korea, Malaysia, Pakistan, the Philippine Islands, Thailand, or Vietnam. *Native Hawaiians or other Pacific Islanders* include persons originating from Hawaii, Guam, Samoa, or other Pacific Islands. *American Indian or Alaska Natives* include persons originating from North and South America (including Central America) who maintain tribal affiliation or community attachment. Nearly 30% of the U.S. population is made up of minorities: black or African American (13.3%), Hispanic or Latino (17.8%), Asian (5.7%), Native Hawaiian or other Pacific Islander (0.2%), American Indian and Alaska Native (1.3%). In addition, 2.6% of the U.S. population identify themselves as being of two or more races (U.S. Census Bureau, 2017).

Significant differences exist across the various racial/ethnic groups on health. Indeed, minority race and ethnicity often serve as a proxy for other factors that are correlated with health status and health care experiences, such as socioeconomic status, language ability, or cultural behaviors. Evidence suggests that racial/ethnic minorities generally have poorer access to health care, receive poorer quality care, and experience worse health outcomes (**EXHIBIT 11.2**).

EXHIBIT 11.2 Racial and Ethnic Disparities

Black Americans

- More likely than whites to be economically disadvantaged.
- Shorter life expectancies than whites.
- Higher age-adjusted death rates than whites for leading causes of death.
- Higher rates of premature death (death before age 75 years) from stroke and coronary heart disease than whites (Centers for Disease Control and Prevention [CDC], 2013).

- More than double the infant mortality rate compared to non-Hispanic white women in both 2005 and 2008 (CDC, 2013).
- More likely than whites to report fair or poor health status.
- Males more likely than white males to smoke cigarettes (National Center for Health Statistics [NCHS], 2015).
- 665% higher homicide rates compared to non-Hispanic whites (CDC, 2013).

Hispanic Americans

- Nearly one-third have less than a ninth-grade education level.
- Among children and adolescents from ages 2 to 19, Hispanics have the highest prevalence of obesity (21.9%) (NCHS, 2016).
- Approximately one-fourth of families live below the poverty line (NCHS, 2015).
- More likely to be uninsured and underinsured than non-Hispanic whites.
- AIDS is the leading cause of death.
- Homicide rate remains the second leading cause of death for young males (NCHS, 2015).
- Among individuals 18 years or older, a higher proportion of Hispanics than whites are overweight or obese.
- Alcohol use is 43.0% among Hispanics (NCHS, 2015).
- Higher homicide rates compared to non-Hispanic whites (CDC, 2013).

Asian Americans

- Bipolar distribution of education, income, and health status.
- The Asian/Pacific Islander category is extremely heterogeneous, encompassing 21 subgroups with different health profiles.
- In 2010, median family income was $64,308; a higher percentage (12.1%) live in poverty compared to non-Hispanic whites (9.9%) (DeNavas-Walt et al., 2011).
- Cambodian refugees have extremely high rates of posttraumatic stress disorder, dissociation, depression, and anxiety.
- As a whole, Asian/Pacific Islanders have the lowest smoking rates in the United States, but certain groups have higher smoking rates:
  - 92% of Laotians
  - 71% of Cambodians
  - 65% of Vietnamese (Yoon & Chien, 1996)
- Korean Americans have a 5 times greater incidence of stomach cancer and an 8 times greater incidence of liver cancer compared to whites.

American Indians and Alaska Natives

- Poverty is associated with a high injury-related mortality rate among these children.
- The rate of death due to alcohol is 7 times greater and the suicide rate is 3.5 times greater than the national averages (Pleasant, 2003).
- Higher rates for drug-induced deaths than among non-Hispanic whites (CDC, 2013).
- Higher homicide rates compared to non-Hispanic whites (CDC, 2013).
- Two to five times higher motor vehicle–related death rates as compared to other races/ethnicities (CDC, 2013).

One of the most consistent findings across decades of research is that minorities have poor access to health services compared to their white counterparts, even after taking into account insurance, socioeconomic, and health status. Various studies have documented that minority Americans experience higher rates of illness and mortality than white Americans. Disparities in health exist between white and nonwhite Americans in measures of perceived health status as well as in traditional indicators of health such as infant mortality rate, general population mortality rate, and birth weight.

Racial/ethnic disparities in quality of care for persons with access to the health care system are equally concerning. A 2002 report from the Institute of Medicine (renamed the National Academy of Medicine in 2015) identified more than 175 studies documenting racial/ethnic disparities in the diagnosis and treatment of various conditions, even when controlled for socioeconomic status, insurance status, site of care, stage of disease, comorbidity, and age, among other potential confounders. These disparities are observed in other empirical studies and reviews of the utilization of preventive and clinical procedures, such as diagnostic and therapeutic procedures (Bolorunduro et al., 2013; Harris et al., 1997), prescription of medication for pain control (Wieder et al., 2014), surgical treatment of lung cancer (Polednak, 2001), referral to renal transplantation (Joshi et al., 2012), treatment of heart failure (Dickson et al., 2015), and the utilization of specific services covered by Medicare, such as immunizations and mammograms (Lees et al., 2005; Mendez-Luck et al., 2016).

One of the most commonly used measures of access to care is whether a person has a regular or usual source of care. A *usual source of care* may be defined as a single provider or place where patients obtain, or can obtain, the majority of their health care. Having a usual source of care is associated with greater coordination of care.

Disparities persist not only in mortality rates, but also in morbidity rates, exposure to environmental hazards, and social determinants of health. Additionally, disparities persist not only between racial/ethnic groups, as most commonly discussed, but also between genders, across socioeconomic strata, and between rural and urban populations. Yet, the majority of federal initiatives have primarily served to draw national attention to racial disparities in health care (see the examples in **EXHIBIT 11.3**). Although federal programs are designed to address the specific needs of minorities, they still use a somewhat fragmented approach to addressing disparities in minority health and health care.

A report from the Agency for Healthcare Research and Quality (AHRQ, 2015) shows that the nation has made progress in improving the health care delivery system to achieve the Triple Aims of better care, smarter spending, and healthier people. Even so, more work needs to be done, particularly in addressing disparities in health care.

EXHIBIT 11.3 Selected Federal Programs to Eliminate Racial and Ethnic Disparities

U.S. Department of Health and Human Services' (DHHS) *Action Plan to Reduce Racial and Ethnic Health Disparities* (2011)

- To reduce disparities in six key areas—infant mortality, cancer screening and management, cardiovascular disease, diabetes, HIV/AIDS, and immunizations—through new opportunities such as the Affordable Care Act, *Healthy People 2020*, Let's Move!, the National HIV/AIDS Strategy, HHS Strategic Action Plan to End the Tobacco Epidemic, Efforts to Reduce Disparities in Influenza Vaccination, and Interagency Working Group on Environmental Justice (DHHS, 2011)

U.S. Office of Minority Health (1985)

- Mission is to improve the health of racial and ethnic minority populations through the development of effective health policies and programs that help eliminate disparities in health (DHHS, 2011)
- Program was launched by the Centers for Disease Control and Prevention in 1999
- Supports the goals of *Healthy People 2020* to eliminate racial disparities in health and health care

Minority Health Initiative (1992)

- Launched by the Office for Research on Minority Health at the National Institutes of Health to improve the national research agenda on minority health issues and strengthen the national commitment and responsiveness to the health and training needs of minority Americans

Indian Health Service

- An agency within the U.S. Department of Health and Human Services with the mission to be the principal advocate and provider of health care services to American Indians and Alaska Natives

Migrant Health Center Program

- Established by the Migrant Health Act (1962) to provide medical and support services to migrant farm workers and their families

Communities Putting Prevention to Work (CPPW)

- Funded by the CDC, the American Recovery and Reinvestment Act, and the Affordable Care Act, with the aim of supporting policy and environmental strategies in 50 communities to address obesity and tobacco use (DHHS, 2011)

Administration of Children and Families Head Start Program

- Serves to promote social and cognitive childhood development through education, health, nutritional, social, and other services for enrollees (DHHS, 2011)

Healthy Start

- Established by the National Institutes of Health to address disparities in the burden of asthma among minority children and children living in poverty (DHHS, 2011)

Women and Children

Although women in the United States now enjoy a life expectancy almost five years longer than that of men, they suffer greater morbidity and poorer health outcomes compared to their male counterparts (NCHS, 2017b). Women also have a higher prevalence of certain health problems than men over the course of their lifetimes. Compared to men of comparable age, women develop more acute and chronic illnesses, resulting in a greater number of short- and long-term disabilities (National Institutes of Health [NIH], 1992; NCHS, 2016). Specifically, women are more likely than men to have obesity or hypertension (NCHS, 2017b). Hospitalized women have higher mortality rates due to heart attacks than men (AHRQ, 2014). Women also have higher cholesterol levels than men at older ages (**FIGURE 11.2**). Women represent the fastest-growing population diagnosed with AIDS as well.

Pronounced health differences between men and women also exist in mental illness. For example, anxiety disorders and major depression affect twice as many women as men (Rodin & Ikovics, 1990). Adolescent females have a higher prevalence of depression, eating disorders, and suicidal thoughts and attempts than adolescent males. However, although females are more likely to have suicidal thoughts than males, overall males have suicide rates that are four times as high as those in women (AHRQ, 2014; Crosby et al., 2011).

The mission of the Office of Research on Women's Health—located under the NIH within the U.S. Department of Health and Human Services—is to stimulate, coordinate, and implement a comprehensive women's health agenda on research, service delivery, and education across the DHHS and other government agencies.

Children's health has unique aspects in the delivery of health care, reflecting children's developmental vulnerability, dependency, and differential patterns of morbidity and mortality. *Developmental vulnerability* refers to the rapid and cumulative physical and emotional changes that characterize childhood, and the potential effects that illness, injury, or untoward family and social circumstances can have on a child's life-course trajectory. *Dependency* refers to the special circumstances that children face that require others to recognize and respond to their health needs. Children depend on their parents, school officials, caregivers, and sometimes neighbors to discover their need for health care, seek health care services on their behalf, authorize treatment, and comply with recommended treatment regimens. These relationships can affect the utilization of health services by children.

Children are increasingly affected by a broad and complex array of conditions that were not very prevalent among previous generations, collectively referred to as *new morbidities*. These new morbidities

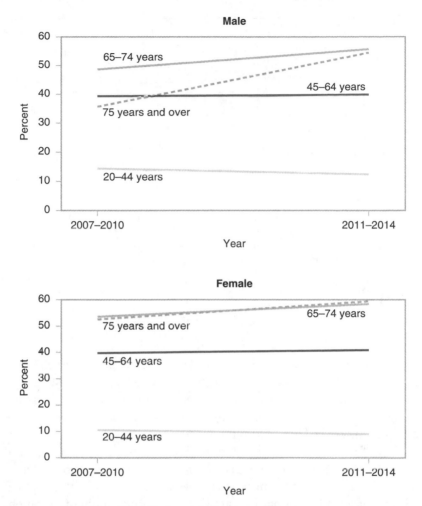

FIGURE 11.2 High Serum Total Cholesterol: Men Versus Women

Data from Centers for Disease Control and Prevention, National Center for Health Statistics. 2017. Health, United States, 2016. Hyattsville, MD. Table 55.

include drug and alcohol abuse, obesity, family and neighborhood violence, emotional disorders, and learning problems. **FIGURE 11.3** provides data on obesity among children. Addressing such conditions requires a continuum of comprehensive services that includes multidisciplinary assessment, treatment, rehabilitation, and community-based prevention strategies.

Geographic Distribution: Rural Health

Poverty is a common dimension of life in rural America. The median household income of rural residents is, on average, $1,910 less than that of their urban counterparts, and 13% of rural children live in poverty

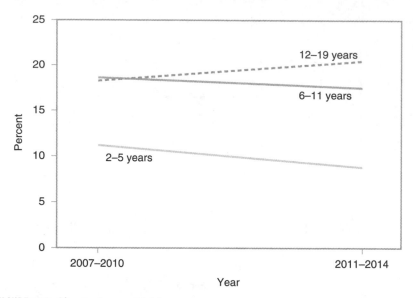

FIGURE 11.3 Obesity Among Children

Data from Centers for Disease Control and Prevention, National Center for Health Statistics. Health, United States, 2016. Hyattsville, MD. 2017, Table 59.

(Bishaw & Posey, 2016). Rural residents face a lack of public health infrastructure and poorer access to health care (Davis et al., 2010). Moreover, rural communities experience an increased burden of heart disease, stroke, diabetes, mental health disorders, tobacco use, and substance abuse (Gamm et al., 2003; Newkirk & Damico, 2014).

One dimension of the barriers to health care access among rural residents is the geographic maldistribution of health care professionals. An estimated 51 million Americans (approximately one-fifth of the total U.S. population) live in places classified as nonmetropolitan, of whom more than 20 million live in areas designated as having primary health care provider shortages. According to the National Rural Health Association, only 10% of all practicing physicians are based in rural areas. Their low population density makes it difficult for such communities to attract physicians and for physicians to establish financially viable practices. Rural residents have particularly low rates of access to specialist physicians.

As a result of these factors, rural populations face greater barriers in access to care. In turn, various measures have been undertaken to improve access to care in rural America, including the promotion of the National Health Service Corps, the designation of health professional shortage areas and medically underserved areas, the development of community and migrant health centers, and the passage of the Rural Health Clinics Act.

▶ Enabling Characteristics

Enabling characteristics include socioeconomic status, individual assets, and various mediating factors. *Socioeconomic status* is associated with social position, access to resources, and variations in health status (e.g., income, education, employment status, and occupation). Individual assets, or human capital, contribute to an individual's ability to be economically self-sufficient (e.g., possessing inheritance, wealth, or certain skills). *Mediating factors* are associated with the use of health care services (e.g., health insurance, access to health care, quality of health care). The following section discusses enabling characteristics such as insurance status and homelessness.

The Uninsured

Even though a large percentage of previously uninsured people have received health insurance coverage under the Affordable Care Act (ACA), a significant number of Americans remain uninsured. In general, uninsured individuals are likely to be poorer and less educated than insured individuals, and tend to work in part-time jobs and/or be employed by small firms. The uninsured also tend to be younger (age 25 to 40 years), because most of the elderly (age 65 and older) are covered by Medicare. Ethnic minorities are also more likely to lack health insurance.

Uninsured persons face greater barriers to accessing essential health care and are more likely to report delays in seeking essential medical care or dental care (**FIGURE 11.4** and **FIGURE 11.5**). The plight of the

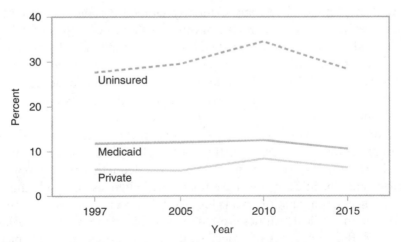

FIGURE 11.4 Delay in Seeking Needed Medical Care by Insurance Status

Data from Centers for Disease Control and Prevention, National Center for Health Statistics. Health, United States, 2016. Hyattsville, MD. 2017, Table 63.

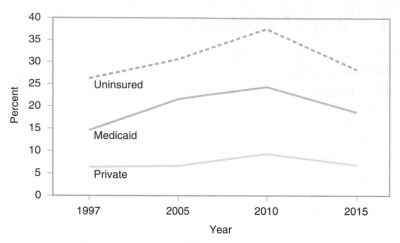

FIGURE 11.5 Delay in Seeking Needed Dental Care by Insurance Status

Data from Centers for Disease Control and Prevention, National Center for Health Statistics. Health, United States, 2016. Hyattsville, MD. 2017, Table 63.

uninsured also affects the insured. For example, community hospitals provide uncompensated care to the uninsured through emergency care; since 2000, hospitals of all types have provided more than $538 billion in uncompensated care to their patients (American Hospital Association, 2016). Much of this cost is currently shared by Medicaid, federal grants to nonprofit hospitals, and charitable organizations, although these costs are likely to be (at least partly) passed on to society if the level of uncompensated care remains the same.

Homelessness

Across the United States, approximately 549,928 people are homeless on a given night. More than 20% of this population consists of families with children or unaccompanied children and youth (U.S. Department of Housing and Urban Development, 2016). War veterans comprise approximately 10.5% of this population. Single women account for nearly 17% of the U.S. homeless adult population. Approximately 26% of all homeless persons have a severe mental illness, yet only 5% to 7% require institutionalization; the rest can live in the community with the appropriate help (National Coalition for the Homeless, 2007a, 2007b).

The homeless face several barriers to adequate and appropriate health care. Specifically, they have financial challenges and problems in satisfying eligibility requirements for health insurance. Accessible transportation to medical facilities is often unavailable to them. The homeless usually suffer from a lack of proper sanitation, do not have a stable place to store medications safely, and are unable to obtain the proper food for the medically indicated diet necessary to treat conditions such as diabetes or hypertension. In addition, the homeless suffer from a high prevalence of untreated acute and chronic medical, mental health, and substance abuse problems. Such persons are also at a greater risk of assault and victimization, as well as exposure to harsh environmental elements.

▶ Need Characteristics

Need attributes of individuals include their self-perceived or professionally evaluated health status and quality-of-life indicators. Self-perceived or professionally evaluated health status refers to the individual's own beliefs about his or her physical and mental health status or the diagnoses of disease made by health professionals, respectively. *Quality-of-life indicators* include such factors as the ability to perform instrumental activities of daily living, social limitations, cognitive limitations, and limitations in the ability to complete work, housework, or schoolwork.

Certain subpopulation groups are at higher health risks. These potential threats include risks to physical health (e.g., high-risk mothers and infants, chronically ill and disabled individuals, and persons with HIV/AIDS), mental health (e.g., the mentally ill and disabled, alcohol or substance abusers, the suicide- or homicide-prone), and social well-being (e.g., abusive families, the homeless, and immigrants and refugees).

Mental Health

Mental disorders are common psychiatric illnesses that affect both adults and children; they represent a serious public health problem in the United States. According to national studies, the most common mental disorders include phobias, substance abuse (including alcohol and drug dependence), and affective disorders (including depression). Schizophrenia is considerably less common, affecting approximately 1.1% of the U.S. population.

Mental illness ranks second, after ischemic heart disease, as a leading nationwide burden on health and productivity. According to 2014 data, an estimated 17.9% of the U.S. adult population has at least one diagnosable mental disorder in any given year. Only 41% of persons with a disorder receive any treatment (Substance Abuse and Mental Health Services Administration, 2016). Serious mental illness costs the United States an estimated $193.2 billion in lost earnings annually. Mood disorders, including major depression, dysthymic disorder, and bipolar disorder, are the third leading cause of hospitalization in the United States for both youth and adults. Mental illness is a risk factor for death from suicide, cardiovascular disease, and cancer. In addition, mental health problems are frequently associated with social problems. For example, due to the easy access to guns in the United States, persons with mental health issues often contribute to gun violence in both public and private settings.

Most mental health services are provided in the general medicine sector—a concept described by Regier and colleagues (1988) as the de facto mental health service system—rather than through formal mental health specialist services. The de facto mental health service system combines specialty mental health services with general counseling services, such as those provided in primary care settings, nursing homes, and community health centers by ministers, counselors, self-help groups, families, and friends. The U.S. mental health system is composed of two subsystems— one primarily for individuals with insurance coverage or private funds and the other for those persons without private means of coverage.

Chronic Illness/Disability

One of the greatest challenges for health systems globally in the 21st century is the increasing burden of chronic diseases and their resulting disabilities. An illness is considered chronic if there is a disease or injury with long-term (i.e., noticed for 3 months or more) conditions or symptoms. Other illnesses—namely, congenital anomalies, asthma, diabetes, and heart disease—are classified as chronic by the National Center for Health Statistics, regardless of their duration (NCHS, 1999, p. 5). Chronic illness and disability also pose unique challenges to a health care system that is primarily focused on treating acute illness.

In its report on the global challenges of chronic diseases, the World Health Organization (WHO) noted that noncommunicable conditions— including cardiovascular diseases, diabetes, cancers, and chronic respiratory diseases—accounted for nearly two-thirds of deaths worldwide (WHO, 2011). The most recent Global Burden of Disease Study (2010) provides further documentation of the continued shift from communicable to noncommunicable diseases around the world, and from premature death to years lived with disability (Murray et al., 2012). Related research indicates the scope of and key risk factors causing these global trends, including high blood pressure, tobacco use and second-hand smoke exposure, high body mass index (BMI), physical inactivity, excessive alcohol use, and diets low in fruits and vegetables and high in sodium and saturated fats (e.g., artificial trans fats) (Lee et al., 2012; Lim et al., 2012; Murray et al., 2012).

The Institute of Medicine reported that the United States is less healthy in key areas—including obesity, diabetes (**FIGURE 11.6**), heart disease, chronic lung disease, and disability—as compared with 16 high-income or similarly developed countries (Committee on Population, National Research Council, 2013; National Research Council & Institute of Medicine, 2013; Woolf

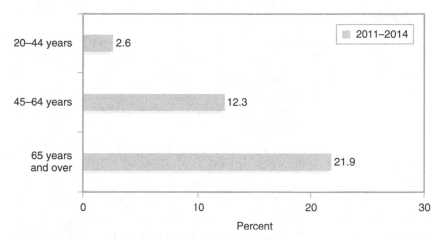

FIGURE 11.6 Diabetes Prevalence in the United States

Data from Centers for Disease Control and Prevention, National Center for Health Statistics. Health, United States, 2016. Hyattsville, MD. 2017, Table 40. 2015, Table 44.

& Aron, 2013). Most Americans are vulnerable to *chronic illness* and disability during their lifetime. Almost half of all Americans currently have at least one chronic condition, and chronic diseases are responsible for 7 of 10 deaths in the United States every year—deaths that are largely attributable to preventable illnesses. Tobacco use, physical inactivity, poor nutrition or diet, excessive alcohol consumption, uncontrolled high blood pressure, and hyperlipidemia contribute to the major chronic disease killers—namely, cardiovascular disease, cancer, diabetes, and chronic obstructive pulmonary disease (CDC, 2010a; Mokdad et al., 2010).

Moreover, people with lower education or income, of specific races or ethnic backgrounds, and in specific geographical locations, among other factors, are disproportionately affected by chronic diseases, often as a result of social disadvantages and vulnerability (Braveman et al., 2011). For example, death rates from stroke are highest in the southeastern states; smoking prevalence is highest in certain Native American tribes, particularly in the northern Plains; cardiovascular disease death rates are highest in African Americans; and obesity rates are highest in persons with low education or low income (Frieden, 2013).

Chronic diseases and noncommunicable conditions are increasingly common, costly, and debilitating. In 2010, total spending for the Medicare population (largely people age 65 years and older) was over $300 billion, with almost all (93%) of that spending going towards support for people with two or more chronic conditions. Similarly, lost productivity from chronic diseases, other chronic conditions, and their risk factors is associated with enormous costs for both those remaining in the workforce and those who prematurely exit the workplace due to disability (DeVol & Bedroussian, 2007).

HIV/AIDS

AIDS is caused by infection with HIV, a retrovirus that represses the immune system. Certain widely recognized risk factors promote the transmission of HIV, including male-to-male sexual contact, male-to-female sexual contact, drug use by injection, exposure to contaminated blood, and perinatal transmission from mother to infant during pregnancy, delivery, or breastfeeding.

At the end of 2015, an estimated 1.1 million persons age 13 and older were living with HIV infection in the United States, including an estimated 162,500 (15%) persons whose infections had not been diagnosed (CDC, 2017). Reporting and surveillance efforts have been more successful in recent years; more people infected with HIV know their positive status and a higher numbers of cases are being reported to the CDC. This trend can largely be traced to increased and more widespread HIV testing.

With the advent of combination antiretroviral therapy, AIDS surveillance data no longer reflects trends in HIV transmission because such therapy has been effective in delaying the progression of HIV to AIDS (CDC, 1999). Advancements in diagnosis and treatment have led to an increase in the number of people living with HIV/AIDS, although the incidence of new cases has remained relatively stable (CDC, 2010b).

The average cost of antiretroviral therapy is at least $15,000 per year, making treatment difficult for many patients in the United States to obtain and keeping it out of reach of patients in developing countries, where more than 90% of new HIV infections occur (Long et al., 2010). Some patients temporarily quit treatment because the complicated drug regimen requires the coordination of many pills and doses, making it easier to skip medications or doses. Other problems associated with HIV in the United States include issues related to urban home health care; HIV infection in rural communities, children, and women; lack of HIV prevention programs; late diagnosis; general discrimination; and the need for more HIV/AIDS-related research and health care provider training.

▶ Eliminating Disparities

Health disparities are not inevitable; actions that reduce social disadvantages can also reduce gaps in health outcomes, quality of care, and access to care. For example, progress in reducing health inequities between blacks and whites was made in the late 1960s and 1970s after the passage of major civil rights legislation (Almond et al., 2006; Kaplan et al., 2008; Krieger et al., 2008). Recent data suggests that inequality in mortality has decreased among the young but increased among older adults (Currie & Schwandt, 2016).

Health insurance coverage also plays an important role in eliminating health care disparities. People without health insurance receive less care than those with health insurance, including preventive care and screening services (Baicker et al., 2013; Sommers et al., 2014), and their health may suffer as a result. Further efforts are needed to ensure coverage, including encouraging states to opt into Medicaid expansion and determining which areas have relatively low enrollment in health insurance exchanges and requiring targeted enrollment efforts.

Policies that improve the overall social and economic well-being of individuals and families will reverberate across a variety of health outcomes and help achieve health equity. Policies that enable individuals and families to cope with challenging periods and life events may be especially effective. Most countries support people for time spent in caring for family members, and the availability of sick leave and parental leave is associated with better health. Across 141 countries, neonatal, infant, and child mortality rates are lower in nations that offer longer paid maternal leave (Heymann et al., 2011).

The *Action Plan to Reduce Racial and Ethnic Health Disparities*, created by the DHHS, outlines goals and actions to reduce health disparities among racial and ethnic minorities in the United States. The *Action Plan* includes a continuous assessment of the impact of all policies and programs on racial and ethnic health disparities and promotes integrated approaches, evidence-based programs, and best practices to reduce disparities. The *Action Plan* builds on the foundation of the ACA and aligns with other programs and initiatives such as *Healthy People 2020* and the national HIV/AIDS strategy. The *Action Plan* has five main goals: (1) to transform health care; (2) to strengthen the nation's health and human services infrastructure and workforce; (3) to advance the health, safety, and well-being of the American people; (4) to advance scientific knowledge and innovation; and (5) to increase the efficiency, transparency, and accountability of health and human services programs.

The ACA also includes provisions for disparities reduction, data collection and reporting, quality improvement, and prevention. In addition, this law is expected to reduce health disparities by investing in prevention and wellness and giving individuals and families more control over their own care.

Other prominent public-sector initiatives to eliminate disparities are highlighted here:.

- One of the four overarching goals of the *Healthy People 2020* initiative is "to achieve health equity, eliminate disparities, and improve the health of all groups" (DHHS, 2010). The *Healthy People 2020* initiative will assess health disparities in the U.S. population by tracking rates of death, chronic and acute diseases, injuries, and other health-related behaviors for subpopulations defined by race, ethnicity, gender identity, sexual orientation, disability status or special health care needs, and geographic location.

- Home-visiting programs, especially during pregnancy and early childhood, have demonstrated multiple benefits.
- Programs such as Healthy Families America, Nurse–Family Partnership, and Parents as Teachers address threats to the social, emotional, and cognitive health of children of low-income families by assessing family needs, educating and supporting parents, and referring and coordinating services as needed. They can help parents and children to build better relationships, strengthen family support networks, and link families to community resources, although results have not been consistent across implementations (Olds, 2016).
- The Let's Move! initiative proposed to create a healthy start in life for children from pregnancy through early childhood, serve healthier food in schools, and increase physical activity.
- President Barack Obama's national HIV/AIDS strategy envisioned that the United States would become a place where new HIV infections are rare and when they do occur, every person—regardless of age, gender, race and ethnicity, sexual orientation, gender identity, or socioeconomic circumstances—would have unfettered access to high-quality, life-extending care, free from stigma and discrimination (National HIV/AIDS Strategy for the United States, 2010).
- The DHHS has announced a strategic action plan to end the tobacco epidemic.
- The DHHS has launched efforts to maximize vaccinations in targeted racial and ethnic minority groups through coordinated efforts as well as private–public partnerships.
- The Interagency Working Group on Environmental Justice under Executive Order 12898 charges each federal agency to identify and address disproportionately high adverse human health or environmental effects on minority and low-income populations.
- The Office of Minority Health (2010) has launched the National Partnership for Action to End Health Disparities.
- An earlier program, Vaccines for Children, implemented in 1994, was effective in reducing disparities in vaccination coverage among U.S. children.

High-burden chronic conditions—such as diabetes, hypercholesterolemia, hypertension, and obesity—can be addressed at both the individual and population levels through policy and environmental approaches to change the context of health behaviors, through early detection and better management in the health care system to improve outcomes, and through community programs linked to the health care system to slow disease progression, mitigate complications, and avert adverse outcomes. For people who have or who are at high risk for chronic conditions, community-deployed, evidence-based, disease self-management regimens can help improve their quality of life and reduce the number of health care visits needed to maintain good health (Administration on Aging, 2017). The combination of whole-population and individual approaches, including targeted resources and support for population subgroups with the greatest burden, can reduce the prevalence of chronic disease and narrow health disparities.

Over time, community-based and clinically based prevention strategies may be developed to address the root causes of chronic conditions such as social conditions and physical environments and manage their existing burden. These prevention strategies seek to create community conditions that support health, such as community water fluoridation and smoke-free air laws, and strengthen links between community settings and health care systems to ensure that patients and caregivers have the means to better manage their health outside the clinical setting (Pearson et al., 2013).

Collaborations between health care systems and public health efforts are needed to bundle strategies and interventions, address combinations of risk factors and conditions, create population-wide changes, help the most affected subgroups, and ensure implementation of measures undertaken in many sectors, including public–private partnerships where all stakeholders are involved. The magnitude of the chronic disease issue in the United States requires a sustained policy and program focused on high-value prevention targets that draw upon strengthened links between public health and clinical care. Historically, major improvements in population health were achieved through collaborations with other sectors, such as investments in water and sewage systems, and policies and regulations establishing housing and transportation safety standards (Cutler & Miller, 2005). The existing burden of chronic conditions underscores the urgent need to intensify upstream policy and environmental approaches to prevent chronic diseases by reducing tobacco use, improving nutrition, increasing physical activity, and strengthening community programs that are connected to clinical settings.

Furthermore, health care financing strategies can be employed to reduce health disparities. Traditional financing models in the United States deliver suboptimal population health outcomes, allow substantial health disparities to arise and persist, and exacerbate the burgeoning costs of medical care. Instead, payment mechanisms that value prevention over acute care should encourage providers to address social factors that drive the need for services (National Academies of Science, Engineering, and Medicine, 2016).

Public health surveillance data provide essential information to guide these strategies by measuring the burden of chronic diseases (i.e., downstream indicators), informing priority setting for interventions, and monitoring progress for the whole population and across population subgroups (Brownson & Bright, 2004; Wegner et al., 2010). Key risk factors and indicators of the epidemiology and burden of chronic diseases are monitored in surveillance and data systems at the state and national levels. For example, the Behavioral Risk Factor Surveillance System (BRFSS) measures the prevalence of lifestyle risk factors at the state level (Li et al., 2011), while the National Health and Nutrition Examination Survey (NHANES) and the National Health Interview Survey (NHIS) (Adams et al., 2011) measure the prevalence of selected chronic conditions and health indicators at the national level. These systems also allow monitoring of conditions and risk behaviors by education, income, race or ethnic origin, and other variables related to health disparities. The National Vital Statistics System (NVSS) measures national cause-specific death rates, and state vital records offices register statewide deaths that together produce national mortality data. Analyses of national survey data (Anderson, 2010) and, particularly for those age 65 years and older, Medicare fee-for-service claims data produce estimates of expenditures associated with chronic conditions.

▶ Conclusion

This chapter has examined the major characteristics of certain vulnerable U.S. population groups that face challenges and barriers in accessing health care services. These groups may be organized along predisposing, enabling, and need characteristics and include racial/ethnic minorities, children and women, persons living in rural areas, the homeless, the mentally ill, and individuals with HIV/AIDS. Current gaps between these groups and the rest of the population demonstrate the need for significant efforts to address the unique health concerns of vulnerable U.S. subpopulations.

References

1. Adams PF, et al. 2011. Summary health statistics for the U.S. population: National Health Interview Survey, *Vital Health Stat.* 10(2012):1–102.
2. Aday LA. 1994. Health status of vulnerable populations. *Ann Rev Public Health.* 15:487–509.
3. Aday LA. 1999. Vulnerable populations: A community-oriented perspective. In: Sebastian JG, Bushy A, eds. *Special populations in the community*. Gaithersburg, MD: Aspen, 313–330.
4. Administration on Aging. 2017. American Recovery and Reinvestment Act communities putting prevention to work: Chronic disease self-management program. https://www.federalgrantswire.com/arra---communities-putting-prevention-to-work -chronic-disease-self-management-program.html. Accessed April 16, 2018.

5. Agency for Healthcare Research and Quality (AHRQ). 2014. Healthcare quality and disparities in women: Selected findings from the 2010 national healthcare quality and disparities reports. Pub. No. 11-0005-1-EF. http://www.ahrq.gov/research/findings/nhqrdr/nhqrdr10/women.pdf. Accessed June 20, 2015.

6. Agency for Healthcare Research and Quality (AHRQ). 2015. 2014 national healthcare quality & disparities report: Executive summary. http://www.ahrq.gov/research/findings/nhqrdr/nhqdr14/exsumm.html. Accessed August 10, 2015.

7. Almond D, et al. 2006. *Civil rights, the war on poverty, and black–white convergence in infant mortality in the rural South and Mississippi.* MIT Department of Economics Working Paper 07-04.

8. American Hospital Association. 2016. Uncompensated hospital care costs. https://www.aha.org/statistics/2018-01-03-uncompensated-hospital-care-cost-fact-sheet-december-2017-update. Accessed April 16, 2018.

9. Anderson G. 2010. *Chronic care: Making the case for ongoing care.* Princeton, NJ: Robert Woods Johnson Foundation. http://www.rwjf.org/content/dam/web-assets/2010/01/chronic-care. Accessed December 11, 2017.

10. Avendano M, et al. 2009. Health disadvantage in US adults aged 50 to 74 years: A comparison of the health of rich and poor Americans with that of Europeans. *Am J Public Health.* 99(3):540–548.

11. Baicker K, et al. 2013. The Oregon experiment: Effects of Medicaid on clinical outcomes. *N Engl J Med.* 368(18):1713–1722.

12. Bishaw A, Posey KG. 2016, December 8. A comparison of rural and urban America: Household income and poverty. U.S. Census Bureau. https://www.census.gov/newsroom/blogs/random-samplings/2016/12/a_comparison_of_rura.html. Accessed December 11, 2017.

13. Bolorunduro OB, et al. 2013. Disparities in trauma care: Are fewer diagnostic tests conducted for uninsured patients with pelvic fracture? *Am J Surg.* 205(4):365–370. doi: 10.1016/j.amjsurg.2012.10.026.

14. Braveman PA, et al. 2011. Health disparities and health equity: The issue is justice. *Am J Public Health.* 101(suppl 1):S149–S155.

15. Brownson RC, Bright FS. 2004. Chronic disease control in public health practice: Looking back and moving forward. *Public Health Rep.* 119:230–238.

16. Centers for Disease Control and Prevention (CDC). 1999. Guidelines for national human immunodeficiency virus case surveillance, including monitoring for human immunodeficiency virus infection and acquired immunodeficiency syndrome. *MMWR.* 48(RR-13):2–7.

17. Centers for Disease Control and Prevention (CDC). 2010a. Chronic disease overview. https://www.cdc.gov/chronicdisease/overview/index.htm. Accessed August 10, 2015.

18. Centers for Disease Control and Prevention. 2010b. HIV in the United States: An overview. https://www.cdc.gov/hiv/statistics/overview/ataglance.html. Accessed April 16, 2018.

19. Centers for Disease Control and Prevention (CDC). 2013, November 22. Health disparities & inequalities report—United States, 2013. *MMWR.* 62(suppl 3):1–187.

20. Centers for Disease Control and Prevention (CDC). 2017. *HIV surveillance report: Diagnoses of HIV infection in the United States and dependent areas, 2016.* Vol. 28. Atlanta, GA: CDC.

21. Committee on Population, National Research Council. 2013. *U.S. health in international perspective: Shorter lives, poorer health. Report brief.* Washington, DC: National Academies Press.

22. Crosby AE, et al. 2011, October 21. Suicidal thoughts and behaviors among adults aged ≥ 18 years—United States, 2008–2009. *MMWR Surveill Summ.* 60(no. SS-13):1–22.

http://www.cdc.gov/mmwr/preview/mmwrhtml/ss6013a1.htm. Accessed April 6, 2018.

23. Currie J, Schwandt H. 2016. Inequality in mortality decreased among the young while increasing for older adults, 1990–2010. *Science.* May 6;352(6286):708-12. doi: 10.1126/science.aaf1437. Epub 2016 Apr 21.

24. Cutler D, Miller G. 2005. The role of public health improvements in health advances: The twentieth-century. *US Demography.* 42:1–22.

25. Davis JR, et al. 2010. The impact of disasters on populations with health and health care disparities. *Disaster Med Public Health Prep.* 4(1):30–38.

26. DeNavas-Walt C, et al. 2011. *Income, poverty, and health insurance coverage in the United States: 2010.* Washington, DC: U.S. Census Bureau, Current Population Reports, P60-239, U.S. Government Printing Office.

27. DeVol R, Bedroussian A. 2007. An unhealthy America: The economic burden of chronic disease charting a new course to save lives and increase productivity and economic growth. http://www.milkeninstitute.org/publications/view/321. Accessed April 16, 2018.

28. Dickson VV, et al. 2015. Racial differences in clinical treatment and self-care behaviors of adults with chronic heart failure. *J Am Heart Assoc.* 4(4). pii: e001561. doi: 10.1161/JAHA.114.001561.

29. Frieden TR. 2013. Centers for Disease Control and Prevention. CDC health disparities and inequalities report—United States, 2013. Foreword. *MMWR Surveill Summ.* 62(suppl 3):1–2.

30. Gamm LD, et al. 2003. *Rural Healthy People 2010: A companion document to Healthy People 2010.* Vol. 1. College Station, TX: Texas A&M University System Health Science Center, School of Rural Public Health.

31. Harris DR, et al. 1997. Racial and gender differences in use of procedures for black and white hospitalized adults. *Ethn Dis.* 7:91–105.

32. Heymann J, et al. 2011. Creating and using new data sources to analyze the relationship between social policy and global health: The case of maternal leave. *Public Health Rep.* 126:127–134.

33. Institute of Medicine. 2002. *Unequal treatment: Confronting racial and ethnic disparities in health care.* Washington, DC: National Academies Press.

34. Joshi S, et al. 2012. Review of ethnic disparities in access to renal transplantation. *Clin Transplant.* 2012 Jul-Aug;26(4):E337-43. doi: 10.1111/j.1399-0012.2012.01679.x. Epub 2012 Jul 9.

35. Kaplan GA, et al. 2008. Lifting gates, lengthening lives: Did civil rights policies improve the health of African American women in the 1960s and 1970s? In: *Making Americans healthier: Social and economic policy as health policy.* New York, NY: Russell Sage Foundation, 145–169.

36. Krieger N, et al. 2008. The fall and rise of US inequities in premature mortality: 1960–2002. *PLoS Med.* 5(2):e46.

37. Lasser KE, et al. 2006. Access to care, health status, and health disparities in the United States and Canada: Results of a cross-national population-based survey. *Am J Public Health.* 96(7):1300–1307.

38. Lee I-M, et al. 2012. For *The Lancet* Physical Activity Series Working Group. Effect of physical inactivity on major non-communicable diseases worldwide: An analysis of burden of disease and life expectancy. *Lancet.* 380:219–229.

39. Lees KA, et al. 2005. Comparison of racial/ethnic disparities in adult immunization and cancer screening. *Am J Prev Med.* 29(5):404–411.

40. Li C, et al. 2011. Centers for Disease Control and Prevention surveillance of certain health behaviors and conditions among states and selected local areas—behavioral risk factor surveillance system, United States, 2009. *MMWR Surveill Summ.* 60:1–250.

41. Lim SS, et al. 2012. A comparative risk assessment of burden of disease and injury attributable to 67 risk factors and risk factor clusters in 21 regions, 1990–2010: A systematic analysis for the Global Burden of Disease Study 2010. *Lancet.* 380:2224–2260.

42. Long EF, et al. 2010. The cost-effectiveness and population outcomes of expanded HIV screening and antiretroviral treatment in the United States. *Ann Intern Med.* 153:778–789.

43. Mendez-Luck CA, et al. 2016. Preventive services use among African American and Latino adult caregivers in South Los Angeles. *Med Care.* 54(12):1098–1104.

44. Mokdad AH, et al. 2004. Actual causes of death in the United States, 2000. *JAMA.* 291:1238–1245.

45. Murray CJL, et al. 2012. Disability-adjusted life-years (DALYs) for 291 diseases and injuries in 21 regions, 1990–2010: A systematic analysis for the Global Burden of Disease Study 2010. *Lancet.* 380:2197–2223.

46. National Academies of Science, Engineering, and Medicine. 2016. *Accounting for social risk factors in Medicare payment: Criteria, factors, and methods.* Washington, DC: The National Academies Press.

47. National Center for Health Statistics (NCHS). 1999. *Healthy People 2000 review, 1998–99.* Hyattsville, MD: Public Health Series, 163–167.

48. National Center for Health Statistics (NCHS). 2015. *Health, United States, 2014: With special feature on adults aged 55–64.* Hyattsville, MD: U.S. Department of Health and Human Services.

49. National Center for Health Statistics (NCHS). 2016. NBK367640 [bookaccession].

50. National Center for Health Statistics (NCHS). 2017b. *Women's health.* Hyattsville, MD: U.S. Department of Health and Human Services.

51. National Coalition for the Homeless. 2007a, August. NCH fact sheet #2: How many people experience homelessness? http://www.nationalhomeless.org/publications/facts/How_Many.pdf. Accessed August 10, 2015.

52. National Coalition for the Homeless. 2007b, August. NCH fact sheet #3: Who is homeless? http://www.nationalhomeless.org/publications/facts/Whois.pdf. Accessed August 10, 2015.

53. National HIV/AIDS Strategy for the United States. 2010. The White House. https://obamawhitehouse.archives.gov/administration/eop/onap/nhas. Accessed April 16, 2018.

54. National Institutes of Health, Office of Research on Women's Health. 1992. *Report of the National Institutes of Health: Opportunities for research on women's health* (NIH Publ. No. 92-3457). Washington, DC: Government Printing Office.

55. National Research Council, Institute of Medicine. 2013. *U.S. health in international perspective: Shorter lives, poorer health. Panel on understanding cross-national health differences among high-income countries.* Woolf SH, Aron L, eds., Committee on Population, Division of Behavioral and Social Sciences and Education, and Board on Population Health and Public Health Practice, Institute of Medicine. Washington, DC: National Academies Press, 1–9.

56. Newkirk V, Damico A. 2014, May 29. *The Affordable Care Act and insurance coverage in rural areas.* Kaiser Commission on Medicaid and the Uninsured. Washington, DC.

57. Olds D. 2016. Building evidence to improve maternal and child health. *Lancet.* 387(10014):105–107.

58. Pearson TA, et al. 2013. American Heart Association guide for improving cardiovascular health at the community level, 2013 update: Scientific statement for public health practitioners, healthcare providers, and health policy makers. *Circulation.* doi: 10.1161/CIR.0b013e31828f8a94.

59. Pleasant R. 2003. Minority health. In: *The Department of Health and Human Services: 50 years of service*. Washington, DC: U.S. Department of Health and Human Services, 92–95.

60. Polednak AP. 2001. Disparities in surgical treatment of early-stage non-small-cell lung cancer. *Yale J Biol Med.* 74(5):309–314.

61. Regier DA, et al. 1988. One month prevalence of mental disorders in the United States: Based on five epidemiologic catchment area sites. *Arch Gen Psychiatr.* 45(11):977–986.

62. Rodin J, Ikovics J. 1990. Women's health: Review and research agenda as we approach the 21st century. *Am Psychol.* 45:1018–1034.

63. Siddiqi A, et al. 2015. Cross-national comparison of socioeconomic inequalities in obesity in the United States and Canada. *Int J Equity Health.* 14(1):1.

64. Sommers BD, et al. 2014. Changes in mortality after Massachusetts health care reform: A quasi-experimental study. *Ann Intern Med.* 160(9):585–593.

65. Substance Abuse and Mental Health Services Administration. 2016. Results from the 2015 National Survey on Drug Use and Health: Mental health findings. https://www.samhsa.gov/samhsa-data-outcomes-quality/major-data-collections/reports-detailed-tables-2015-NSDUH. Accessed April 16, 2018.

66. U.S. Census Bureau. 2017. Quick facts: United States. https://www.census.gov/quickfacts/fact/table/US/PST045217. Accessed December 11, 2017.

67. U.S. Department of Health and Human Services (DHHS). 2010. *Healthy People 2020.* https://www.healthypeople.gov/sites/default/files/HP2020_brochure_with_LHI_508_FNL.pdf. Accessed August 11, 2015.

68. U.S. Department of Health and Human Services (DHHS). 2011. HHS action plan to reduce racial and ethnic health disparities: A nation free of disparities in health and health care. http://minorityhealth.hhs.gov/npa/files/Plans/HHS/HHS_Plan_complete.pdf. Accessed June 20, 2015.

69. U.S. Department of Housing and Urban Development. 2016. The 2016 Annual Homeless Assessment Report (AHAR) to Congress. https://www.hudexchange.info/resources/documents/2016-AHAR-Part-1.pdf. Accessed April 16, 2018.

70. U.S. Office of Minority Health. 2010. *Racial and ethnic approaches to community health.* Rockville, MD: U.S. Office of Minority Health.

71. van Hedel K, et al. 2014. The contribution of national disparities to international differences in mortality between the United States and 7 European countries. *Am J Public Health.* 105(4):e112–e119.

72. Wegner MV, et al. 2010. Chronic disease surveillance. In: Remington PL, et al., eds. *Chronic disease epidemiology and control.* 3rd ed. American Public Health Association, Washington DC.

73. Wieder R, et al. 2014. Prescription coverage in indigent patients affects the use of long-acting opioids in the management of cancer pain. *Pain Med.* 15(1):42–51. doi: 10.1111/pme.12238.

74. Woolf SH, Aron LY. 2013. The US health disadvantage relative to other high-income countries: Findings from a National Research Council/Institute of Medicine report. *JAMA.* 309:771–772.

75. World Health Organization (WHO). 2011. Global status report on non-communicable diseases 2010. http://www.who.int/nmh/publications/ncd_report2010/en/. Accessed April 16, 2018.

76. Yoon E, Chien F. 1996. Asian American and Pacific Islander health: A paradigm for minority health. *JAMA.* 275(9):736–737.

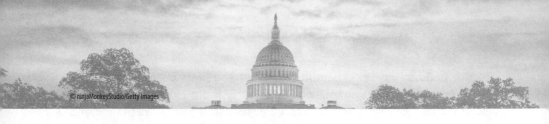

CHAPTER 12

Cost, Access, and Quality

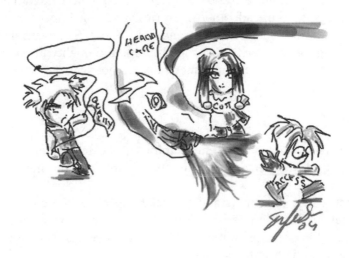

▶ Introduction

The effectiveness of a health care delivery system is typically evaluated in terms of cost, access, and quality. All three major outcomes of health care delivery continue to be considered by various stakeholders. Yet, unless costs are brought down to a reasonable level, any achievements in the other two domains will remain elusive, because cost, access, and quality are interrelated.

From a macro prospective, costs are commonly viewed in terms of national expenditures for health care. A widely used measure for national health expenditures is the proportion of its gross domestic product (GDP) that a country spends on the delivery of health care services. In simple terms, national health expenditures refer to the proportion of national income that a country spends on health care. From a micro perspective, health care costs refer to the cost of purchasing health insurance and the out-of-pocket costs incurred by individuals when they receive health care services. Costs must be contained at both the macro and micro levels. Increased access generally leads to higher utilization and, in turn, higher costs, assuming there are no significant structural changes in how health care is delivered (e.g., prevention versus treatment, primary care versus tertiary care, and community versus institutional orientation). High-quality care should also be the most cost-effective care. Hence, cost is an important factor in the evaluation of quality of health care services delivered.

This chapter discusses some key reasons for the dramatic rise in health care expenditures. Costs of health care in the United States are compared with those of other countries, and the impact of various cost-containment measures is examined. The U.S. government has played a significant role in cost containment and quality improvement, but access to health care by all Americans has not yet been achieved.

▶ Cost of Health Care

The term *cost* can carry different meanings in the delivery of health care, depending on the perspective one takes. Three distinct meanings are presented here.

First, when consumers and financiers speak of the cost of health care, they are usually referring to the price of health care, such as the physician's bill or the premiums that both employers and employees pay when purchasing health insurance.

Second, from a national perspective, health care costs refer to how much a nation spends on health care services, commonly referred to as *health care expenditures* or *health care spending*. These terms primarily reflect the consumption of economic resources in the delivery of health care. Such economic resources include health insurance, skills of health care professionals, organizations and institutions of health care delivery, pharmaceuticals, medical equipment and supplies, public health functions, and new medical discoveries. Because expenditures equal price multiplied by quantity ($E = P \times Q$), growth in health care spending can be accounted for by growth in the prices charged by providers as well as by increases in the utilization of services.

A third perspective is that of the providers. From their viewpoint, cost refers to staff salaries, capital costs for building and equipment, rental of space, purchase of supplies, and other costs of production.

It is useful to understand which factors drive costs, as this can help identify which costs can be controlled to ensure that health care is delivered at an optimal value.

▶ The High Cost of U.S. Health Care

Health care spending spiraled upward at double-digit rates during the 1970s due to the massive expansion in access to health care created by the Medicare and Medicaid programs in 1965. By 1970, U.S. government expenditures for health care services and supplies had grown by 140%, from $7.9 billion to $18.9 billion (National Center for Health Statistics [NCHS], 1996). During the 1980s, the growth rate began slowing down. Then, in the 1990s, medical inflation was finally brought under control to a single-digit rate of growth, mostly because medical care costs and utilization were controlled through managed care. The average annual rate of growth in health spending slowed to 5.7% between 1993 and 2000 as managed care proliferated; however, the growth rate then started to accelerate again. The recent economic recession slowed health care spending growth substantially, with only a 4.1% increase in 2008 and a 4.0% increase in 2009—the slowest growth rate in more than 50 years. Simultaneously, however, federal health spending increased as more people became eligible for benefits and government revenues declined, increasing spending from 37.6% of federal revenues in 2008 to 54.2% in 2009 (Martin et al., 2011). In 2015, total U.S. health care spending reached $3.2 trillion, or $9,990 per person (Centers for Medicare and Medicaid Services [CMS], 2015b, 2017). In 2016, 17.9% of the U.S. GDP was consumed by health care (CMS, 2017).

Trends in national health expenditures are commonly evaluated by comparing medical inflation to general inflation in the economy, measured by annual changes in the consumer price index and by comparing changes in national health spending to changes in the GDP. Typically, the rates of change in medical inflation have remained consistently above the rates of change in the consumer price index, and health care spending growth rates have consistently surpassed growth rates in the general economy. When health care spending grows at a faster rate than GDP, a growing share of the country's total economic resources is devoted to health care delivery.

TABLE 12.1 compares U.S. health spending with that of 30 other developed countries. In 2016, the United States spent $9,892 per capita on health—approximately $2,400 more than the country with the second highest spending, Luxembourg.

TABLE 12.1 Health Spending in Organization for Economic Cooperation and Development Countries

	Total Health Spending per Capita, 2016			GDP per Capita, 2016			Health Spending as a Percentage of GDP, 2016	
	U.S. $PPP	% of U.S. Level	AAG, 2009–2016 (%)	U.S. $PPP	% of U.S. Level	AAG, 2009–2016 (%)	% of GDP	% of U.S. Level
United States	9,892	100	2.1	57,591	100	1.5	17.2	100
Luxembourg	7,463	75.4	0.9	102,019	177.1	2.3	6.3	36.6
Norway	6,647	67.2	1.8	58,792	102.1	1.1	10.5	61.0
Switzerland	7,919	80.1	2.8	63,889	110.9	1.3	12.4	72.1
Austria	5,227	52.8	1	50,503	87.7	2.5	10.4	60.5
Iceland	4,376	44.2	1	50,012	86.8	1.4	8.6	50.0
Belgium	4,840	48.9	1	46,607	80.9	0.9	10.4	60.5
France	4,600	46.5	0.9	41,364	71.8	0.6	11	64.0
Canada	4,753	48.0	1.1	44,793	77.8	1.6	10.6	61.6
Germany	5,551	56.1	1.8	48,947	85.0	1.1	11.3	65.7

Australia	4,708	47.6	2.7	48,243	83.8	0.7	9.6	55.8
Denmark	5,205	52.6	0.3	49,012	85.1	0.6	10.4	60.5
Netherlands	5,385	54.4	1	50,540	87.8	0.5	10.5	61.0
Greece	2,223	22.5	–5	26,746	46.4	–3.7	8.3	48.3
Ireland	5,528	55.9	0.1	72,485	125.9	5.1	7.8	45.3
Sweden	5,488	55.5	0.9	48,905	84.9	1.8	11	64.0
United Kingdom	4,194	42.4	0.9	42,622	74.0	1.2	9.7	56.4
Italy	3,391	34.3	–0.3	38,370	66.6	–0.8	8.9	51.7
Japan	4,518	45.7	1.8	42,293	73.4	0.6	10.9	63.4
New Zealand	3,590	36.3	0.6	38,346	66.6	2.3	9.2	53.5
Finland	4,033	40.8	1	43,378	75.3	–0.5	9.3	54.1
Spain	3,248	32.8	0.3	36,318	63.1	–0.1	9	52.3
Portugal	2,734	27.6	–1.3	30,606	53.1	–0.5	8.9	51.7

(continues)

TABLE 12.1 Health Spending in Organization for Economic Cooperation and Development Countries *(continued)*

	Total Health Spending per Capita, 2016			GDP per Capita, 2016			Health Spending as a Percentage of GDP, 2016	
	U.S. $PPP	% of U.S. Level	AAG, 2009–2016 (%)	U.S. $PPP	% of U.S. Level	AAG, 2009–2016 (%)	% of GDP	% of U.S. Level
Czech Republic	2,544	25.7	0.1	34,753	60.3	1.1	7.3	42.4
Hungary	2,101	21.2	2.7	26,701	46.4	0.8	7.6	44.2
Korea	2,729	27.6	5.7	36,532	63.4	3.1	7.7	44.8
Slovak Republic	2,150	21.7	1.9	30,460	52.9	1.9	6.9	40.1
Poland	1,798	18.2	3.1	27,058	47.0	3.1	6.4	37.2
Mexico	1,080	10.9	1.1	18,535	32.2	2.2	5.8	33.7
Turkey	1,088	11.0	1.7	25,655	44.5	5.3	4.3	25.0
Organization for Economic Cooperation and Development Median	4,003	40.5	1.4	42,162	73.2	1.4	9	52.3

Abbreviations: AAG: annual average growth; PPP: purchasing power parity.
Data from Organization for Economic Cooperation and Development (OECD). OECD Statistics, https://stats.oecd.org. Accessed February 17, 2018.

▶ Reasons for High Health Care Costs

The rise in health care expenditures has been attributed to the complex interaction of many factors. General inflation in the economy is a prominent cause of health care spending, because it affects the cost of producing health care services through such tangibles as higher wages and costs of supplies. Apart from general inflation, numerous other factors influence medical cost inflation (**EXHIBIT 12.1**).

Third-Party Payment

Health care is among the few services for which a third party—not the consumer—pays the lion's share for most of the services used. Whether the government or a private insurance company foots the bill, individual patients pay a price that is far lower than the actual cost of the service (Altman & Wallack, 1996). As a result, the propensity to utilize greater quantities of health care than one would if services were fully paid out of pocket—moral hazard—leads to excessive utilization. Actually, the parties representing both demand (patient) and supply (provider) have little incentive to be cost-conscious when someone else is paying the bill.

Growth of Technology

In the adoption and diffusion of intensive medical procedures, the United States follows an early-start, fast-growth pattern (TECH Research Network, 2001). The introduction and intensive use of technology directly impacts the escalation of health care costs. Developing new technology is expensive, and research and development costs are included in the total health care expenditures. Once technology is developed, its mere availability creates demand for its use. The introduction of new technology raises consumer expectations about the ability of medical science to diagnose and treat disease and prolong life. Unsurprisingly, attempts to

---

EXHIBIT 12.1 Main Reasons for the High Cost of Health Care

- Third-party payment
- Growth of technology
- Increase in the elderly population
- Medical model of health care delivery
- Multipayer system and administrative costs
- Defensive medicine
- Waste and abuse
- Variations in practice

limit the diffusion of certain expensive technologies in the United States have proved largely unsuccessful. Medical technology assessment—that is, the systematic evaluation of new methods in medical care delivery in terms of their efficacy—still lags behind in development and remains unevenly applied.

Increase in the Elderly Population

During the past 100 years, life expectancy in the United States has increased significantly. Life expectancy at birth increased by almost 30 years, from 47.3 years in 1900 to nearly 78.8 years in 2015 (NCHS, 2017). The increased life expectancy of the aging baby boomer population has added to the notable increase in the total U.S. elderly population. The elderly consume more health care services compared to other age groups, incurring costs that are nearly three times as high as those for the general population. In 2007, the average medical expenses for a person 65 years or older amounted to $9,696 per person, compared to $3,499 per person for individuals younger than 65 (NCHS, 2010, p. 377). Personal health care spending for the 65 and older population was $18,988 per capita in 2012, more than 5 times greater than the spending per child ($3,552) and approximately 3 times the spending per working-age person ($6,632) (CMS, 2018).

Medical Model of Health Care Delivery

The *medical model* emphasizes medical intervention after a person has become sick, rather than focusing on prevention or lifestyle/behavior changes to promote health. Although health promotion and disease prevention are not the answer to every health problem, these principles have yet to be accorded their rightful place in the U.S. health care delivery system. Consequently, more costly health care resources must be used to treat many health problems that could have been prevented or delayed in onset.

Multipayer System and Administrative Costs

Administrative costs include costs associated with health insurance marketing and enrollment, contracting with providers, claims processing, utilization monitoring, and handling of denials and appeals. Because of the complexity inherent in a multipayer system, costs are often duplicated and account for as much as 25% of total health care expenditures in the United States. A single-payer health care system may have lower administrative costs.

Defensive Medicine

The U.S. health care delivery system is riddled with legal risks for providers that encourage the use of defensive medicine. The practice of *defensive medicine* involves tests and services that are not medically justified but, rather, performed or ordered by physicians to protect themselves against potential malpractice lawsuits. Unrestrained malpractice awards by the courts and increased malpractice insurance premiums for physicians significantly add to the cost of health care.

Waste and Abuse

Health care fraud is a major problem in Medicare and Medicaid programs. It may also occur when more services are provided than are medically necessary, or when services that were not actually provided are billed to third-party payers. The latter practice may entail billing for a higher-priced service than is actually delivered, or picking a more favorable diagnosis as in a diagnosis-related groups (DRG) payment scheme.

Practice Variations

The work of John Wennberg and others brought to light a disturbing aspect of physician behavior that accounted for wide variations in treatment patterns for similar patients. These differences in practice are referred to as *small-area variations*, in recognition of the fact that the observed differences in practice patterns were associated only with certain geographic areas of the country. Such a variation in practice intensity, which can be as great as twofold, cannot be explained by age, gender, race, pricing variations, demand inducements, or health status (Baucus & Fowler, 2002). Small-area variations signal gross inefficiencies in the U.S. health care delivery system because they increase costs without appreciably improving outcomes.

▶ Cost Containment

Even though rising health care expenditures may seem innocuous to some, they must be controlled for several reasons. First, rising health care costs mean that Americans must forgo other basic goods and services such as education, housing, road, public transportation, safety. Second, economic resources should be directed to their highest-valued uses, even though consumers decide how much to spend on purchasing a product or service based on their perception of its expected value (Feldstein, 1994, p. 13).

The United States has made many attempts to control health care spending, through a combination of government regulation and market-based competition. Most undertakings have met with limited success, mainly because implementing a system-wide cost-control initiative has not proved feasible in such a fragmented system. Cost-containment measures in the United States can be applied only in a piecemeal fashion and can affect only specific targeted sectors of the health care delivery system at one time. In contrast, national health care programs in other countries have *single-payer systems* in which effective centralized controls are feasible.

Another reason that cost-control efforts in the United States have not proved very successful is cost-shifting between programs and sectors. *Cost-shifting* refers to the ability of providers to make up for lost revenues in one area by increasing utilization or charging higher prices in other areas that are free of controls. Only system-wide controls can prevent cost-shifting.

Health Planning

Health planning refers to an undertaking by the government to align and distribute health care resources in order to achieve desired health outcomes for all people. Health planning employs supply-side rationing to control health care expenditures. This kind of central planning function does not fit well in a system that is largely private, without a central administrative agency to monitor the system. In the United States, the types of health care services, their geographic distribution, access to these services, and the prices charged by providers develop independently of any preformulated plans.

Price Controls

In 1971, President Richard Nixon created the Economic Stabilization Program, which limited the amount by which hospitals could raise their prices from year to year (Williams & Torrens, 1993). The Economic Stabilization Program controlled moderated influence on price increases for most medical services; however, the program placed no limits on the quantity of services or costs of production, and inflation returned to its pre-control levels once the controls were lifted (Altman & Eichenholz, 1976).

Perhaps the most important initiative to control prices for inpatient hospital care was the transformation of hospital Medicare reimbursement from a retrospective plan to a prospective system based on diagnosis-related groups as authorized by the Social Security amendments of 1983. This change reduced the growth in inpatient hospital spending, but had little impact on total per capita Medicare cost inflation; costs mainly shifted from the inpatient to the outpatient sector.

Another rate-setting mechanism was the Omnibus Budget Reconciliation Act of 1989, which helped establish a national Medicare fee schedule. With this fee schedule, known as the *resource-based relative value scale*, physicians are paid according to relative value units established for more than 7,000 covered services. In addition, a volume performance standard was implemented to contain the annual rate of growth in Medicare physician payments.

Peer Review

The term *peer review* refers to the general process of medical review of utilization and quality carried out directly by, or under the supervision of, physicians (Wilson & Neuhauser, 1985, p. 270). Under the Medicare program, peer review organizations were established in 1984 to determine whether care is reasonable, necessary, of adequate quality, and provided in the most appropriate setting. Now called quality improvement organizations, these statewide private organizations are composed of practicing physicians and other health care professionals who are paid by the federal government to review the care provided to Medicare beneficiaries. They can deny payment if the care does not meet certain standards.

Competitive Approaches

Competition refers to rivalry among sellers for customers (Dranove, 1993). In the context of health care delivery, health care providers try to attract patients who can choose from several different providers. Although competition more commonly refers to price competition, it may also be based on technical quality, amenities, access, or other factors (Dranove, 1993). In the United States, competitive reforms are preferred because of the growing interest in market-oriented approaches across many sectors of the economy during the Ronald Reagan presidency in the 1980s. Market-oriented reforms were accompanied by mounting cost-containment efforts in the private sector and the rise of managed care. Competitive strategies can be classified into four broad types: demand-side incentives, supply-side regulation, payer-driven price competition, and utilization controls.

Demand-side incentives refer to cost-sharing mechanisms that place a larger cost burden on consumers, thereby encouraging consumers to be more cost-conscious in selecting the insurance plan that best serves their needs and more judicious in utilizing services. *Supply-side regulation* typically refers to U.S. antitrust laws, which prohibit business practices that stifle competition among providers, such as price fixing, price discrimination, exclusive contracting arrangements, and mergers deemed anticompetitive by the Department of Justice. Such restrictions force health care organizations to be cost-efficient in order to survive. *Payer-driven price competition* occurs when employers shop for the best value in terms of the cost of premiums and the benefits package (competition among insurers), and when managed care organizations (MCOs) shop for the best value from providers of health services (competition among providers). In managed care, *utilization controls* have eliminated some of the unnecessary or inappropriate services provided to consumers by intervening in provider decisions, in an effort to ensure that only appropriate and necessary services are provided.

Chronic Disease Prevention and Management

Approximately 70% of all U.S. health care costs are generated by 10% of patients, who typically have one or more chronic diseases; thus, there is enormous potential for cost containment through improving the delivery of care for chronic conditions. So far, steering the system toward a preventive and chronic disease–oriented model has proved difficult. But new approaches, such as the medical home model and accountable care organizations, are being investigated as a means to nudge the health care system in this direction. There is also a notable regulatory push for providers to adopt electronic health records. The effectiveness of these approaches in controlling costs remains uncertain.

▶ Unequal Access to Health Care

In broad terms, *access* to care can be defined as the ability to obtain personal health services that are needed, affordable, convenient, acceptable, and effective in a timely manner. Access to appropriate health care services is one of the key determinants of health status, along with environment, lifestyle, and heredity factors. Access to care also helps assess the effectiveness of the care delivery system and is increasingly linked to quality of care and the efficient use of necessary services.

Although *access* is a familiar term used in both popular and academic media, it is associated with many differing concepts. It may refer to the availability or unavailability of a usual source of care for an individual, the actual utilization of health services, or the acceptability of particular services. **FIGURE 12.1** illustrates the system, provider, and individual characteristics that influence access to care.

Data on Access

Population-based surveys supported by federal statistical agencies are the major data sources for analyses on access to care. Large national

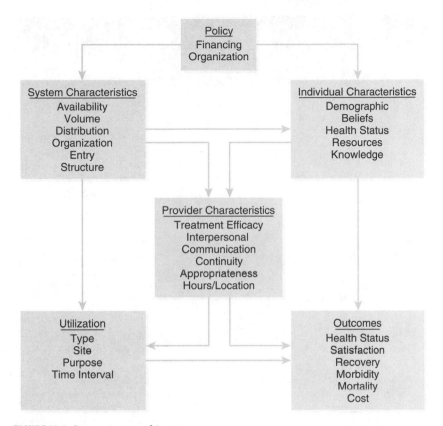

FIGURE 12.1 Determinants of Access

surveys such as the National Health Interview Survey and the Medical Expenditure Panel Survey are the leading data sources used to monitor access trends as well as other issues related to health care. The latter comprises a series of surveys on health care use and expenditures (e.g., inpatient, outpatient, and office-based care; dental care; and prescription medications), health insurance coverage, access to care, sources of payment, health status and disability, medical conditions, health care quality, and measures of socioeconomic and demographic characteristics.

Other well-known national surveys are listed in **TABLE 12.2**. They include national surveys and surveys on special topics.

The federal government also collects data on special topics such as community health centers (e.g., Bureau of Common Reporting Requirement and Uniform Data System), human immunodeficiency virus/acquired immunodeficiency syndrome (HIV/AIDS; e.g., HIV Cost and Services Utilization Study 1994–1998), managed care (e.g., Consumer Assessment of Health Plans Study 1996), and mental health (e.g., Mental Health Care Services Study). The Medicare Current Beneficiary Survey, the Medicare Statistical System, the Medicaid Data System, and

TABLE 12.2 Selected National Surveys of Health Care

Survey Title	Survey Author	Survey Function
Current Population Survey and Survey of Income and Program Participation	U.S. Census Bureau	Information on population characteristics
Area Resource File	Bureau of Health Professions	Pools information on characteristics of population and health care delivery system
National Health and Nutrition Examination Survey	NCHS	Information on demographics, prevalence of selected diseases, nutrition, and behavioral risk factors
National Hospital Discharge Survey	NCHS	Data on short-stay hospital discharges and utilization
Ambulatory Medical Care Survey	NCHS	Data on ambulatory medical encounters
National Hospital Ambulatory Medical Care Survey	NCHS	Data on ambulatory hospital encounters
National Nursing Home Survey	NCHS	Data on nursing homes and utilization, nursing home residents, and nursing home staff
Behavioral Risk Factor Survey	CDC	Data on health practices and behavioral risks of illness
National Health Provider Inventory	CDC	Data on inpatient facilities
Longitudinal Survey on Aging	CDC	Data on older individuals
National Nursing Home Survey Follow-Up	CDC	Data on nursing homes

| National Employer Health Insurance Survey | CDC | Data on insurance |
| Vital Statistics of the United States | CDC | Vital statistics information |

Abbreviations: CDC: Centers for Disease Control and Prevention; NCHS: National Center for Health Statistics.
Data from Centers for Disease Control and Prevention; NCHS, National Center for Health Statistics. http://www.cdc.gov /nchs/surveys.htm

the Medicaid Demonstration Projects (1983–1984, 1992–1996) have collected data relevant to Medicare and Medicaid.

States, associations, and research institutions also regularly collect data on topics of interest. Examples include state health services utilization data (e.g., all-payer hospital discharge data systems), state-managed care data (e.g., managed care encounter data), state Medicaid enrollee satisfaction data (e.g., Medicaid enrollee satisfaction surveys), physician data from the American Medical Association's Physician Masterfile, and hospital data from the American Hospital Association's Annual Survey of Hospitals 1946 to present. Examples of research institution–based initiatives include data collection on the health care delivery system (e.g., Center for Evaluative Clinical Sciences: Dartmouth Atlas of Health Care in the United States), women's health (e.g., Commonwealth Fund: Women's Health Survey 1993), minority health (e.g., Commonwealth Fund: Health Care Services and Minority Groups: A Comparative Survey of Whites, African Americans, Hispanics, and Asian Americans 1994), health insurance (e.g., Mathematica Policy Research/Robert Wood Johnson Foundation: Family Survey on Health Insurance 1993–1994), and access to care (e.g., Robert Wood Johnson Foundation National Access Surveys, Mathematica Policy Research: Access to Care Pilot Survey of Medicaid Beneficiaries 1994).

With the growth of managed care, encounter databases have become critical in recording and evaluating access to care. In addition to the federal government, private nonprofit research centers collect information on managed care. Examples include the National Health Maintenance Organization Census (1977 to the present, sponsored by Interstudy) and the Healthcare Effectiveness Data and Information Set (sponsored by the National Committee for Quality Assurance).

Access Disparities

Access to care is best predicted by race, income, and occupation. These three factors are interrelated: Individuals belonging to minority groups tend to be poorer, less educated, and more likely to work in job environments that pose greater health risks. In the United States, both low socio-economic status and minority group membership are associated with lower overall health care access and utilization. Racial/ethnic minorities are less likely than their white counterparts to have a specific source of ongoing care. A similar trend is observed among lower-income individuals as compared to their higher-income counterparts. Among persons with a usual source of care, blacks and Hispanics are more likely than whites to have hospital-based (as opposed to office-based) care. Hispanics, in particular, are less likely than their non-Hispanic white counterparts to have a usual primary care provider (36% versus 21%). Nonwhite beneficiaries of Medicare have fewer cancer screenings, fewer flu shots, less mental health care, and fewer ambulatory and physician visits than their white counterparts (Almario et al., 2016; Daly et al., 2017; Gornick, 2000; Jackson et al., 2016; Nadruz et al., 2017; Saadi et al., 2017).

Geographic disparities in access are also present, such that individuals in rural areas face greater barriers to access than those residing in urban areas. Rural Americans have higher mortality and morbidity rates and shorter life expectancies than their urban counterparts (Cordes, 1989; DeFriese & Ricketts, 1989; Rowland & Lyons, 1989; Sherman, 1991). Although rural residents have a greater need for health care services, services to address their needs are often sorely lacking. The main challenges in rural health care delivery include shortage and maldistribution of physicians, lack of both primary and specialty care services, and inability to pay for services.

Access Initiatives

Access to care has been incrementally addressed by the U.S. government through a variety of public programs. Efforts to increase access for disadvantaged populations have been undertaken periodically throughout U.S. legislative history. The Sheppard-Towner Act of 1921 exemplifies early federal attempts to provide direct primary care health services to economically disadvantaged mothers and children. Government interest in ensuring access to care for other lower-income populations grew during World War II, when comprehensive care was extended to the wives and children of low-rank armed forces personnel. Concern for the health care access for disadvantaged populations paved the way for the Great Society programs of the 1960s to help the elderly and poor through the Medicare and Medicaid programs.

Later, services such as cancer screening and immunizations were added to Medicare, and states were allocated $24 million in 1997 to create the Children's Health Insurance Programs (CHIP) for children in low-income families who do not otherwise qualify for Medicaid.

Several states have expanded their Medicaid programs under the Affordable Care Act (ACA), although the mandate for all states to expand Medicaid was struck down by the U.S. Supreme Court.

▶ Health Care Quality

Quality can be interpreted from both a micro perspective and a macro perspective. **EXHIBIT 12.2** provides examples of micro- and macro-level quality indicators. The micro view focuses on services at the point of delivery and their effects, and is associated with the performance of caregivers and health care organizations. The macro view looks at quality from the view of populations and reflects the performance of the entire health care delivery system.

The Institute of Medicine defines *quality* as "the degree to which health services for individuals and populations increase the likelihood of desired health outcomes and are consistent with current professional knowledge" (McGlynn, 1997, p. 8). This definition has several implications:

1. Quality performance occurs on a continuum, theoretically ranging from unacceptable to excellent.
2. Quality focuses on the services provided by the health care delivery system, as opposed to individual behaviors.
3. Quality may be evaluated from the perspective of individuals, populations, or communities.
4. Quality emphasizes desired health outcomes, and evidence must be used to identify the services that improve health outcomes.
5. In the absence of evidence regarding appropriateness of care, professional consensus can be used to develop the definition and measurement of quality (McGlynn, 1997).

EXHIBIT 12.2 Selected Quality Indicators

Micro level

- Small-area variations
- Medical errors
- Patient satisfaction
- Quality of life
- Health outcomes

Macro level

- Costs of care
- Access to care
- Population health

Although comprehensive in many respects, the definition of quality proposed by the Institute of Medicine fails to include the roles of cost and access in the evaluation of quality. Even though the United States spends more of its GDP on health care than other nations, Americans are not the healthiest people in the world. The main reasons that the United States trails behind other industrialized nations in population measures of health include inadequate emphasis on disease prevention and health promotion, poor access to primary health care, and prevailing socioeconomic and racial/ethnic disparities in health and health care. Greater health care expenditures and more intensive use of medical technology do not necessarily produce better health. In other words, more is not better and does not imply better quality.

In his well-known model for defining and measuring quality in health care organizations, Donabedian (1980) proposed three domains in which to examine health care quality: structure, process, and outcomes, which are all important in measuring the quality of care.

The domains of structure, process, and outcomes are closely linked (**FIGURE 12.2**). They are also hierarchical. Specifically, structure is the foundation of quality of care; good processes require good structure. Deficiencies in structure generally have a negative effect on health care delivery processes (defined in the "Process" subsection later in this section). Together, structure and processes influence quality outcomes. This model views quality strictly from the perspective of the delivery system, and it does not account for social and individual lifestyle and behavioral factors that may also have a significant influence on health status.

Structure

Structure is defined as "the relatively stable characteristics of the providers of care, of the tools and resources they have at their disposal, and of the physical and organizational settings in which they work" (Donabedian, 1980, p. 81). Structural measures indicate the extent to which health care organizations can provide adequate levels of care (Williams & Torrens, 1993). Hence, structure is an indirect measure of quality, assuming that a good structure enables health care delivery professionals to employ good processes that lead to good outcomes.

A significant initiative geared toward improving structure is the use of electronic health records (EHR)—digitally formatted medical records that provide real-time patient medical information for authorized personnel (HealthIT, 2013). However, their effectiveness in improving quality is not yet clearly established.

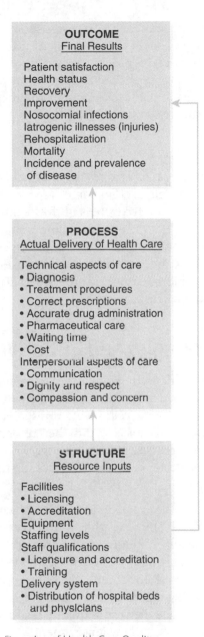

OUTCOME
Final Results

Patient satisfaction
Health status
Recovery
Improvement
Nosocomial infections
Iatrogenic illnesses (injuries)
Rehospitalization
Mortality
Incidence and prevalence
 of disease

PROCESS
Actual Delivery of Health Care

Technical aspects of care
• Diagnosis
• Treatment procedures
• Correct prescriptions
• Accurate drug administration
• Pharmaceutical care
• Waiting time
• Cost
Interpersonal aspects of care
• Communication
• Dignity and respect
• Compassion and concern

STRUCTURE
Resource Inputs

Facilities
• Licensing
• Accreditation
Equipment
Staffing levels
Staff qualifications
• Licensure and accreditation
• Training
Delivery system
• Distribution of hospital beds
 and physicians

FIGURE 12.2 The Three Domains of Health Care Quality

Process

Process refers to the specific manner in which care is provided. Examples of process include diagnostic tests, prescriptions, drug administration, pharmaceutical care, waiting time to see a physician, and interpersonal aspects of care delivery. As with structure, it is important to relate process to care outcomes, and structures and processes should be employed with the objective of achieving better outcomes. Significant initiatives toward improving process have taken place in recent years, including clinical practice guidelines, cost-efficiency analysis, critical pathways, and risk management (discussed in the "Developments in Process Improvement" section later in this chapter).

Outcome

Outcome refers to the effects or final results of utilizing the structure and processes of health care delivery. Outcomes are viewed by many as the bottom-line measure of the effectiveness of the health care delivery system (McGlynn & Brook, 1996). Positive outcomes suggest recovery from disease and improvement in health as well as an overall improvement in population's health. Outcome measures include postoperative infection rates, nosocomial infections, iatrogenic illnesses, rates of hospitalization readmission, and patient satisfaction.

▶ Quality Strategies and Initiatives

Several government agencies, individual organizations, and collaborative initiatives have helped shape the national health care agenda with respect to quality improvement, cost-saving transparency, accountability, improvement, and informed choice. Within their respective areas of focus, they have helped to advance technical knowledge, resources, and tools.

The CMS Quality Strategy strives to achieve the three broad aims of the National Quality Strategy (CMS, 2013):

- *Better care*: Improve the overall quality of health care by making care more patient-centered, more reliable, more accessible, and safer.
- *Healthy people, healthy communities*: Improve the health of the U.S. population by supporting evidence-based interventions to address behavioral, social, and environmental determinants of health in addition to delivering higher-quality care.
- *Affordable care*: Reduce the cost of quality health care for individuals, families, employers, and the government.

The ACA requires the U.S. Department of Health and Human Services to develop quality-focused data collection and reporting tools such as a quality rating system, a quality improvement strategy, and an enrollee satisfaction survey system. Information obtained with these tools will inform consumer selection of a Quality Health Plan (QHP), decisions about QHP certification, and the monitoring of QHP performance by federal and state marketplaces (CMS, 2015a).

Formerly known as the Physician Quality Reporting Initiative, the Physician Quality Reporting System (PQRS) encourages eligible individual professionals and group practices to report information on the quality of care to Medicare. PQRS allows participating professionals and group practices to assess the quality of care they provide. In 2015, the program applied a negative payment adjustment to eligible individual professionals and group practices that failed to satisfactorily report data on quality measures for Medicare Part B Physician Fee Schedule–covered professional services via PQRS in 2013. Those who report satisfactorily for the 2015 program year will avoid the 2017 PQRS negative payment adjustment (CMS, 2015c).

The Agency for Healthcare Research and Quality (AHRQ) developed a set of Quality Indicators (QIs)—standardized, evidence-based measures of health care quality that can be used with readily available hospital inpatient administrative data. The 101 Quality Indicators are organized into four main modules and two stand-alone modules that measure quality associated with care delivery. To use the QIs, organizations may download and use free software from AHRQ in SAS or Windows format. The software output of QI results can be used to highlight potential quality concerns, identify areas for further investigation, and track changes in quality over time (AHRQ, 2017a).

Surveys for the Consumer Assessment of Healthcare Providers and Systems (CAHPS) ask consumers and patients to report and evaluate their health care experiences. These surveys focus on topics of relevance to consumers and aspects of quality that consumers are best qualified to assess, such as provider communication skills and ease of access to care. All CAHPS surveys and related documents are free to anyone who wishes to use these surveys to assess patients' experiences of care. Among the users of CAHPS survey results are patients and consumers, health care providers, quality monitors and regulators, health plans, community collaboratives, and public and private purchasers of health care. These individuals and organizations use survey results to evaluate and compare health care providers and to improve the quality of health care services (AHRQ, 2017b).

My Own Network, Powered by AHRQ (MONAHRQ) is a free software product for health care performance and quality reporting that enables an organization to input its own hospital administrative data and generate an interactive, data-driven querying website. The MONAHRQ software tool, developed by AHRQ, supports public, web-based reporting of health care quality measures. It enables host users to automatically generate their own interactive health care reporting website, which they then host as they choose. Some sections of the reporting website are designed for health care consumers, while other sections are designed for more sophisticated data users. Although the MONAHRQ software is available to anyone, its primary host users—those interested in generating and hosting a MONARHQ reporting website—may be state data organizations, chartered value exchanges, and hospital organizations. To generate the website, host users must provide input data—hospital administrative data and/or another publicly available measure result that MONAHRQ can load and report. Minimal technical knowledge is required to use MONAHRQ (AHRQ, 2017c).

The Aligning Forces for Quality (AF4Q) program is a signature effort of the Robert Wood Johnson Foundation to enhance the overall quality of health care in selected communities, reduce racial and ethnic disparities, and provide models for national health care reform. AF4Q asks the people who receive care, the people who provide care, and the people who pay for care to work together toward common, fundamental objectives for better care. The 16 participating communities are geographically, demographically, and economically diverse and, together, cover 12.5% of the U.S. population. After eight years, AF4Q communities have built transformative partnerships. Data on quality, cost, and patient experience measures are collected and publicly reported. Through this project, practice coaches are deployed in hundreds of primary care practices, hospitals are improving care from the emergency department to the bedside, patients are playing a crucial role in transforming health care, new models for delivery and organization are being tested and implemented, and innovative payment reform is becoming a reality (Robert Wood Johnson Foundation, 2017a).

The Consumer–Purchaser Alliance is a collaboration among leading consumer, employer, and labor groups to promote the use of performance measurement in health care to inform consumer choice, value-based purchasing, and payment. Funded by the Robert Wood Johnson Foundation and supported by participating organizations, the collaboration envisions a future in which data on meaningful measures of performance—clinical and patient-reported outcomes, coordination of care across the health system, affordability, and patient experience— are used by consumers to make informed choices about health care, by purchasers to make good decisions about the health benefits they offer, and by physicians, hospitals, and other health care providers to continuously improve the care they deliver. The result would be a system that delivers top-quality, affordable care. The mission of the Consumer–Purchaser Alliance is to strengthen the role of consumers and purchasers in the quest for higher-quality, more affordable health care (Robert Wood Johnson Foundation, 2017b).

The Informed Patient Institute (IPI) is an independent nonprofit organization that provides credible online information for consumers about health care quality, patient safety, and health care costs. IPI rates the usefulness of online doctor, hospital, and nursing home report cards and provides Tip Sheets about what to do in case of concerns about quality in a hospital, nursing home, or physician's office. Rollout of these services began in California, Connecticut, Maine, New York, Pennsylvania, and South Carolina. IPI also advocates for making quality and cost information available to consumers (IPI, 2017).

The Joint Commission has a longstanding commitment to providing meaningful information about the performance of accredited organizations to the public. Its Quality Check website (www.qualitycheck.org), launched in 1996, fulfills this commitment. On the site, consumers can search for accredited and certified organizations by city and state, name, zip code, and organization Joint Commission ID number, if known. Consumers can also find organizations by type of service provided in a geographic area, with results filtered by accreditation decision, provider type, setting of care, or patient population, if preferred. Users can download free hospital performance measure results by clicking on the Quality Data Download tab, and print a list of Joint Commission–certified disease-specific care and health care staffing programs, in addition to programs with add-on certification in behavioral health home, memory care, primary care medical home, and other areas (Joint Commission, 2017).

The Measure Applications Partnership (MAP), a public–private partnership convened by the National Quality Forum (NQF), provides input to the U.S. Department of Health and Human Services (DHHS) on selecting performance measures. Since 2011, the DHHS has called upon MAP to recommend the most appropriate measures for public reporting, performance-based payment, and other uses. One of MAP's key initiatives is to have stakeholders conduct an intensive annual review of the quality measures being considered by the DHHS for more than 20 federal health programs. More recently, MAP provided input to the DHHS on assessing the quality of care for the nearly 10 million Americans who are enrolled in both Medicare and Medicaid due to their very low income and complex healthcare needs. Another recent MAP initiative is recommending core measures of quality of care for adults in Medicaid and ensuring that the measure set evolves over time. In 2014, MAP began to work on a core set of measures for children enrolled in Medicaid. The DHHS is guided by the recommendations from all of these projects as it finalizes measures for programs, which help improve the quality of care for the more than 100 million Americans covered by these federal health programs.

In convening MAP, the NQF brings together representatives of consumers, businesses and purchasers, labor, health plans, clinicians and providers, communities and states, and suppliers. MAP's balance of these stakeholder interests ensures that the federal government receives varied, thoughtful input on the selection of performance measures. As of 2018, MAP gathered approximately 150 health care leaders and experts, representing nearly 90 private-sector organizations, as well as liaisons from 7 federal agencies. MAP's work is intended to foster the use of a more uniform set of measures among federal programs and across public and private sectors. This uniformity is intended to help providers better identify key areas for improving quality; reduce wasteful data collection for hospitals, physicians, and nurses; and curb the proliferation of redundant measures that could confuse patients and payers (NQF, 2017).

▶ Developments in Process Improvement

Clinical Practice Guidelines

In response to findings of small-area variations, various professional groups, MCOs, and the U.S. government have developed standardized practice guidelines. *Clinical practice guidelines* (also called *medical practice guidelines*) are explicit descriptions of preferred clinical processes for managing a clinical problem based on research evidence, where possible, and on consensus in the absence of evidence (Larsen, 1996). Hence, clinical practice guidelines are designed to provide evidence-based or well-researched protocols to guide physicians' clinical decisions and to promote lower costs of care and better health outcomes. Currently, the National Guideline Clearinghouse works within the Agency for Healthcare Research and Quality to compile, update, and disseminate objective, detailed clinical practice guidelines for various conditions, diseases, and treatments in the U.S. (AHRQ, 2015).

Cost-Efficiency

Cost-efficiency, also referred to as cost-effectiveness, is an important concept in quality assessment. A service is *cost-efficient* when the benefit received is greater than the cost incurred in providing the service. In economic terms, services beyond the optimal point produce diminishing marginal returns. This point also represents optimal quality, which serves as a point of demarcation between underutilization and overutilization. On the one hand, *underutilization* (underuse) occurs when the benefits of an intervention outweigh its risks or costs, yet the intervention is not used (Chassin, 1991). On the other hand, *overutilization* (overuse) occurs when the costs or risks of treatment outweigh the benefits, yet additional care is delivered. When health care is overused, precious resources are wasted.

Critical Pathways

Critical pathways are interdisciplinary, outcome-based, patient-centered tools for clinical management that facilitate care coordination among multiple departments and caregivers in a health care facility, such as a hospital. A critical pathway is a timeline that identifies planned medical interventions and expected patient outcomes for a specific diagnosis or class of medical conditions, often defined by a diagnosis-related group. Pathways may also measure factors such as patient satisfaction, self-reported health status, mental health, and daily activities. Using these tools reduces costs and improves quality by reducing errors, improving coordination among different players, streamlining clinical management, providing systematic data for assessing care, and reducing variation in practice patterns (Abrahams et al., 2017; Giffin & Giffin, 1994).

Risk Management

Risk management consists of proactive efforts to prevent adverse events related to clinical care and facilities operations, with a special focus on avoiding medical malpractice (Orlikoff, 1988). Initiatives by a health care organization to review clinical processes and establish protocols for the purpose of reducing malpractice litigation can actually enhance quality of care. Malpractice concerns cause defensive medicine; thus, risk-management approaches should employ cost efficiency principles along with standardized practice guidelines and critical pathways. Unfortunately, fear of litigation may lead to reluctance on the part of hospitals and physicians to disclose preventable harm and actual medical errors. In this respect, fear of litigation may actually conceal problems that compromise patient safety (Lamb et al., 2003).

▶ Patient Safety

Patient safety and quality are two sides of the same coin. Quality indicates higher performance and better clinical and health outcomes, while safety emphasizes the absence of medical errors that could compromise performance and reduce clinical and health outcomes. A patient safety event is any process, act of omission, or commission that causes hazardous health care conditions or unintended harm to the patient. Patient safety has become a major concern of society and policymakers. A report by the Institute of Medicine,[1] *To Err Is Human: Building a Safer Health,*

---

1 The Institute of Medicine was renamed the National Academy of Medicine in 2015.

highlighted the risks of medical care in the United States. A primary focus of patient safety research has been to analyze data to identify problems and prove that a new practice will lead to improved quality or safety.

First, the key safety issues that contribute to patient risk can be classified as process errors in domains such as diagnosis, prescribing, communication, policy, and administration. Pace et al. (2005) identified medical errors and their relationship to harm in the U.S. health care system by analyzing medical errors reported to the Patient Safety Reporting System. From 357 reports, 608 errors were identified and subjected to univariate, bivariate, and multivariate logistic analysis. The study found that harm was associated with the therapeutic intent of an activity (odds ratio [OR], 2.71; 95% confidence interval [CI], 1.75–4.17), language barriers (OR, 8.35; 95% CI, 2.52–27.65), errors of judgment (OR, 2.36; 95% CI, 1.34–4.16), communication from another office (OR, 2.11; 95% CI, 1.20–3.73), mistiming of procedures (OR, 1.95; 95% CI, 1.28–2.95), and medication errors (OR, 4.14; 95% CI, 2.69–6.39) (Pace et al. 2005).

Second, a failure to capture and maintain accurate, comprehensive clinical information may present a risk in U.S. primary care. Primary care coordination or management is information-intensive and may be impeded if relevant clinical information is missing. In a cross-sectional survey conducted by Smith et al. (2005) among U.S. ambulatory care physicians, missing clinical information was reported in 13.6% of visits. Important missing information included laboratory results, letters, radiology results, history and physical examination documentation, and information relating to patient medications. The authors reported that this missing information was likely to adversely affect patients in 44% of cases and had resulted in delayed care or a need for additional services in 60% of cases (Smith et al., 2005).

Third, the failure to maintain medical equipment is a risk to patient safety. A wide range of equipment is used in primary care settings, and potential errors in maintaining or using such equipment may result in patient harm. Daniel and Rupert (2003) conducted a cross-sectional survey study of the calibration of ultrasound units in physical therapy communities. They found that a large percentage (44% of the 45 machines tested) of ultrasound machines in chiropractic physicians' offices delivered too much or too little dosage to the patient. Electrical safety inspections also revealed a significant failure rate, as only 2 of the 45 machines tested had been checked for safety in the previous 12 months (Daniel & Rupert, 2003).

Fourth, processes associated with ordering, transcribing, dispensing, administering, or monitoring medications are sources of potential risk to patient safety. The role of pharmacists in potential medication errors, unregulated alternative therapy, and patient risk has been investigated.

Evidence suggests that high prescription volumes, pharmacist fatigue, pharmacist overwork, interruptions to dispensing, similarity or confusion in drug names, lack of systematic dispensing workflow, or lack of regulatory guidelines may result in dispensing errors that compromise patient safety (Davis et al., 2004; Franks et al., 2009; Persell et al., 2004).

Finally, diagnostic errors pose a particular risk to patient safety. In a descriptive cross-sectional analysis of malpractice databases of the Physician Insurers Association of America (PIIA) conducted by Philips et al. (2004), one-third of the underlying causes of malpractice claims were due to diagnostic errors, followed by medication errors, improper performance, failure to communicate with patients, and failure in referral.

As for solutions to reduce patient safety risk, current efforts can be summarized as follows. First, pharmacist-led reviews of medication can help reduce hospital admissions. Krska et al. (2001) conducted a randomized controlled trial in a primary care setting to determine whether a multidisciplinary approach (pharmacist and general practitioner) could reduce medication-related problems in patients with chronic diseases who took multiple drugs. Such problems included adverse drug reactions, poor compliance with therapy, and inappropriate drug selection. Pharmacists reviewed the medications of 332 patients with at least two chronic health conditions who took at least four prescribed medications daily. The intervention group had their medications reviewed and a pharmaceutical care plan drawn up, whereas the control group received usual care. After 3 months, 70% of the medication problems in the intervention groups were resolved, compared to 14% in the control groups. The authors reported that pharmacist-led medication review may substantially reduce medication-related errors, and any patient 65 years or older should have a pharmaceutical review. Although this is only a single study, it provides evidence that regular review of medication is one way to reduce the risk of medication errors (Krska et al., 2001).

Second, evidence suggests that accuracy in electronic prescriptions is improving, but could improve further. Steele et al. (2005) confirmed the benefit of automated alerts on provider ordering behavior in a U.S. outpatient setting. As prescribers ordered medications on a computer, an alert was automatically displayed for any relevant drug–laboratory result interactions. Drug–laboratory interaction refers to clinically relevant laboratory-determined values associated with medication use. The number and type of laboratory tests a prescriber ordered were monitored in response to automated drug alerts. This study focused on interactions related to medication use that could lead to hyperkalemia or hypokalemia, among other interactions. As providers ordered medications on a computer, any "abnormal" or "missing" laboratory values were identified and an automatic alert was provided (Steele et al., 2005). This study concluded that providers tended to adhere to alerts and use this feedback to improve patient care.

Third, educational interventions may increase awareness of patient safety risk among both medical students and medical practitioners. Wallace et al. (2007) examined interventions within the English health authority that were designed to improve risk management in general practice. Educational interventions included the practices' own initiatives, significant event audits (SEAs), and workshops with the Medical Defence Union which included significant event analysis of reported errors. The authors reported that promoting education among general practitioners, practice nurses, practice managers, and administrative staff yielded improved competence in identifying and managing patient risk over the period of the study, particularly through widening the breadth of staff involved in patient safety and using formal recording systems (Wallace et al., 2007).

Fourth, reporting patient safety events appears to be an effective approach for improving patient safety. The mechanism of event reporting was first introduced in high-risk industries, such as the aviation, nuclear, and rail industries, to improve safety and enhance organizational learning from errors. The mechanism was then extended to health care systems, with additional features such as anonymous reporting, meaningful feedback, and greater ease of reporting. By collecting data on adverse events and near misses in health care, the reporting systems enable safety specialists to analyze events, identify underlying factors, and generate actionable knowledge to mitigate risks. Since the emergence of electronic patient safety reporting (e-reporting) systems, the collection and analysis of events has been conducted more efficiently than with traditional paper-based systems (Kou et al., 2012; Pronovost et al., 2008).

Finally, more recent studies have examined the relationships among the safety culture, patient safety, and quality of care outcomes in hospital settings and identified directions for future research. In a systematic review of patient safety culture and patient outcomes, DiCuccio (2015) observed inconsistent findings regarding significant relationships between safety culture and nursing-sensitive patient outcomes. For example, one study found that a strong safety culture was related to fewer medication errors (Chang & Mark, 2011), whereas other investigators found that a strong safety culture was associated with more medication errors (Mark et al., 2008). Similarly, Mark et al. (2008) found a positive relationship between safety culture and patient falls, whereas Obrien (2009) found nonsignificant results. It is possible that a heightened safety culture may yield greater awareness and sensitivity in measurement, leading to a positive correlation between safety culture and safety issues.

▶ Conclusion

Increasing costs, lack of access, and concerns about quality of health care constitute the greatest challenges to health care delivery in the United States. To some extent, these three issues are interrelated. Increasing costs limit the ability of the health care delivery system to expand access. However, without universal health insurance coverage for all Americans, the United States is unlikely to ever match other developed countries in population health outcomes.

Health care costs in the United States are the highest in the world. The shift toward prospective payments and the growth of managed care helped curb the rise in health care spending during the 1990s. Even so, current forecasts predict accelerated spending growth in the future, as a larger share of U.S. economic resources will be spent on health care.

Access to appropriate medical care is one of the determinants of health status, along with environmental, lifestyle, and heredity factors. Access is also regarded as a benchmark in assessing the effectiveness of the medical care delivery system, and is explained in terms of enabling and predisposing factors as well as factors related to health policy and health care delivery.

One reason that the effort to pursue quality in health care has trailed behind the emphasis on cost and access to care is the challenge of defining and measuring quality. Nevertheless, the growth of managed care and the emphasis on cost containment have raised interest in quality because of the intuitive concern that control of costs may negatively impact quality. Much work remains to be done in specifying what constitutes good quality in medical care, how to guarantee good quality in patient care, and how to reward providers and health plans whose outcomes indicate successes in quality improvement. One challenge to achieving this goal is that patients, providers, and payers may define quality differently, translating into different expectations of the health care delivery system and, therefore, differing evaluations of quality (McGlynn, 1997).

References

1. Abrahams E, et al. 2017, June 26. Clinical pathways: Recommendations for putting patients at the center of value-based care. *Clin Cancer Res.* 23(16):4545–4549. doi: 10.1158/1078-0432.CCR-17-1609.
2. Agency for Healthcare Research and Quality (AHRQ). 2015. National Guideline Clearinghouse. http://www.guideline.gov/about/index.aspx. Accessed August 12, 2015.
3. Agency for Healthcare Research and Quality (AHRQ). 2017a. Quality Indicators overview. http://www.qualityindicators.ahrq.gov. Accessed December 16, 2017.

4. Agency for Healthcare Research and Quality (AHRQ). 2017b. Consumer Assessment of Healthcare Providers and Systems. https://www.ahrq.gov/cahps/index.html. Accessed December 16, 2017.

5. Agency for Healthcare Research and Quality (AHRQ). 2017c. MONAHRQ. https://www.ahrq.gov/professionals/systems/monahrq/index.html. Accessed December 16, 2017.

6. Almario CV, et al. 2016, June 29. Persistent racial and ethnic disparities in flu vaccination coverage: Results from a population-based study. *Am J Infect Control.* 44(9):1004–1009. doi: 10.1016/j.ajic.2016.03.064.

7. Altman SH, Eichenholz J. 1976. Inflation in the health industry: causes and cures. In: Zubkoff M, ed. *Health: A victim or cause of inflation?* New York, NY: Milbank Memorial Fund, 1–32.

8. Altman SH, Wallack SS. 1996. Health care spending: Can the United States control it? In: Altman SH, Reinhardt UE, eds. *Strategic choices for a changing health care system.* Chicago, IL: Health Administration Press.

9. Baucus M, Fowler EJ. 2002. Geographic variation in Medicare spending and the real focus of Medicare reform. *Health Aff.* 2002 Jul-Dec;Suppl Web Exclusives:W115-7.

10. Centers for Medicare and Medicaid Services (CMS). 2013. CMS quality strategy 2013—beyond. Washington DC. https://www.ahrq.gov/sites/default/files/wysiwyg/workingforquality/cms-quality-strategy.pdf. Accessed April 16, 2018.

11. Centers for Medicare and Medicaid Services (CMS). 2015a. Health insurance marketplace quality initiatives. http://www.cms.gov/Medicare/Quality-Initiatives-Patient-Assessment-Instruments/QualityInitiativesGenInfo/Health-Insurance-Marketplace-Quality-Initiatives.html. Accessed August 15, 2015.

12. Centers for Medicare and Medicaid Services (CMS). 2015b. *National health expenditures 2015 highlights.* Author, Washington DC.

13. Centers for Medicare and Medicaid Services (CMS). 2015c. Physician Quality Reporting System. https://www.cms.gov/Medicare/Quality-Initiatives-Patient-Assessment-Instruments/PQRS/index.html. Accessed August 11, 2015.

14. Centers for Medicare and Medicaid Services (CMS). 2017. Historical. https://www.cms.gov/Research-Statistics-Data-and-Systems/Statistics-Trends-and-Reports/NationalHealthExpendData/NationalHealthAccountsHistorical.html. Accessed December 11, 2017.

15. Centers for Medicare and Medicaid Services (CMS). 2018. National health expenditure data. https://www.cms.gov/research-statistics-data-and-systems/statistics-trends-and-reports/nationalhealthexpenddata/nhe-fact-sheet.html. Accessed April 9, 2018.

16. Chang Y, Mark B. 2011. Effects of learning climate and registered nurse staffing on medication errors. *Nurs Res.* 60:32–39.

17. Chassin MR. 1991. Quality of care: Time to act. *JAMA.* 266:3472–3473.

18. Cordes SM. 1989. The changing rural environment and the relationship between health services and rural development. *Health Serv Res.* 23(6):757–784.

19. Daly MC, et al. 2017. Surviving rectal cancer: Examination of racial disparities surrounding access to care. *J Surg Res.* 211:100–106. doi: S0022-4804(16)30564-9.

20. Daniel DM, Rupert RL. 2003. Calibration and electrical safety status of therapeutic ultrasound used by chiropractic physicians. *J Manipulative Physiol Ther.* 2003 Mar-Apr;26(3):171–175.

21. Davis TC, et al. 2006. Literacy and misunderstanding prescription drug labels. *Ann Intern Med.* 145(12):887–894.

22. DeFriese GH, Ricketts TC. 1989. Primary health care in rural areas: An agenda for research. *Health Serv Res.* 23(6):931–974.

23. DiCuccio MH. 2015. The relationship between patient safety culture and patient outcomes: A systematic review. *J Patient Saf.* 11:135–142.

24. Donabedian A. 1980. *Explorations in quality assessment and monitoring: The definition of quality and approaches to its assessment.* Vol. 1. Ann Arbor, MI: Health Administration Press.

25. Dranove D. 1993. The case for competitive reform in health care. In: Arnould RJ, et al., eds. *Competitive approaches to health care reform.* Washington, DC: Urban Institute Press, 67–82.

26. Feldstein P. 1994. *Health policy issues: An economic perspective on health reform.* Ann Arbor, MI: AUPHA Press/Health Administration Press.

27. Franks AS, et al. 2009, December 17. Do medication samples jeopardize patient safety? *Ann Pharmacother,* 43(1). http://journals.sagepub.com/doi/abs/10.1345/aph.1L362. Accessed April 16, 2018.

28. Giffin M, Giffin RB. 1994. Market memo: Critical pathways produce tangible results. *Health Care Strat Manage.* 12(7):1–6.

29. Gornick ME. 2000. *Vulnerable populations and Medicare services: Why do disparities exist?* New York, NY: Century Foundation Press.

30. HealthIT. 2013. What is an electronic health record (EHR)? http://www.healthit.gov /providers-professionals/faqs/what-electronic-health-record-ehr. Accessed August 11, 2015.

31. Informed Patient Institute (IPI). 2017. About IPI. https://www.informedpatientinstitute .org/about.php. Accessed December 16, 2017.

32. Jackson CS, et al. 2016. Health disparities in colorectal cancer among racial and ethnic minorities in the United States. *J Gastrointest Oncol.* 7(suppl 1):S32–S43. doi: 10.3978/j.issn.2078-6891.2015.039.

33. Joint Commission. 2017. Facts about Quality Check and Quality Reports. https:// www.jointcommission.org/facts_about_quality_check_and_quality_reports/. Accessed December 16, 2017.

34. Krska J, et al. 2001. Pharmacist-led medication review in patients over 65: A randomized, controlled trial in primary care. *Age Aging.* 30:205–211.

35. Kuo YH, et al. 2012. The evaluation of a web based incident reporting system. *Computers Informatics Nurs.* 30(7):386–394.

36. Lamb RM, et al. 2003. Hospital disclosure practices: Results of a national survey. *Health Aff.* 22(2):73–83.

37. Larsen RR. 1996. Narrowing the gray zone: How clinical practice guidelines can improve the decision-making process. *Postgrad Med.* 100(2):17–24.

38. Mark BA, et al. 2008. Exploring organizational context and structure as predictors of medication errors and patient falls. *J Patient Saf.* 4:66–77.

39. Martin A, et al. 2011. National Health Expenditure Accounts Team. Recession contributes to slowest annual rate of increase in health spending in five decades. *Health Aff.* 30(1):11–22.

40. McGlynn EA. 1997. Six challenges in measuring the quality of health care. *Health Aff.* 16(3):7–21.

41. McGlynn EA, Brook RH. 1996. Ensuring quality of care. In: Andersen RM, et al., eds. *Changing the U.S. health care system: Key issues in health services, policy, and management.* San Francisco, CA: Jossey-Bass.

42. Nadruz W Jr, et al. 2017. Racial disparities in risks of stroke. *N Engl J Med.* 376(21):2089–2090. doi: 10.1056/NEJMc1616085.

43. National Center for Health Statistics [NCHS], 1996. *Health, United States, 1996.* Hyattsville, MD: U.S. Department of Health and Human Services.

44. National Center for Health Statistics (NCHS). 2010. *Health, United States, 2010.* Hyattsville, MD: U.S. Department of Health and Human Services.

45. National Center for Health Statistics (NCHS). 2017. *Health, United States, 2016: With chartbook on long-term trends in health.* Hyattsville, MD: U.S. Department of Health and Human Services.

46. National Quality Forum (NQF). 2017. Measure Applications Partnership. http://www.qualityforum.org/map/. Accessed December 16, 2017.

47. Obrien RL. 2009. *Keeping patients safe: The relationship between patient safety climate and patient outcomes* [Doctoral dissertation]. University of California, San Francisco.

48. Orlikoff JE. 1988. *Malpractice prevention and liability control for hospitals.* 2nd ed. Chicago, IL: American Hospital Publishing.

49. Pace W, et al. 2005. Developing a taxonomy for coding ambulatory medical errors: A report from the ASIPS Collaborative. *Adv Patient Saf.* 2:63–73.

50. Persell SD, et al. 2004. Understanding of drug indications by ambulatory care patients. *Am J Health-System Pharmacy.* 61(1):2523–2527.

51. Phillips RL Jr, et al. 2004. Learning from malpractice claims about negligent, adverse events in primary care in the United States. *Qual Saf Health Care.* 13:121–126.

52. Pronovost PJ, et al. 2008. Improving the value of patient safety reporting systems. In: Henriksen K, et al., eds. *Advances in patient safety: New directions and alternative approaches. Vol. 1: Assessment.* Rockville (MD): Agency for Healthcare Research and Quality; 2008 Aug.

53. Robert Wood Johnson Foundation. 2017a. Aligning Forces for Quality (AF4Q). http://forces4quality.org/about-us.html. Accessed December 16, 2017.

54. Robert Wood Johnson Foundation. 2017b. Consumer–Purchaser Alliance. http://www.consumerpurchaser.org/who-we-are-menu/about-cpdp-menu. Accessed December 16, 2017.

55. Rowland D, Lyons B. 1989. Triple jeopardy: Rural, poor, and uninsured. *Health Serv Res.* 23(6):975–1004.

56. Saadi A, et al. 2017. Racial disparities in neurologic health care access and utilization in the united states. *Neurology.* 88(24):2268–2275. doi: 10.1212/WNL.0000000000004025.

57. Sherman A. 1991. *Falling by the wayside: Children in rural America.* Washington, DC: Children's Defense Fund.

58. Smith PC, et al. 2005. Missing clinical information during primary care visits. *JAMA.* 293(5):565–571.

59. Steele AW, et al. 2005. The effect of automated alerts on provider ordering behavior in an outpatient setting. *PLoS Med.* 2(9):e255.

60. TECH Research Network. 2001. Technology change around the world: Evidence from heart attack care. *Health Aff.* 20(3):25–42.

61. Wallace LM, et al. 2007. Organizational interventions to promote risk management in primary care: the experience in Warwickshire, England. *Health Serv Manage Res.* 20(2):84–93.

62. Williams SJ, Torrens PR. 1993. Influencing, regulating, and monitoring the health care system. In: Williams SJ, Torrens PR, eds. *Introduction to health services.* 4th ed. Albany, NY: Delmar, 421–429.

63. Wilson FA, Neuhauser D. 1985. *Health services in the United States.* 2nd ed. Cambridge, MA: Ballinger.

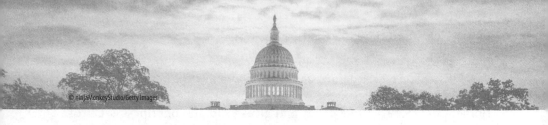

CHAPTER 13
Health Policy

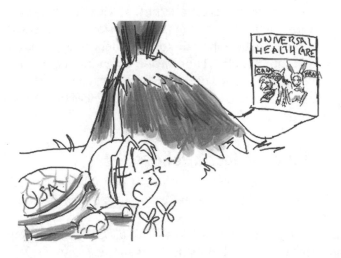

▶ Introduction

Although the United States does not have a centrally controlled
system of health care delivery, the nation does have a history of
federal, state, and local government involvement in health and
social policy. Perhaps the most well-known policy efforts were the social
programs created under Social Security legislation during Franklin Roosevelt's presidency in the 1940s. These paved the way for the creation
of the Medicare and Medicaid programs through amendments to the
Social Security Act in 1965. Recently, the Affordable Care Act (ACA)
has brought about multifaceted changes to the U.S. health care system,
yielding some benefits such as insurance expansion and use of information technology, but not yet achieving other impacts such as those on
cost containment and quality improvement.

This chapter first defines health policy and explores the principal features of health policy in the United States. Next, it describes the development of U.S. legislative policy and gives examples of critical issues of health policy. Finally, an overview of the ACA and subsequent events is provided.

▶ What Is Health Policy?

Public policies are authoritative decisions that are made in the legislative (congressional), executive (presidential), or judicial (courts, including the Supreme Court) branches of government with the intention to direct or influence the actions, behaviors, or decisions of others (Longest, 2002). When public policies pertain to or influence the pursuit of health, they become health policies. Thus, *health policy* can be defined as "the aggregate of principles, stated or unstated, that … characterize the distribution of resources, services, and political influences that impact on the health of the population" (Miller, 1987, p. 15).

Different Forms of Health Policies

Health policies often arise as a by-product of public social policies created by the government. A relevant example is the expansion of health insurance coverage. Previously, policies that excluded fringe benefits from income or Social Security taxes—and a U.S. Supreme Court ruling that employee benefits, including health insurance, could be legitimately included in the collective bargaining process—led to important changes in the U.S. health care system. As a result, employer-provided health insurance benefits grew rapidly in the mid-20th century (Health Insurance Association of America, 1992). In 1965, adoption of Medicare and Medicaid legislation expanded the health sector by providing publicly subsidized health insurance to the elderly and indigent. More recently, the ACA has reduced the number of uninsured Americans by several million.

The American health care system has developed under exceedingly favorable public policies. For example, the federally funded National Institutes of Health (NIH) had a budget of approximately $10 million when it was established in the early 1930s. Today, following exponential growth in funding, the NIH's annual budget exceeds $30 billion (NIH, 2017). In addition, private industry spends a significant amount on biomedical research and development, encouraged by governmental policies that permit businesses to recoup investments in research and development.

Health policies pertain to health care at all levels, including the production, delivery, and financing of health care services. Such policies may affect groups or classes of individuals, such as physicians, the poor, the elderly, or children. They can also affect organizations—such as medical schools, health maintenance organizations (HMOs), nursing homes, producers of medical technology, or employers. In the United States, each branch and level of government can influence health policy. For example, both the executive and legislative branches at the federal, state, and local levels can establish health policies, and the judicial branch can uphold, strike down, or modify existing laws affecting health and health care at any level.

Statutes or laws are also considered policies—for example, the statutory language in the 1983 amendments to the Social Security Act that authorized the prospective payment system (PPS) for reimbursing hospitals for Medicare beneficiaries. Another example is the certificate-of-need programs through which many states seek to regulate capital expansion in their health care systems.

Regulatory Tools

Health policies can be used as *regulatory tools* (Longest, 2002). They may call upon the government to prescribe and control the behavior of a particular target group by monitoring the group and imposing sanctions for failure to comply. Federally funded organizations for quality improvement, for instance, develop and enforce standards for appropriate care under Medicare. State insurance departments across the country regulate health insurance companies in an effort to protect customers from excessive premiums, mendacious practices, and defaults on coverage in case of the financial failure of an insurance company.

Some health policies are self-regulatory. For example, physicians set standards of medical practice, and schools of public health decide which courses are part of their graduate programs in public health (Weissert & Weissert, 1996).

Allocative Tools

Health policies can also be used as *allocative tools* (Longest, 2002), involving the direct provision of income, services, or goods to certain groups of individuals or institutions. Allocative tools in health care are of two main types: distributive and redistributive. *Distributive policies* spread benefits throughout society and include NIH funding of medical research, the construction of facilities (e.g., hospital construction under the Hill-Burton Act program during the 1950s and 1960s), and the establishment of new institutions (e.g., HMOs). *Redistributive policies*, in contrast, obtain resources from one group and allocate them to another group—a system that often creates visible beneficiaries and payers. As a consequence, health policy is often most visible and politically charged when it performs redistributive functions. Redistributive policies include Medicaid, which spends public taxes on the poor in the form of free health insurance.

▶ Principal Features of U.S. Health Policy

Several distinct features characterize U.S. health policy, including the role of the government as a subsidiary to the private sector; fragmented, incremental, and piecemeal reform; pluralistic (interest group) politics; a decentralized role for the states; the impact of presidential leadership; and, to a lesser extent, the role of the research community. These interrelated features often influence the development and evolution of health policies.

Government as Subsidiary to the Private Sector

In the United States, health care is not regarded as a right of citizenship nor as a primary responsibility of government. Instead, the private sector plays a dominant role in providing health care. As with many other public policy issues, Americans generally prefer market solutions over government intervention in health care financing and delivery and thus have a strong preference for minimizing the government's role in health care delivery. One result is that Americans are far more reluctant than their counterparts in most other industrialized democracies to develop social insurance programs. Public opinion in the United States often presumes such programs to be overly generous.

Generally, the role of government in U.S. health care has grown incrementally, mainly in response to perceived problems and negative consequences. The most widely cited problems associated with government involvement include escalating costs, bureaucratic inflexibility and red tape, excessive regulation, irrational paperwork, arbitrary and sometimes conflicting public directives, inconsistent enforcement of rules and regulations, fraud and abuse, inadequate reimbursement, arbitrary denial of claims, insensitivity to local needs, consumer and provider dissatisfaction, and charges that such efforts tend to promote welfare dependence rather than a desire to seek employment (Longest, 2002).

The most credible argument for policy intervention begins with identifying situations in which markets fail or function inefficiently. Health care in the United States is a large industry, but certain characteristics and conditions of the health care market distinguish it from other types of businesses. Notably, the market for health care services in the United States violates the conditions of a competitive market in several ways.

For example, the complexity of health care services renders consumers almost unable to make informed decisions without guidance from the sellers (providers). In addition, the entry of sellers into the health care market is heavily regulated. Widespread insurance coverage also affects the decisions of both buyers and sellers in these markets. Therefore, markets for health care services do not operate competitively, which invites policy intervention to rectify perceived inequities.

Government spending for health care has been mostly confined to filling gaps in the private sector. Such interventions have included environmental protection, preventive services, communicable disease control, care for special groups, institutional care for the mentally and chronically ill, provision of medical care to the indigent, and support for research and training. Health coverage is considered a privilege for those offered insurance through employers, and the government is left to take on a gap-filling role for the most vulnerable of the uninsured population.

Fragmented, Incremental, and Piecemeal Reform

The subsidiary role of the government and the attendant mixture of private and public approaches to the delivery of health care also result in a complex, fragmented pattern of health care financing. Under this scheme, (1) the employed are predominantly covered by voluntary insurance provided through contributions made by themselves and their employers; (2) the aged are insured through a combination of coverage financed out of Social Security tax revenues (Medicare Part A), voluntary insurance for outpatient and prescription drug coverage (Medicare Part B and Part D), and voluntary purchase of Medigap plans; (3) the poor are covered through Medicaid via federal, state, and local revenues; and (4) special population groups, such as veterans, Native Americans, and members of the armed forces, have coverage that is provided directly by the federal government.

Health policies in the United States have been introduced in an incremental, piecemeal fashion. One example is the gradual reforms in Medicaid since it was established in 1965. In 1984, the first steps were taken to mandate coverage of pregnant women and children in two-parent families who met income eligibility requirements and to mandate coverage for all children age 5 years or younger who met financial eligibility requirements. In 1986, states were given the option of covering pregnant women and children up to 5 years of age in families with incomes below 100% of federal poverty income guidelines. In 1988, that option was expanded to cover families with incomes at 185% of the federal poverty level. In 1988, as part of the Medicaid Catastrophic Act, still in effect today, Congress mandated coverage for pregnant women and infants in families with incomes below 100% of federal poverty guidelines. (In 1989, this criterion was expanded to 133% of the federal poverty income, and coverage of children was extended to include children up to 6 years of age.) In 1988, Congress required that Medicaid coverage continue for 6 months for families leaving the Aid to Families with Dependent Children program and allowed states the option of adding another 6 months to that extension. The Children's Health Insurance Program (CHIP) lets states use Medicaid expansion to extend insurance coverage to uninsured children who do not otherwise qualify for existing Medicaid programs.

These examples illustrate how a program may be reformed and expanded through successive legislative enactments over several years. In characteristic American fashion, Medicaid has been reformed through incremental change, but has not ensured access to care for all uninsured people in the nation. Among the uninsured are millions of Americans who are not categorically eligible for services—mostly adults younger than age 65 with no dependent children. Congress has demonstrated the desire and political will to address the needs of a small number of the uninsured who are considered to be the most vulnerable (e.g., pregnant women and children), but did not develop a consensus on more dramatic steps until the passage of the ACA. The ACA greatly increased insurance options for previously uninsured Americans, including a Medicaid expansion for adults with incomes up to 133% of the federal poverty level (in states that chose to expand their Medicaid programs), the creation of state and federal health insurance exchanges for better regulation of private plans, and a prohibition on insurers against denying coverage due to preexisting medical conditions.

The development process of legislative health policy offers another vivid case of institutional fragmentation. Thirty-one different congressional committees and subcommittees try to claim a fragment of jurisdiction over health legislation. Reform proposals that emerge from these various committees face a daunting political challenge, because proposals must go through separate consideration and passage in each chamber of Congress, are subject to negotiations in a joint conference committee to reconcile bills passed by the two houses, and then return to each chamber for approval. In the Senate, 41 of the 100 members can thwart the process at any stage.

Even after a bill has passed in Congress, its journey is far from over. Multiple levels of federal and state bureaucracy must interpret the legislation, and rules and regulations must be written for its implementation. During this process, the ultimate design of the program may be influenced by political actors, interest groups, or project beneficiaries.

At times, the final result may differ significantly from the initial intent of the congressional sponsors of the bill.

This complex and seemingly disorganized process of policy formulation and implementation makes fundamental, comprehensive policy reform extremely difficult to achieve. Traditional ideology and the hierarchical organization of government reinforce the tendency to maintain the status quo. It usually takes a great political event—a landmark election, a mass popular upheaval, a war, or a domestic crisis—to shake off (even if only temporarily) the tilt toward inaction. The passage of the ACA was a notable feat in this regard, but it remains to be seen how effectively the law will be in reducing health care costs while increasing coverage and access to care.

Pluralistic and Interest Group Politics

Perhaps the most common explanation for health policy outcomes in the United States is the role of interest groups and the incremental policies that result from compromises to satisfy their demands. Traditionally, policy community members have included (1) the legislative committees with jurisdiction in a policy domain, (2) the executive branch agencies responsible for implementing policies in the public domain, and (3) the interest groups in the private domain. The first two categories are the suppliers of the policies demanded by the third category.

Innovative, non-incremental health policies are resisted by established groups, because they undermine the bargaining practices designed to reduce threats to established interests. The system is stable, because overall most groups are satisfied with the benefits they receive; however, the satisfaction for any single group is less than optimal.

The most effective demanders of health policies are the well-organized interest groups. The pluralism of interest groups affects health policy discussions, as it does any other policy debate in American politics. Powerful interest groups involved in health care politics are adamant about resisting major change (Alford, 1975), and each group fights hard to protect its own interests.

By combining and concentrating the resources of their members, organized interest groups can dramatically change the ratio between the costs and benefits of participation in the political arena for policy change. Interest groups represent a variety of individuals and entities, such as physicians in the American Medical Association, senior citizens allied with AARP (formerly the American Association of Retired Persons), institutional providers such as hospitals belonging to the American Hospital Association, nursing homes belonging to the American Health Care Association or the American Association of Homes and

Services for the Aging, and member drug companies in the Pharmaceutical Research and Manufacturers of America. In recent years, physicians have often found it difficult to find a unified voice to lobby for their interests, due to the sheer variety of physician specialty groups.

The policy agenda of interest groups is typically reflective of their interests. For example, AARP advocates programs to expand financing for long-term care for the elderly. Organized labor was among the staunchest supporters of national health insurance during the 1950s and again in the 1990s. Universities, medical schools, and teaching hospitals would like more funding (e.g., from the NIH) for research. Educational institutions and accrediting organizations have primary concerns embedded in policies that enable them to receive more funding to educate health care professionals.

Employers

The health policy concerns of American employers are mostly shaped by the degree to which employers help provide health insurance benefits for their employees, their employees' dependents, and their retirees. Many small business owners oppose health policies that require them to provide employees coverage, believing they cannot afford to do so. Health policies affecting the health of workers, or the health of labor–management relations as experienced by employers, also attract their attention. For example, employers must comply with federal and state regulations for the health and well-being of their employees and engage in measures to prevent job-related illnesses and injuries. Employers are often subject to inspection by regulatory agencies to ensure that they adhere to health and safety policies for the workplace.

Consumer Groups

Consumer interests are not uniform, nor are the policy preferences of their interest groups. Often, consumers have insufficient financial means to organize and advocate for their own interests. Because most Americans already have private or public health insurance, consumer concerns are directed more toward lowering premiums and copayments or having more covered benefits, than toward expanding insurance to the uninsured, especially if it imposes higher taxes or premiums for their own insurance.

The health policy concerns of consumers and the groups representing them reflect the rich diversity of the American people. African Americans and, more recently, a growing number of Hispanics experience unique health problems. Both groups are underserved for many health care services and underrepresented in all health professions in the

United States. Their health policy interests include having their unique health problems be adequately addressed—including higher infant mortality, higher exposure to violence among adolescents, higher levels of substance abuse among adults, and earlier deaths from cardiovascular disease and various other causes.

Manufacturers of Technology

The health policy concerns of medical technology and pharmaceutical organizations include discerning changes in health policy areas and exerting influence over the formulation of policies. Health policy concerns for medical technology (including pharmaceuticals) are driven by three main factors: (1) Medical technology plays an important role in rising health costs, (2) medical technology often provides health benefits (albeit not always), and (3) medical technology provides economic benefits in addition to health benefits. These factors are likely to remain important determinants of the nation's policies toward medical technology.

Another factor that is driving current policy for medical technology in the United States is the interest of policymakers in developing cost-saving technology and expanding its access. To this end, the government spends an increasing amount of money on technology assessment of the relative values of alternative technologies, presumably so it can support the best values in technology.

Alliances

To overcome pluralistic interests and optimize health policy outcomes, diverse interest groups may create alliances among themselves and with members of the legislative body to protect and enhance the interests of those benefitting from government programs. Members of the alliances receive benefits from current programs. Meanwhile, legislators can show their constituencies the economic benefits from government spending in their districts, agencies can expand their programs, and interest groups directly receive benefits bestowed by government programs.

Decentralized Role of the States

In the United States, individual states play a significant role in developing and implementing health policies. The importance of the role of individual states can be seen in programs focused on the following concerns:

- Financial support for the care and treatment of the poor and chronically disabled, including primary responsibility for the administration of federal/state Medicaid and CHIP programs

- Quality assurance and oversight of health care practitioners and facilities (e.g., state licensure and regulation)
- Regulation of insurance, including health insurance
- Control of Medicaid costs
- Health personnel training (states cover most of the cost for training health care professionals)
- Authorization of local government health services

States are vested with broad legal authority to regulate almost every facet of the health care system. They license and regulate health care facilities and health professionals; restrict the content, marketing, and price of health insurance (including professional liability or malpractice insurance); set and enforce environmental quality standards; and enact a variety of controls on health care costs. All states bear a large responsibility for financing health services for the poor, primarily through Medicaid, for which financing is shared with the federal government. In addition, most states subsidize some of the costs of delivering health services to persons with neither public nor private coverage. Personal health services that are funded or provided by states, often in cooperation with local governments, include a range of services, such as public health nursing, communicable disease control, family planning and prenatal care, nutrition counseling, and home health services.

Most of the incremental policy actions of recent years originated in state governments. One such action was the creation of insurance risk pools—a measure intended to help persons who were otherwise unable to acquire private insurance because of the medical risks they posed to insurance companies. Most of these programs are financed by a combination of individual premiums and taxes on insurance carriers. Other state-initiated programs have addressed additional vulnerable populations. For example, New Jersey developed a program to ensure access to care for all pregnant women. Florida began the Healthy Kids Corporation program to link health insurance to schools. Massachusetts, Hawaii, and Oregon experimented with more comprehensive programs designed to provide universal access to care within their jurisdictions. Under the ACA, all states have to decide whether to expand Medicaid and whether to establish a state-run health insurance exchange.

Arguments have been made against excessive state control over health policy decisions. The more control states have, the more difficult it is to develop a coordinated national strategy. For example, it is difficult to plan a national disease control program if not all states participate in the program or if they do not all collect and report data in the same manner. Moreover, some critics argue that disparities among states may cause inequalities in access to health services. This, in turn, may lead to increased migration from states offering poor health benefits to states providing more generous programs.

Impact of Presidential Leadership

Americans often look to strong presidential leadership to catalyze major change in health policies. In turn, presidents have key opportunities to influence congressional outcomes by achieving political compromises that allow for the passage of bills with at least some of their preferred agendas.

President Lyndon Johnson's role in the passage of Medicare and Medicaid is often cited as a prime example. Johnson shepherded the passage of Medicare and Medicaid legislation through Congress in 1965 in the context of an unusually favorable political opportunity and by effectively using his leadership skills.

The major piece of health legislation that was passed under President Harry Truman was the Hill-Burton Hospital Construction Act. Two other major pieces of health legislation were passed during Richard Nixon's presidency: (1) the actions leading to federal support of HMOs in 1973 and (2) the enactment of the National Health Planning and Resources Development Act of 1974. Under President Ronald Reagan, new approaches to Medicare cost control for hospitals and physicians were created, as well as additional Medicare coverage for the elderly. Although President Bill Clinton's efforts at comprehensive health care reform failed, many of his incremental initiatives succeeded, including the Health Insurance Portability and Accountability Act (HIPAA) of 1996 and CHIP.

Many political lessons can be learned from the failure of Clinton's health care reform initiative (Litman & Robins, 1997). Presidential leadership in achieving landmark changes in health policies can be successful only when political opportunity, political skill, and commitment converge. Opportunities were uniquely abundant for Johnson in 1965, so he effectively handled his legislative role. Presidents Harry Truman, John Kennedy, and Jimmy Carter might have promoted their proposals with greater skill, but were fundamentally thwarted by the absence of a true window of opportunity. Clinton enjoyed uniquely high public interest in health care reform but failed in part due to other weaknesses related to opportunity, especially his failure to act within the first 100 days after his inauguration. The complexity of the ever-changing details of his proposal was another major flaw and ultimately proved too much for the public to comprehend and too easy for adversaries to distort.

The 2008 presidential race, from which President Barack Obama emerged victorious, offered another opportunity for Democrats to take up health care reform. While campaigning for the presidency, Obama presented a framework for health care reform to achieve three goals: (1) modernize the U.S. health care system to improve quality and reduce costs, (2) expand health insurance coverage to all Americans, and

(3) improve prevention and public health. The ACA is the most ambitious expansion of insurance since the creation of Medicare and Medicaid.

Research and Policy Development

The research community can influence health policymaking through documentation, analysis, and prescription (Longest, 2002). The first role of research in policymaking is documentation—the gathering, cataloging, and correlating of facts about the state of the world that policymakers face. Documentation may help define a given public policy problem or raise its political profile.

A second way in which research informs, and influences, policymaking is through the analysis of what does and does not work. Program evaluation and outcomes research fall under this domain. Analysis often takes the form of demonstration projects intended to provide a factual basis for determining the feasibility, efficacy, or practicality of a policy intervention, and can help shape the solutions to health policy problems.

The third way in which research influences policy making is through prescription. Research that demonstrates that a particular course of action being contemplated by policymakers may (or may not) lead to undesirable or unexpected consequences can contribute significantly to policymaking.

▶ Development of Legislative Health Policy

The making of health policy in the United States is a complex process involving both the private and public sectors, including multiple levels of government.

Policy Cycle

The formation and implementation of health policy occur in a policy cycle comprising five components: (1) issue raising, (2) policy design, (3) building of public support, (4) legislative decision-making and building of policy support, and (5) policy implementation. These activities are likely to be shared in varying degrees with Congress and interest groups.

The first component, issue-raising, is clearly essential in the policy formation cycle. Before a new policy is enacted, various issue-raising actions typically create widespread awareness of a problem and the need for it to be addressed. The president may form policy concepts from a variety of sources, including campaign information; party ideology; recommendations from advisers, cabinet members, and agency chiefs; personal views; expert opinions; and public opinion polls.

The second component of policy-making activity involves the design of specific policy proposals. Presidents have substantial resources for developing new policy proposals. For example, they may call on segments of the executive branch of government, such as the Centers for Medicare and Medicaid Services (CMS), or policy staff within the U.S. Department of Health and Human Services.

In building public support, presidents can choose from a variety of strategies. For example, they may make major addresses to the nation, mobilize their administrations to make public appeals, and organize attempts to increase support among interest groups.

In order to facilitate legislative decision-making and building of policy support, presidents, key staff, and department officials interact closely with Congress. Presidents generally meet with legislative leaders several times a month in an effort to shape upcoming legislative agenda and identify possible problems as bills move through different committees.

Legislative Process

When a bill is introduced in the House of Representatives, the speaker assigns it to an appropriate committee. The committee chair forwards the bill to the appropriate subcommittee, which then forwards proposed legislation to agencies that will be affected by the legislation, holds hearings and debates (markup), receives testimony, and may add amendments. The subcommittee and committee may recommend or not recommend the bill, or recommend that the bill be tabled. Diverse interest groups, individuals, experts in the field, and business, labor, and professional associations often exert influence over the bill at this stage through campaign contributions and intense lobbying. The full House then hears the bill and may add amendments. The bill can be approved with or without amendments, and the approved bill is sent to the Senate.

In the Senate, the bill is sent to an appropriate committee and then forwarded to an appropriate subcommittee, which may send the bill to agencies that will be affected and also holds hearings and receives testimony from interested parties (e.g., private citizens, business, labor, agencies, experts). The subcommittee votes on and forwards the proposed legislation with appropriate recommendations. Amendments may or may not be added. Then, the full Senate hears the bill and may add amendments. If the bill and House of Representatives amendments are accepted, the bill goes to the president. If the Senate adds amendments that have not been voted on by the House, then the bill must go back to the floor of the House for a vote.

If the amendments are minor and noncontroversial, the House may vote to pass the bill. If the amendments are significant and controversial, the House may call for a conference committee to review the amendments. The conference committee consists of members from the equivalent committees of the House and Senate. If their recommendations are not accepted, another conference committee is called.

After the bill has passed both the House and the Senate in identical form, it is forwarded to the president for signature. If the president signs the legislation, it becomes law. If the president does not sign it, after 10 days (excluding Sundays), it becomes law unless it is vetoed by the president. If fewer than 10 days remain in the congressional session, inaction on the part of the president results in a veto—a situation called a pocket veto. The veto can be overturned by a two-thirds majority vote of the Congress; otherwise, the bill is dead.

After legislation has been signed into law, it is forwarded to the appropriate agency for implementation. The agency publishes proposed regulations in the *Federal Register* and holds hearings regarding how the law is to be implemented. A bureaucracy, only loosely controlled by the president or Congress, writes regulations—namely, it publishes, gathers comments about, and rewrites them. At that point, the program goes on to all 50 states for enabling legislation, if appropriate. At the state level, organized interest groups hire local lawyers and lobbyists, and a whole new political cycle begins. Finally, to settle disputed issues, all parties may adjourn to the courts, with potentially long rounds of litigation shaping the final outcome.

▶ Critical Policy Issues

Government health policies have been enacted to resolve or prevent perceived deficiencies in health care delivery. Over the last four decades, most health policy initiatives and legislative efforts have focused on access to care (e.g., expanding insurance coverage, outreach programs in rural areas), cost of care (e.g., PPS, resource-based relative value scale), quality of care (e.g., creating the Agency for Health Care Policy and Research, later renamed the Agency for Healthcare Research and Quality [AHRQ]), and calling for clinical practice guidelines.

Access to Care

Policies on access to care are intended primarily for health care providers and financing mechanisms, with the purpose of expanding care to the most needy and underserved populations, including the elderly, minorities, rural residents, individuals with low income, and persons with acquired immunodeficiency syndrome (AIDS). In addition to the coverage provisions of the ACA, other programs, such as an expansion of the Community Health Center program by 263 new centers (serving a total of 1.25 million additional patients), aim to increase access to health care services (Bureau of Primary Health Care, 2011).

Providers

Several groups of providers are involved in delivering health care. Policy issues include ensuring a sufficient number of providers with a desirable geographic distribution. The debate over the supply of physicians is an important public policy issue, because policy decisions influence the number of persons entering the medical profession which, in turn, has implications for other policies. The number of new entrants into the profession is influenced by government assistance programs for individual students and by government grants given directly to educational institutions. On the negative side, an increasing supply of physicians may result in increased health care expenditures because of provider-induced demand. On the positive side, an increasing supply of physicians may help alleviate shortages in certain regions of the country. Policy approaches to expand access have included the National Health Service Corps, legislation supporting rural health clinics to expand geographic access to care, student assistance programs to expand the pool of health care workers, and legislation to expand the system of emergency medical services.

Public Financing

In the United States, public financing has largely been used to help vulnerable groups obtain health care. Vulnerable groups include the elderly (Medicare), poor children (Medicaid), poor adults (Medicaid and local or state general assistance), the disabled (Medicaid and Medicare), veterans (Veterans Health Administration), Native Americans (Indian Health Service), and patients with end-stage renal disease (Medicare and Social Security benefits for kidney dialysis and transplants). Inadequate access to care continues to be a problem in many communities, however, partly because policies enacted since 1983 have focused on narrowly defined elements of the delivery system.

Access and the Elderly

Two main concerns dominate the debate about Medicare policy. First, spending must be restrained to keep the program solvent. Second, the program must be made truly comprehensive by adding services that are currently not covered or covered inadequately, such as comprehensive nursing home coverage. These concerns create a paradox, however, since their goals are at odds.

Access and Minorities

Minorities are more likely than whites to face health care access problems. Hispanics, blacks, Asian Americans, and Native Americans, to name the most prevalent minorities, all experience difficulties accessing the U.S. health care delivery system. In some instances, the combination of low income and minority status creates further difficulties; in others, the interaction of distinct cultural habits and minority status causes problems in accessing health care. Resolving the problems confronting these groups will require policies to encourage professional education programs that are sensitive to the unique needs of minorities as well as programs to expand the delivery of services to areas populated by minorities. Many of these areas have been designated as having shortages of health care workers.

Access in Rural Areas

Delivery of health care services in rural communities has always posed the problem of making advanced medical care available to residents of sparsely settled areas. Purchasing high-tech equipment to serve a few people is not cost-efficient, and finding physicians who want to reside in rural areas is difficult. Thus, specialists and expensive diagnostic equipment are not readily available in rural medical practices. Furthermore, reimbursement systems based on average costs make financial survival difficult for rural hospitals that serve few patients.

Funding the National Health Service Corps is one step toward addressing the problem of personnel shortages in rural areas; however, the Corps affects only those graduating physicians who practice in workforce-shortage areas, and only for a limited time for each student. Additional programs are needed to increase the total supply of physicians and create incentives for permanent practice in rural areas.

Access and Low Income

Low-income mothers and their children have problems accessing the health care system, both because they lack insurance and because they generally live in medically underserved areas. Pregnant women in low-income families are far less likely to receive prenatal care than are women in higher-income categories. CHIP, created in 1997, has given states some flexibility in how they spend federal funds allocated for investment in children's health coverage ("States Face a Welcome Dilemma," 1997).

Smoking and Tobacco Use

In the United States, lung cancer is the leading cause of death from cancer, killing 156,000 people annually (American Cancer Society, 2017).

Overall, tobacco use causes almost 1 in 5 deaths in the United States and is responsible for approximately 480,000 premature deaths every year (Centers for Disease Control and Prevention [CDC], 2016). In 2007, the Institute of Medicine[1] released a report entitled *Ending the Tobacco Problem: A Blueprint for the Nation*, with the stated goal of reducing smoking rates in the United States. This goal is to be achieved through a two-pronged strategy that strengthens and fully implements traditional tobacco control measures and modifies the regulatory landscape to permit policy innovations. The report concluded that, if states maintain a comprehensive integrated tobacco control strategy at the CDC-recommended funding level of $15 to $20 per capita, tobacco use could be effectively reduced.

Research has shown that more capital and time invested in tobacco control programs result in greater and quicker impact. For example, in California, the state with the longest-running tobacco control program, smoking rates fell from 22.7% in 1988 to 13.2% in 2008. Residents of the state now buy approximately half the number of cigarettes as the rest of the nation. California was the first state to pass electronic tax stamp laws, making it easier to collect sales taxes and prevent tax evasion. The program adopted a novel "de-normalization" strategy to reduce the social acceptability of tobacco use and exposure to second-hand smoke in California communities. This approach shifted public attitudes, changed social norms, and is saving lives (California Tobacco Control Program, 2010, 2017).

In addition to supporting control programs, the U.S. government has teamed up with national partners to run nationwide campaigns directed at smoking cessation. The American Legacy Foundation administers the "truth" campaign, which supports state-based youth prevention efforts. The Americans for Nonsmokers' Rights group provides states and municipalities with assistance and guidance in passing and implementing smoke-free indoor air policies. The American Cancer Society, American Heart Association, and American Lung Association provide advocacy on tobacco control policy issues, while also providing community-level support through offices across the nation.

Cost Containment

To a large extent, the strengths of the U.S. health care delivery system also contribute to its weaknesses. The United States boasts both the

---

1 The Institute of Medicine was renamed the National Academy of Medicine in 2015.

latest developments in medical technology and an ample supply of well-trained specialists, but these advances collectively create the most expensive means possible to provide care to patients, making the U.S. health care system the costliest health care system in the world. No other aspect of health care policy has received more attention during the past 30 years than efforts to contain increases in health care costs. Two major policy initiatives enacted by the federal government have targeted hospitals (PPS) and physician services (resource-based relative value scale) for price controls.

The National Health Planning and Resources Development Act of 1974 marked the transition from improving access to containing cost as the principal theme of U.S. federal health policy. Through certificate-of-need review, health planning was used as a policy tool to contain hospital costs. One major change in health policy that strives to hold down costs was the launch of the prospective payment system (PPS) of paying hospitals for Medicare clients, enacted in 1983 (Mueller, 1988). The PPS method of reimbursement has proved to be the most successful tool for controlling hospital expenditures (Wennberg et al., 1984). Government programs—especially Medicare and Medicaid—federal employee benefit programs, and Veterans Health Administration and armed services programs face constant pressure from Congress to keep costs down.

Expenditures are a function of the price of services multiplied by the quantity of services delivered. In the past, most policies that were enacted focused on the price of services. Policymakers are reluctant to consider restricting the quantity of services, fearful of a backlash if they are perceived as "rationing care."

Increasing debate over the right to die and the value of life-extending services provides an opportunity to discuss limiting reimbursable services. So far, the federal government has been reluctant to adopt an explicit rationing strategy to contain expenditures, but state governments can be expected to experiment with other means of cost containment.

The private sector also influences the policy focus on cost containment. Major corporations are now aggressively pursuing methods to restrain the growth of health insurance costs for their employees. Large employers have started to offer discounts toward the purchase of health insurance when employees enroll in healthy lifestyle programs and achieve certain health goals. In early 2018, three corporate behemoths—Amazon, Berkshire Hathaway, and JPMorgan Chase—announced that they would form an independent health care company for their employees in the United States. The alliance was another sign of just how disappointed American businesses are with the state of the nation's health care system and the upwardly spiraling costs of medical treatment.

Quality of Care

Along with access and cost, quality of care is another main concern of health care policy. The Health Care Quality Act of 1986 mandated the creation of a national database within the U.S. Department of Health and Human Services to provide data on legal actions against health care providers. This information allows people recruiting physicians in one state to discover actions against those physicians in other states, thereby helping ensure they choose the best possible employees.

Under the Omnibus Budget Reconciliation Act (OBRA) of 1989, Congress created a new agency, the National Center for Health Services Research (now called the Agency for Healthcare Research and Quality [AHRQ]), and mandated it to conduct and support research with respect to the outcomes, effectiveness, and appropriateness of health care services and procedures (U.S. House of Representatives, 1989). AHRQ has established funding for patient outcomes research teams that focus on particular medical conditions. These research teams are part of a broader effort—the medical treatment effectiveness program, which "consists of four elements: medical treatment effectiveness research, development of databases for such research, development of clinical guidelines, and the dissemination of research findings and clinical guidelines" (Salive et al., 1990). The development of clinical guidelines was carried out by AHRQ from 1992 to 1996; this effort has now broadened to become the National Guideline Clearinghouse, which is responsible for the analysis and dissemination of clinical guidelines across the United States (National Guideline Clearinghouse, n.d.). AHRQ also focuses on improving quality of care through comparative effectiveness research, health information technology initiatives, preventive medicine (through the U.S. Preventive Services Task Force in particular), and health care value analyses. Other initiatives introduced to further improve the quality of care include Consumer Assessment of Healthcare Providers and Systems (CAHPS), National Healthcare Quality and Disparities Reports (QDR), and My Own Network, Powered by AHRQ (MONAHRQ) (AHRQ, 2017).

Mental Health

Mental health policy encompasses a variety of areas pertaining to people with a diagnosis or possible diagnosis of a mental health condition, and to those providers involved in managing or treating these patients. In the past, mental health care in the United States experienced four major periods of reform: the American asylum movement led by Dorothea Dix in 1843; the "mental hygiene" movement inspired by Clifford Beers in 1908; the deinstitutionalization started by Action for Mental Health in

1961; and the community support movement called for by the CMCH Act Amendments of 1975.

In 1843, Dorothea Dix submitted a Memorial to the Massachusetts legislature, describing the abusive treatment and horrible conditions received by the mentally ill patients in jails, cages, and almshouses. In 1866, the New York state legislature was presented with a recommendation to establish a separate asylum for chronic, mentally ill patients. Some hospitals placed patients with chronic mental illness into separate wings or wards, or different buildings, though their care was not necessarily improved by these measures (Luchins, 1989). In *A Mind That Found Itself* (1908), Clifford Whittingham Beers described the humiliating treatment he received and the deplorable conditions he encountered while in a mental hospital. In 1909, the National Committee for Mental Hygiene (NCMH) was founded by a small group of reform-minded scholars and scientists—including Beer himself—which marked the beginning of the "mental hygiene" movement (Cohen, 1983).

In 1961, the Joint Commission on Mental Health published the *Action for Mental Health*, a call that recommended that community clinics take on the burden of prevention and early intervention of mental illness. Soon, courts started to rule in favor of patients on the topic of involuntary committal, stating that they could not necessarily be forced into mental health treatment (Koyanagi & Goldman, 1991).

However, simply changing the location of mental health care from state hospitals to nursing homes was insufficient to implement the idea of deinstitutionalization. In 1975, the National Institute of Mental Health created the Community Support Program (CSP) to provide funds for communities to set up comprehensive mental health services and supports to help mentally ill patients become integrated successfully in society. The program stressed the importance of other supports in addition to medical care, including housing, living conditions, employment, transportation, and education, and it established a new national priority for assisting people with serious mental disorders. In 1980, Congress enacted the Mental Health Systems Act to prioritize the provision of services to the mentally ill and to emphasize the expansion of services beyond just clinical care alone (Koyanagi & Goldman, 1991).

Later in the 1980s, under the influence of Congress and the Supreme Court, many programs started to help mentally ill patients reclaim their benefits. A new Medicaid service was also established to assist people who were diagnosed with a chronic mental illness. People who were temporarily hospitalized were provided with aid and care, and a pre-release program was created to enable people to apply for Medicaid reinstatement prior to discharge. Not until 1990, about 35 years after the start of the deinstitutionalization, did the first state hospital begin to close.

The number of such hospitals eventually dropped from around 300 to approximately 40 in the 1990s (Koyanagi, 2007).

Some critics maintain that deinstitutionalization has, from a mental health point of view, been a total failure. Many seriously mentally ill individuals are either homeless or in prison; in either case (especially the latter), they typically receive little or no mental health care. This failure may be attributable to lack of funding for community support programs and a shortage of mental health providers (Torrey, 2005).

In 1990, Congress passed the Americans with Disabilities Act (ADA). Title I of this civil rights law protects individuals with depression, post-traumatic stress disorder (PTSD), and other mental health conditions from discrimination in the workplace. It prohibits employers with 15 or more employees from firing, refusing to hire, or taking other adverse actions against a job applicant or employee based on real or perceived mental health conditions. It also strictly limits the circumstances under which an employer can ask for information about medical conditions, including mental health conditions, and imposes confidentiality requirements on any medical information the employer has (U.S. Public Health Service, 1999).

The Paul Wellstone and Pete Domenici Mental Health Parity and Addiction Equity Act of 2008 (MHPAEA) is a federal law that prevents group health plans and health insurance issuers providing mental health and substance use disorder (MH/SUD) benefits from imposing less favorable limitations on such benefits than on medical/surgical coverage benefits. CMS further applies these rules to Medicaid and CHIP, preventing inequities between beneficiaries who have mental health or substance use disorder conditions in the commercial market (including the state and federal marketplace) and those who have such conditions and are covered by Medicaid or CHIP. This also promotes greater cross-state consistency for patients (Substance Abuse and Mental Health Services Administration, 2011).

The 2011 National Prevention Strategy included goals for mental and emotional well-being. In particular, implementing better parenting and early intervention programs increases the likelihood that such prevention programs will be included in future U.S. mental health policies and research funding will be broadened to include longitudinal prevention studies (National Institute of Mental Health, 2012).

In recent years, public policies have focused on support for rigorous addiction rehabilitation programs and an improved mental health safety net. Efforts include promoting federal initiatives that support public education on mental illness and addiction, such as the Mental Health First Aid Act; ensuring that federal funding is implemented and expanded for community behavioral health organizations, as outlined in the Excellence in Mental Health Act; promoting and funding incentives to help states and local governments expand drug treatment, prevention, and recovery efforts, as emphasized in the Comprehensive Addiction and Recovery Act; preserving funding for other important behavioral health programs, such as the Substance Abuse Prevention and Treatment Block Grant and other programs funded by the Substance Abuse and Mental Health Services Administration; ensuring that behavioral health providers are eligible for health information technology incentives, as expressed in the Behavioral Health IT Act; protecting federal funding for Medicaid and protecting Medicaid beneficiaries and providers; and ensuring the full inclusion of behavioral health in health reform implementation (National Council for Behavioral Health, 2016).

▶ National Health Reform

Health reform in the United States has a long history. In only the past ten years, landmark reform has been passed through two federal statutes enacted in 2010: the Patient Protection and Affordable Care Act (ACA), signed on March 23, 2010, and the Health Care and Education Reconciliation Act of 2010 (H.R. 4872), which amended the ACA and became law on March 30, 2010 (Blumenthal et al., 2015). The years following the ACA's passage have witnessed intense implementation efforts, and new opportunities for policy making have emerged, such as the bipartisan passage of the Medicare Access and the CHIP Reauthorization Act (MACRA) in 2015 (Blumenthal et al., 2015; Obama, 2016).

A central goal of the ACA is to significantly reduce the number of uninsured Americans by providing affordable coverage through Medicaid and the health insurance marketplaces. The ACA offers states the opportunity to expand Medicaid coverage for adults to those with incomes that are up to 138% of the federal poverty level, and indeed 33 states have done so as of April 2018 (Kaiser Family Foundation 2018). The ACA also extended funding for CHIP through fiscal year 2015 and has reauthorized for the program through 2019. As of 2017, 15 states (including the District of Columbia) have opted to use CHIP funds to expand their Medicaid programs. The other 36 states used CHIP funds to run a combination or separate health insurance program. During fiscal year 2016, 8.9 million children were enrolled in CHIP-funded coverage, while 37.1 million children were enrolled in Medicaid-financed coverage (CMS, 2018).

Under the ACA's provisions for employer-shared responsibility, certain employers—called applicable large employers [ALEs]—must offer minimum essential health benefits to full-time employees or else make an employer-shared responsibility payment to the Internal

Revenue Service. As a result, approximately 94% of all U.S. companies with 50 to 199 employees and 98% of all U.S. companies with 200 or more employees now offer health insurance coverage (Kaiser Family Foundation, 2017a).

In addition to Medicaid expansion and reform of individual health insurance markets, the ACA contains numerous provisions aimed at reforming health care delivery and payment in the United States. These provisions focus on three broad aspects: (1) testing new delivery models and promoting successful ones (e.g., the development of accountable care organizations [ACOs], the patient-centered medical home [PCMH]), (2) encouraging the shift toward value-based payment (e.g., shared savings, pay-for-performance, bundled payment), and (3) developing resources for system-wide improvement (e.g., meaningful use of health information system, precision medicine).

According to the Commonwealth Fund (2015), there are three major challenges related to fully implementing the ACA:

- The Supreme Court made it optional for states to expand Medicaid eligibility, resulting in significant consequences for residents in states that opted out. Millions of people in those states are now trapped in a coverage gap, earning too much to qualify for Medicaid but not enough for marketplace subsidies (Commonwealth Fund, 2015).
- Undocumented immigrants are excluded from the law; consequently, they cannot purchase marketplace coverage or qualify for Medicaid (Commonwealth Fund, 2015). The Congressional Budget Office estimates that 30% of the remaining uninsured people will consist of unauthorized immigrants by 2020 (Commonwealth Fund, 2015).
- Some individuals with higher incomes are having difficulty affording their premiums and deductibles, due to subsidies becoming less generous with higher household income (Commonwealth Fund, 2015).

In 2017, under the administration of President Donald Trump, the American Health Care Act (AHCA) was introduced in the House of Representatives. On May 4, 2017, the House voted to pass this act by a narrow margin of 217–213, sending the bill to the Senate for deliberation. The Senate developed several amendments and bills to modify the AHCA bill that had passed in the House, but none received enough votes to win passage. On July 28, 2017, the bill was returned to the calendar after the Senate rejected several amendments (*Congressional Record*, 2017).

Although Congress was unable to pass a comprehensive national health reform bill in 2017, many other reforms are playing out in

Congress, regulatory agencies, and state capitals that could profoundly impact the health care landscape over the coming years. These changes include efforts by Congress to reform the federal tax code (which could repeal ACA's insurance mandate); efforts by the Department of Health and Human Services to reshape how the ACA is administered and how government pays for value over volume; and efforts by individual states to control Medicaid and drug spending thus limiting coverage (Kaiser Family Foundation, 2017b).

▶ Conclusion

Health policies are developed to serve the public's interests; however, public interests are diverse, and members of the public often hold conflicting views. Although the U.S. public consistently supports the goal of national health insurance, it rejects the idea of the federal government running the health care delivery system. Similarly, although the American public wants the government to control health care costs, many people believe the federal government already exerts too much control over their daily lives. The challenge for policymakers is to find a balance between governmental provisions (i.e., control) and the private health care market to improve coverage and affordability of care. Successful health policies are more likely to be couched in terms of cost containment—a market justice, economic, business, and middle-class concern—than in terms of improved or expanded access and reduction or elimination of health disparities (a social justice, liberal, labor, low-income issue). Nevertheless, cost-related health policies will likely have little impact on improving the quality of care or reducing health disparities.

References

1. Alford RR. 1975. *Health care politics: Ideology and interest group barriers to reform.* Chicago, IL: University of Chicago Press.
2. Agency for Healthcare Research and Quality (AHRQ). 2017. TalkingQuality: Key quality initiatives. https://www.ahrq.gov/professionals/quality-patient-safety/talkingquality /resources/initiatives/index.html. Accessed December 15, 2017.
3. American Cancer Society. 2017. Key statistics for lung cancer. https://www.cancer.org /cancer/non-small-cell-lung-cancer/about/key-statistics.html. Accessed December 15, 2017.
4. Blumenthal D, et al. 2015. The Affordable Care Act at 5 years. *N Engl J Med.* 372(25):2451–2458. doi: 10.1056/NEJMhpr1503614.
5. Bureau of Primary Health Care. 2011. HHS awards Affordable Care Act funds to expand access to health care. https://wayback.archive-it.org/3926/20140108162109 /http://www.hhs.gov/news/press/2011pres/08/20110809a.html. Accessed August 12, 2015.

6. California Tobacco Control Program. 2010. Two decades of the California Tobacco Control Program: California tobacco survey, 1990–2008. https://library.ucsd.edu/dc/object/bb5086895c/_5_1.pdf. Accessed April 16, 2018.
7. California Tobacco Control Program. 2017. California Tobacco Control Program overview. https://www.cdph.ca.gov/Programs/CCDPHP/DCDIC/CTCB/CDPII%20Document%20Library/AboutUS/ProgramOverview/AboutUsProgramOverview081216.pdf. Accessed December 15, 2017.
8. Centers for Disease Control and Prevention (CDC). 2016. Tobacco-related mortality. https://www.cdc.gov/tobacco/data_statistics/fact_sheets/health_effects/tobacco_related_mortality/index.htm. Accessed December 15, 2017.
9. Centers for Medicare and Medicaid Services (CMS). 2018. Children's Health Insurance Program. https://www.medicaid.gov/affordable-care-act/chip/index.html. Accessed April 9, 2018.
10. Cohen S. 1983. The mental hygiene movement, the development of personality and the school: The medicalization of American education. *Hist Educ Q*. 23(2):123–149.
11. Commonwealth Fund. 2015. The Affordable Care Act at five years: How the law is changing health coverage in the U.S. http://www.commonwealthfund.org/ACAat5/coverage-reform/. Accessed August 12, 2015.
12. *Congressional Record*. 2017, July 27. p. S4415. https://www.congress.gov/crec/2017/07/27/CREC-2017-07-27-pt1-PgS4415-2.pdf. Accessed April 9, 2018.
13. Health Insurance Association of America. 1992. *Source book of health insurance data*. Washington, DC: Health Insurance Association of America.
14. Institute of Medicine. 2007. *Ending the tobacco problem: A blueprint for the nation*. Washington, DC: Institute of Medicine.
15. Kaiser Family Foundation. 2017a. 2012 employer health benefits survey. http://www.kff.org/report-section/ehbs-2012-section-2/. Accessed April 9, 2018.
16. Kaiser Family Foundation. 2017b. Home page. https://www.kff.org. Accessed December 2017.
17. Kaiser Family Foundation. 2018. https://www.kff.org/health-reform/state-indicator/state-activity-around-expanding-medicaid-under-the-affordable-care-act/?currentTimeframe=0&sortModel=%7B%22colId%22:%22Location%22,%22sort%22:%22asc%22%7D. Accessed April 16, 2018.
18. Koyanagi C. 2007. *Learning from history: Deinstitutionalization of people with mental illness as precursor to long-term care reform*. Menlo Park, CA: Kaiser Family Foundation, 1–22.
19. Koyanagi C, Goldman H. 1991. The quiet success of the national plan for the chronically mentally ill. *Hosp Commun Psychiatry*. 42(9):899–905. https://www.researchgate.net/publication/21411449_The_Quiet_Success_of_the_National_Plan_for_the_Chronically_Mentally_Ill. Accessed April 9, 2018.
20. Litman T, Robins L. 1997. The relationship of government and politics to health and health care: A sociopolitical overview. In: Litman T, Robins L, eds. *Health politics and policy*. 3rd ed. New York, NY: John Wiley and Sons, 3–45.
21. Longest BB. 2002. *Health policymaking in the United States*. Ann Arbor, MI: Health Administration Press.
22. Luchins, AS. 1989. Moral treatment in asylums and general hospitals in 19th-century America. *J Psychol*. 123(6):585–607.
23. Miller CA. 1987. Child health. In: Levine S, Lillienfeld A, eds. *Epidemiology and health policy*. New York, NY: Tavistock, 15.
24. Mueller KJ. 1988. Federal programs do expire: The case of health planning. *Public Admin Rev*. 48:719–735.

25. National Council for Behavioral Health. 2016. Mental health and addiction policy agenda. https://www.thenationalcouncil.org/policy-action/policy-agenda/. Accessed December 16, 2017.

26. National Guideline Clearinghouse. n.d. Help & about. http://www.guideline.gov /about/index.aspx. Accessed August 12, 2015.

27. National Institute of Mental Health. 2012. Priorities for prevention research at NIMH. https://www.nimh.nih.gov/about/advisory-boards-and-groups/namhc/reports /priorities-for-prevention-research-at-nimh.shtml. Accessed December 16, 2017.

28. National Institutes of Health (NIH). 2017. NIH budget. https://www.nih.gov/about -nih/what-we-do/budget. Accessed December 15, 2017.

29. Obama B. 2016. United States health care reform: Progress to date and next steps. *JAMA*. 316(5):525–532. doi: 10.1001/jama.2016.9797.

30. Salive ME, et al. 1990. Patient outcomes research teams and the Agency for Health Care Policy and Research. *Health Serv Res*. 25:697–708.

31. States face a welcome dilemma: How to best spend $24 billion to cover nation's uninsured children. 1997. *State Health Watch*. 4(8):1, 4.

32. Substance Abuse and Mental Health Services Administration. 2011. Implementation of the Mental Health Parity and Addiction Equity Act (MHPAEA). https://www .samhsa.gov/health-financing/implementation-mental-health-parity-addiction -equity-act. Accessed December 16, 2017.

33. Torrey EF. 2005, May 25. Deinstitutionalization: A psychiatric "Titanic." *Frontline*. WGBH Educational Foundation. Excerpts from Torrey EF. 1997. *Out of the shadows: Confronting America's mental illness crisis*. New York, NY: John Wiley & Sons.

34. U.S. House of Representatives. 1989. *Omnibus Budget Reconciliation Act of 1989: Conference Report to Accompany H.R. 3299*. Washington, DC: Government Printing Office.

35. U.S. Public Health Service. 1999. Overview of mental health services. In: *Mental health: A report of the Surgeon General*. Washington DC, Government Printing Office.

36. Weissert C, Weissert W. 1996. *Governing health: The politics of health policy*. Baltimore, MD: Johns Hopkins University Press.

37. Wennberg JE, et al. 1984. Will payment based on diagnosis-related groups control hospital costs? *N Engl J Med*. 311(5):295–300.

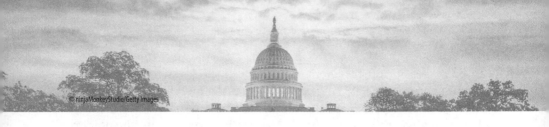

CHAPTER 14

The Future of Health Services Delivery

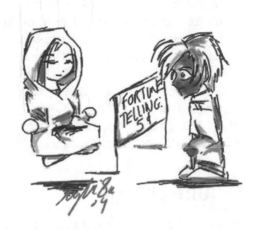

▶ Introduction

F undamental features of U.S. health care delivery, such as the largely private infrastructure and traditional American values, have, in the past, resisted any proposals for a sweeping transformation of health care. How certain forces of change play out in the future will be particularly significant. The main forces affecting the U.S. health care system include social, demographic, and cultural trends; economic conditions; political will and legal rulings; technological innovation; global health issues; and ecological events, such as the emergence of new diseases and catastrophic occurrences. Some of these forces, such as demographic trends, will follow a foreseeable course, based on which some predictions can be made. For other factors, making even short-term predictions is difficult. For instance, it is impossible to predict the future course of the U.S. economy, employment, and family incomes, all of which will affect what individual Americans and the nation may or may not be able to afford in the wake of rising health care costs. It is clear, however, that U.S. health care stands at a tipping point—a convergence of a growing, graying, and highly consumptive population with increasingly limited financial and human capital resources (Frist, 2014).

Despite the intents and promises of the Affordable Care Act (ACA), serious issues remain to be resolved in the areas of coverage, cost, access, and affordability. As of spring 2018, the U.S. Congress had failed to pass a comprehensive reform bill. However, the ACA's individual mandate— which had required all Americans to either have health insurance or pay a tax penalty—was effectively repealed by the Tax Cuts and Jobs Act of 2017. Going forward, it is unclear whether or how the lingering issues of health insurance associated with the ACA—such as the employer mandate, health insurance exchanges,[1] federal subsidies for low-income people to buy health insurance, and Medicaid expansion in the more than 30 states that implemented it—will be addressed. Moreover, a significant number of Americans continue to lack health insurance—an estimated 27 million people in 2016 (Congressional Budget Office [CBO], 2016).

This chapter puts the future of American health care in the larger national and global context. Likely future courses of health care reform, models of care delivery, and clinical technology are discussed.

▶ Forces of Future Change

The framework presented here views health care delivery and policy from a macro perspective. Keen observers of these forces can create opportunities for change. These forces also ensure that the U.S. health care system will continue to evolve.

Social, Demographic, and Cultural Trends

It is no secret that the rising tide of the elderly in America, concomitant with dropping birth rates, will put serious strains on Medicare and Social Security—the government-run medical and retirement programs, respectively, which are funded through workers' payroll taxes.

---

1 Under the ACA, some states, and the federal government in states that opted not to do so, established online marketplaces where people could shop for an approved health insurance plan.

For example, according to recent Medicare trustees reports, this program faces a substantial financial shortfall with looming negative consequences for beneficiaries, providers, and taxpayers, despite the 165-some provisions contained in the ACA to reduce Medicare costs, increase revenues, and combat program fraud and abuse (Centers for Medicare and Medicaid Services [CMS], 2012).

Aging of the population will also affect the supply of and demand for health care workers. The demand for health care services, and hence for health care workers, will increase as the population becomes older because the elderly consume a disproportionately large share of health care services. Yet, the supply of health care workers may decrease as those workers become older themselves and large numbers retire or reduce their working hours. An aging population will also affect the nature of the skills and services the health care workforce must be equipped to provide (Willis Towers Watson, 2016). Rational policies on future immigration may be one factor that affects the supply of health care professionals.

The U.S. society's cultural mix, which also reflects the rate and nature of immigration, will continue to slowly transform health care delivery in the United States. Social and cultural factors affect exposure and vulnerability to disease, risk-taking behaviors, health promotion and disease prevention, and health care–seeking behaviors. For example, rates of health risk behaviors among students in grades 9–12 are generally higher among blacks and Hispanics compared to whites, and emergency department use is disproportionately higher among blacks compared to whites (National Center for Health Statistics [NCHS], 2017). Even though illegal immigrants are technically uninsured, they do get health care through a variety of sources, including emergency rooms, community health centers, and charity from hospitals. Increasing dependency on government assistance and a haphazard immigration policy that does not promote cultural assimilation have the potential to alter the traditional American health care system in important ways in the future.

Economic Forces

Currently, health care expenditures consume one-fifth of the U.S. economic production. Hence, the nation's economic health, to a large extent, depends on the expenses incurred for the delivery of health care. Expenditures can rise as long as people can afford them; in turn, affordability of health care at both individual and national levels is critical. Household income in relation to economic inflation is a fundamental determinant of affordability, and both employment and personal income depend on the nation's economic health and quality of employment. In the past few years, President Donald Trump's economic agenda, relief from some burdensome regulations, and tax cuts have inspired some early signs of a stronger economy and employment growth compared to previous years, but this trend needs to be maintained over the longer term. Following are some of the key elements of Trump's economic agenda:

- A manufacturing recovery within the United States would add to both household incomes and tax revenues.
- Energy self-sufficiency would provide a tremendous boost to the U.S. economy.
- Repeal and replacement of the remaining portions of the ACA that deal with health insurance might help convert many part-time jobs into full-time positions, thereby boosting household incomes. Any new legislation must include policies that make health insurance more affordable.
- Increased spending on national defense and the country's infrastructure could improve employment.
- Despite positive signs in the nation's economy and personal incomes, many unknowns remain. For example, protracted military involvement overseas or even trade wars could produce negative results.

Political Will, Ideologies, and Legal Rulings

The ACA is a textbook case that illustrates the role of political will on the part of the president and his political party in passing and rolling out a substantial piece of legislation. While it has improved health care access across the country to some extent, this legislation has also resulted in rising health insurance premiums for many Americans while still leaving a large number of people uninsured.

The ACA was overwhelmingly supported by Democrats, who held the majority in both houses of Congress in 2010. The political landscape was reversed in 2016, when Republicans captured the majority in Congress. Even so, the American Health Care Act of 2017, which was designed to partially repeal and replace the ACA, failed to pass. Hence, the future direction of health care reform remains unclear.

Nevertheless, based on Republicans' campaign promises, health care reform is not likely to remain a dead issue. In the short term, much will depend on whether the Republican Party gains or loses congressional seats (and its majorities in the House of Representatives and Senate) in the November 2018 elections. As was the case with the ACA, the courts are also likely to play a pivotal role in deciding future challenges to any major reform efforts in the future.

Technological Innovation

The adoption of new medical technology almost invariably increases health care costs. Yet, Americans strongly favor ongoing innovation, availability, and use of new technology. One recent example of this preference is the 21st Century Cures Act of 2016, which is aimed at advancing medical innovation and providing quick access to new treatments. The high cost of research and development and the subsequent costs associated with the use of technology, however, do call into question the unrestrained innovation and use of medical technology. In the future, the health care system is likely to focus on those technologies that promote a greater degree of self-reliance and self-care for patients, with remote monitoring to ensure effectiveness and safety.

Global Health Issues

In many respects, the world has become progressively interconnected and interdependent through greater ease of trade and travel. Globalization presents both opportunities and challenges. For example, manufacture of generic and other drugs by Asian countries for export to Europe, Canada, and the United States helps the economies of both the manufacturing and importing countries. From the developed world's perspective, however, safety can become an issue with remote manufacturing. The Food and Drug Administration (FDA) has warned that consumers may be buying potentially risky drugs over the Internet with no guarantee of their effectiveness or safety. From the developing world's perspective, immigration of trained professionals, such as physicians, nurses, and therapists, results in "brain drains" that leave shortages of skilled health care workers in developing countries while relieving shortages in developed nations. This flow may go in the other direction when it comes to patients: The World Health Organization has estimated that over a 10-year period from 2007 to 2017, the number of Americans traveling abroad to receive cosmetic as well as medical treatments (referred to as medical tourism) increased from 750,000 to 16 million (Saltsman & Lett, 2017).

On other fronts, the prevention and control of infectious diseases globally will continue to pose major challenges. In this young 21st century alone, increased cross-border travel has resulted in the spread to the United States of previously unknown communicable diseases such as severe acute respiratory syndrome (SARS), as well as deadly infections such as the Ebola virus and the Middle East respiratory syndrome (MERS) virus. Current efforts to strengthen global health security include disease surveillance for outbreaks of international importance and urgency, exchange of technical information on new pathogens, and early warning and control of serious animal disease outbreaks. In a rapidly changing world, renewed efforts and cooperation among nations will become necessary. The worldwide shortage of trained health care workers is another area of alarming concern, as lack of treatment and isolation capabilities often result in deadly pandemics, affecting large segments of a population.

Ecological Events

New diseases, natural disasters, and bioterrorism have major implications for public health. Diseases that are communicable—such as new strains of influenza—and those related to environmental agents—such as vector-borne diseases (for example, West Nile virus and Chikungunya virus)—can bring about mass hysteria particularly in large population centers, especially when some diseases remain mysterious and treatments are not readily available, as was the case with Ebola-related illnesses in 2014. Growth of populations and expansion of the human footprint around the globe will intensify interactions at the human–animal–ecosystem interface, raising the probability that new diseases will emerge in the future. Whenever a significant number of people are affected or threatened by disease, research and technological innovation go into high gear. Technologies such as remote biosensing and geographic information systems, therefore, will find ongoing applications in public health and safety.

Natural disasters not only disrupt people's daily lives, but also create conditions that pose serious health risks through contamination of food and water. Health problems and psychological distress often follow in their wake. Initiatives such as biosurveillance and infrastructure upgrades will be constantly needed to cope with the consequences of both natural and human-made disasters. The roles of the Centers for Disease Control and Prevention (CDC) and other partnering agencies will continue to evolve as new challenges emerge. On the downside, the need to combat new ecological threats will divert resources from the quest to provide routine health care to the patients in most need of those services, especially those in developing countries.

▶ Coverage, Cost, and Access Dilemmas

The number of Americans who gained health insurance under the various provisions of the ACA has been estimated at approximately 20 million (Jost & Pollack, 2016), or an estimated 7.3% of the nonelderly U.S. population. Of these, almost 44% were enrolled in Medicaid, 23% in exchange-based plans (with premium subsidies), and 8.8% in other privately purchased health plans (without premium subsidies). Approximately 27 million people remain uninsured (CBO, 2016). It is estimated that the repeal of the ACA's individual mandate will increase the number of uninsured by 13 million in 2027 (CBO, 2017). The rationale for this projection is that healthier people will be less likely to obtain insurance and, especially in the nongroup market, the resulting increases in premiums will cause more people to not purchase insurance. Hence, achieving universal coverage in the United States will remain a challenge well into the future.

One important test of a robust health care system is whether the insured get timely access to health care services. Health insurance *facilitates* access, but it does not *guarantee* it. Alcalá and colleagues (2018) concluded that despite ACA-related gains in insurance coverage, those persons who purchased insurance through government-established exchanges or in the individual health insurance market and those individuals covered by Medicaid encountered more barriers to care than those with employer-based insurance. Hence, costly and inefficient use of hospital emergency departments has persisted among many individuals with health insurance coverage because they cannot find a doctor to serve their medical needs. Finding a primary care physician appears to be the biggest hurdle; finding a specialist or a dentist has been even tougher (Millman, 2014).

For many years, the success of health policy has been measured by the number of insured versus uninsured, under the erroneous assumption that once insured, everyone will somehow be able to get appropriate health care services when needed. Thus, little has been done to address the shortage of health care practitioners. The capacity of the health care system to meet the demand for services is now recognized as a major issue that threatens future access to health care for most Americans. Hospital executives, for example, believe that across the nation there are shortages of physicians, nurses, and advanced practitioners ("Hospital Executives," 2014). Economists estimate that one-third of the current physician workforce and at least half of the nurse workforce could retire by 2021. It is also projected that the United States will require 10 to 12 million new and replacement direct care workers—medical assistants, nursing aides, home health aides, and so on—to meet patients' demands for various types of health care services (Okrent, 2011).

The cost of health care is another critical variable that affects both coverage and access. Under the ACA, the average health insurance premiums in the individual health insurance market were estimated to increase by 25% in 2017 (Herron, 2016) and by 37% in 2018 (Luhby, 2017). By comparison, in the employer-based health insurance market, premiums rose by less than 4% in 2017 (Claxton et al., 2017). Clearly, because of its many regulatory mandates, the ACA failed to control runaway health insurance premiums for those forced to purchase insurance in the government-established exchanges, but who did not benefit from taxpayer-supported federal subsidies.

Unaffordable premiums affect people's ability to obtain coverage, but a second layer of costs—in the form of deductibles—influences their ability to obtain services despite having insurance. For 2018, the annual maximum deductible under the ACA was $14,700 for a family plan.[2] By comparison, in employer-sponsored plans, the average annual deductible varied between $2,503 and $4,527 per family; this included high-deductible health plans (Claxton et al., 2017). According to one report, the "sticker shock" comes not on the front end when purchasing a plan, but on the back end when health care is needed; "sky-high deductibles . . . are leaving some newly insured feeling as vulnerable as they were before they had coverage" (Pear, 2015).

▶ The Future of Health Care Reform

Health care reform in the United States is currently at a crossroads, with an unclear future. It does not appear that any major policy initiatives will emerge until after the November 2018 congressional elections. The Republicans in power have lacked the fortitude to come up with a solution to the problems and issues described in the previous sections. Their Democratic counterparts have opted for the status quo, perhaps hoping that given the opportunity in future they may be able to evolve the ACA into a *single-payer system*, a national health care program in which the financing and insurance functions are taken over by the federal government.

The American Health Care Act

The American Health Care Act (AHCA) of 2017 was crafted by the Republicans in the House of Representatives, but was not supported by all Republicans. It barely squeaked through the House with a 217–213 vote. For the conservatives who wanted to repeal the ACA fully, the AHCA did not go far enough; for moderates, its effects on lower- and middle-income Americans were too harsh. Even President Trump remarked that the proposed legislation did not adequately protect individuals who would buy health insurance through the exchanges (Davis, 2017). Republicans in the Senate then drafted their own version of a health care reform proposal, which failed to pass. As mentioned previously, the individual mandate was later repealed under the Tax Cuts and Jobs Act of 2017, leaving the rest of the ACA mainly intact.

It is noteworthy that public opinion about the AHCA was not positive, even though the ACA drew even more pessimistic ratings in public polls. A greater number of people said that, under the AHCA, costs

---

2 In two years, the deductible increased by more than 11%, from $13,200 in 2015 (Herman, 2015).

would go up and quality of care would go down than those who had positive views about these two issues (Freeman, 2017).

Repeal of some of the ACA's key insurance provisions under the AHCA would have increased the number of uninsured by as many as 24 million people by 2026. At the same time, the projected cost savings under the program would have reduced national budget deficits by $337 billion over the 2017–2026 period (Jost, 2017).

Will a Single-Payer System Emerge?

In an interview, then Senator Harry Reid (Democrat–Nevada), one of the chief architects of the ACA, confessed that a number of Democrat lawmakers were ready to support a single-payer system (McHugh, 2013). Hence, a necessary (though not necessarily sufficient) precondition for development of a single-payer system in the United States in the future would be control of Congress and the White House by the Democratic Party.

In a recent national survey by the Pew Research Foundation, a majority of Americans (60%) said that it was the federal government's responsibility to make sure all Americans have health care coverage— the highest percentage favoring a role for the U.S. government in ensuring health insurance for all in nearly a decade. Overall, one-third of the public supported a single-payer approach run by the government, rather than delivered through a mix of private companies and government programs. Perhaps not surprisingly, support for such a system is highest among liberal Democrats (64%) (Kiley, 2017). Interestingly, such a scenario has occurred in American politics in the past: In 1993, President Bill Clinton's Health Security Act failed to gain traction after the public became disenchanted with the prospects of paying higher taxes to fund a single-payer plan. Earlier polls had shown that the public would be in favor of a national health insurance program run by the government.

A single-payer system in the United States would be fairly similar to today's Medicaid program, in which the beneficiaries get tax-financed health care, but with more controls over how that health care is delivered. Alternatively, a single-payer system might resemble today's Medicare program,[3] in which the beneficiaries get subsidized health care. Over time, however, such a program would likely start leaning toward the Medicaid model, with some out-of-pocket cost sharing still in place.

---

3 This idea was proposed in 2016 by Trump's opponent, Hillary Clinton, during the presidential race.

Unlike Medicaid and Medicare, however, a single-payer system would not have eligibility criteria. Instead, such a scheme aims to provide *universal coverage*—that is, all legal residents get health insurance—and some form of *universal access*—that is, all the insured get some degree of access to health care services. As discussed previously, it remains unknown how a given degree of access would be assured for all.

Throughout the history of health care reform, political forces have taken center stage in the debates. Indeed, for largely political reasons, the central features of the ACA were not scheduled to be implemented until 2014, after Obama's second-term election in 2012. The outcome of the 2014 congressional elections, in which Democrats ceded both houses of Congress to Republican control, may well have hinged on the widespread disenchantment with the promises of the ACA and the experiences of those who lost the coverage they had liked. Following the 2014 elections, Senator Chuck Schumer, an influential Democrat from New York, said that whatever the merits or demerits of health reform, it was "bad politics" (Goodman, 2014). In future, politicians will have to assess the political cost they would personally incur for taking a position in favor of a single-payer system, if it comes to that.

Transitioning the ACA into a single-payer system will also depend on social and economic factors. For example, if health insurance premium costs and out-of-pocket costs rise beyond what most people consider to be affordable, there could be a push for a single-payer system. Conversely, mass dissatisfaction with the ACA might kill the prospects of a single-payer system, unless crafty politicians could put the blame on corporate America and if Americans buy into that spin. Corporations could be accused of being insensitive to the rising cost of health insurance, and insurance companies could be labeled as profit mongers.

The Cost-Control Imperative

The ACA's coverage expansion in 2014 spurred a spike in health care spending, as would be expected. The law enabled millions of people to get subsidized health insurance through the exchanges and "free" coverage through Medicaid expansion. Health care costs increased by 5.3% in 2014, up from a low of 2.9% in 2013. The Office of the CMS Actuary estimated that increased use of health care services accounted for nearly 40% of the increase in per capita health spending. Health costs grew by 5.8% in 2015 (Weiner et al., 2017).

For a system to remain solvent, any expansion of coverage must be accompanied by cost-control measures. To control costs materially, it is necessary to manage utilization, limit reimbursement to providers, and employ some sort of rationing for the supply of health care services. Only the government is in a position to wage war against costs on all three fronts at the same time, particularly in a single-payer national health care system. However, heavy-handed government controls would be strongly opposed by most Americans. Hence, this approach is not seen as a practical alternative for future reforms.

Other factors, such as benefit design and technology innovation, could have some impact on rising health care expenditures, which consumed almost 18% of the United States' total economic production in 2015 (NCHS, 2017). In high-deductible health plans, for example, the insured monitor their own benefit design by seeking value in their health care consumption behavior. Slower adoption of expensive new medical technology and fewer new blockbuster drugs may also be important factors contributing to cost control (Weiner et al., 2017). Going forward, however, there are no easy answers to the health care cost dilemma.

National Debt

Any meaningful health care reform cannot be undertaken in isolation from broader economic realities. U.S. budget deficits (overspending) and the rising national debt (borrowing money to pay for the overspending) will affect all aspects of the economy, including health care. According to the U.S. Department of the Treasury (2018), the country's total outstanding public debt was $20.5 trillion in January 2018. Since the previous edition of this text was prepared, the United States has racked up an additional $2.5 trillion in debt. If at some point in the future (no one knows when, and it may not happen for a few years to come), the United States defaults on its obligation to repay the debt, there would be unimaginable consequences that will reverberate throughout the world's economies. The national debt has consequences for the world's economies and the standard of living that Americans have been taking for granted.

This is what the CBO (2015) has said about the mounting debt:

> The rising debt could not be sustained indefinitely; the government's creditors would eventually begin to doubt its ability to cut spending or raise revenues by enough to pay its debt obligations, forcing the government to pay much higher interest rates to borrow money.

Higher interest rates will only exacerbate the problem because they will increase the cost of borrowing.

Medicare's Generational Impact

The financing of Medicare is essentially a generational transfer system in which current taxpayers pay for the benefits provided to current beneficiaries. Shortfalls in such a financing system must be paid by future generations. Data from the three most recent reports (2014–2016) of the boards of trustees of the Federal Hospital Insurance and Federal Supplementary Medical Insurance Trust Funds (trustees' report) on annual Medicare deficits are presented in **TABLE 14.1**. The short-term trend is in a favorable direction, going from a deficit of $14.1 billion in 2014 to a surplus of $31.5 billion in 2016. Various provisions of the ACA seem to have made an impact on what had been out-of-control Medicare spending. More recently, the Medicare Access and CHIP Reauthorization Act (MACRA) of 2015 seems to have made a difference in cost savings through its payment reform initiatives. Notably, the rate of growth of Medicare expenditures has slowed to 4.8% (Table 14.1), although it remains above the rate of growth of total health care expenditures between 2015 and 2016 (4.3%) (Office of Actuary, 2018).

Even though the estimated date for Medicare's bankruptcy fluctuates from year to year, there is no denial that within the next 10 to 15 years the system will be insolvent, mainly because of the rapid rise in the number of beneficiaries. No meaningful health care reform can ignore the serious steps needed to address this impending disaster that will otherwise affect the lives of not only millions of senior citizens but also all working Americans. Going forward, the solvency of Medicare will depend on the size of the workforce and the level of workers' earnings. Numerous economic and demographic factors will come into play, as well as more efficient methods of care delivery, productivity improvements in the delivery of health care, and elimination of fraud and abuse in the program.

TABLE 14.1 Deficits and Surpluses in Medicare Funding: 2014–2016

	2014	2015	2016
Total income	$599.3	$644.4	$710.2
Total expenditures	$613.3	$647.6	$678.7
Surplus (deficit) (income minus expenditures)	$(14.1)	$(3.2)	$31.5
Rate of growth of expenditures from previous year	—	5.6%	4.8%

Data from Centers for Medicare and Medicaid Services 2015, 2016, 2017 Annual report of the boards of trustees of the federal hospital insurance and federal supplementary medical insurance trust funds.

▶ Future Models of Care Delivery

Accountable care organizations and medical homes—discussed in other chapters of this text—have received much attention since the passage of the ACA. These care delivery models are still in their infancy and, as time progresses, new models of health care delivery will undoubtedly emerge. Indeed, there will be both successes and failures along the way. Yet, certain guiding principles will remain in place to inform the development of new approaches that achieve better health at reduced costs. To serve a variety of needs, several different models of care will find a footing in the U.S. health care delivery system. Even so, having different models of care by no means suggests a dismantling of the traditional infrastructure consisting of hospitals of different types, small and large clinics, and other existing settings of care. Innovative payment systems that reward providers for achieving the desired goals of quality and cost will incentivize newer approaches to care delivery.

Value-Based Shared Savings Payments

Providers respond to incentives built into reimbursement methods— and they will have to be nimble to be able to respond to changes in those reimbursement schemes. To sustain their businesses, they will have to improve their productivity by "doing more with less" while still achieving their desired profit margins. Future payment methods may be based on achievement of health-related goals, management of chronic conditions and prevention of complications, preventing hospitalizations, and reaching population health targets. A payer–provider partnership that will share cost savings will enhance value in the delivery of health care.

Population Health

In the health maintenance organization (HMO) model, the provider assumed the responsibility for meeting all the health care needs of a given population. During the managed care bashing of the 1990s, HMOs were given a bad name by doctors, enrollees, politicians, and the media. Subsequently, HMOs fell out of favor while preferred provider organizations (PPOs) gained popularity. Care delivery through PPOs, however, is fraught with inefficiencies because of the absence of gatekeeping and care coordination. In the future, provider-led organizations, such as ACOs and integrated delivery systems, will likely evolve into risk-bearing entities, somewhat like staff-model HMOs, at first through partnerships with health plans. Eventually, employers and payers such as Medicare and Medicaid are likely to enroll their insured populations into these organizations, which will provide insurance coverage and also manage the total health care needs of the covered populations for a negotiated fee per enrollee. A tighter consolidation within one organization—compared to what exists in today's managed care organizations—of financing, insurance, delivery, and payment functions will achieve synergies and efficiencies that do not currently exist. The end result will be better health at a lower cost.

Community Outreach

The type of organization just described will be in a position to engage in community health programs, such as prevention and/or management of diabetes, stroke, and cardiovascular issues. Health education through community outreach will improve health of the community on the one hand and bring goodwill to the organization on the other hand.

Virtual Care

To some extent, the health care delivery system will evolve to replace periodic encounters between patients and providers with an ongoing relationship that includes remote monitoring and virtual consultations. Virtual video consultations are an effective way to provide timely medical interventions and promise to reduce or eliminate wait times for face-to-face encounters.

Technology-Driven Home Visits

An increasing amount of care will be delivered where patients are, in their own homes. Home care will be used extensively to manage high-risk populations. Biosensors, early warning systems, and remote monitoring will enable the shift from frequent office visits to home care. A major objective of remote monitoring is to keep chronically ill patients connected to necessary clinical expertise in between office visits so as to avert medical crises that might otherwise land these patients in the emergency room (Moore, 2009). Further innovations in remote care may enable just-in-time provider interventions when needed (Kvedar et al., 2011).

▶ Future Workforce Challenges

An adequate and well-trained workforce is a critical component of the health care delivery infrastructure. The impending shortage of health care professionals has been pointed out previously. Hence, the most productive use of existing resources must be emphasized.

According to the recommendations included in a report produced by the National Academy of Sciences (2010), nurses should practice to the full extent of their education and training. Licensing requirements and rules governing the scope of practice across states need to be unified for advanced-practice nurses who have master's or doctoral degrees. Residency programs for nurses need to incorporate training in community health, public health, and geriatrics.

Primary care physicians need training so they can adequately function as "comprehensivists" to address the needs of a growing number of people with complex chronic conditions. They must be prepared to manage complex pharmacology, understand end-of-life issues and medical ethics, and lead health care teams.

A shortage of health care professionals trained in geriatrics is a critical challenge with serious implications, given the anticipated growth in the U.S. elderly population. This problem is compounded by the shortage of faculty in colleges and universities who are trained in geriatrics. The elderly use the majority of home health care services and nursing home care, account for roughly half of all hospital inpatient days, and represent approximately one-fourth of all ambulatory care visits. Many elderly patients suffer from chronic conditions, and their care is often complicated by the presence of comorbidities, the use of multiple prescription drugs, and an increased prevalence of mental conditions and dementia. Evidence shows that care of older adults by health care professionals specifically prepared in geriatrics yields better physical and mental outcomes without increasing costs (H. J. Cohen et al., 2002). The most effective strategies to incentivize future workers to train for geriatric care remain uncertain, however. Under alternative demographic scenarios, an additional 2.5 to 3 million professionals in various occupations (e.g., nurses, assistants, social workers) will be needed to meet the United States' demand for long-term care services by 2030 (Spetz et al., 2015).

Integration of a racially and culturally diverse workforce is also a growing necessity. It is estimated that somewhere near the middle of the 21st century, more than half of all U.S. citizens will be nonwhite (U.S. Census Bureau, 2001). Developing skills in cultural competence will divert some resources from health care. The term *cultural competence* refers to knowledge, skills, attitudes, and behavior required of a practitioner to provide optimal health care services to persons from a wide range of cultural and ethnic backgrounds. To demonstrate cultural competence, health care providers need to understand how and why different belief systems, cultural biases, ethnic origins, family structures, and many other culture-based factors influence the manner in which people experiencing illness comply with medical advice and respond to treatment. Such variations have implications for outcomes of care (J. J. Cohen et al., 2002).

▶ Global Challenges

As pointed out previously, global issues can affect health care at the country level. Each year, more than 350 million foreign travelers arrive in the United States. To safeguard the public's health, the CDC operates quarantine stations at several major entry points. In addition, American businesses have spread worldwide, so the CDC has become actively involved in global surveillance and early detection of health threats and works closely with U.S. embassies overseas. The CDC operates more than 60 Global Disease Detection Centers and other offices worldwide.

Even though international cooperation is absolutely critical for combating health threats, achieving this lofty goal has proved to be an ongoing challenge. Since 2007, International Health Regulations (IHRs) have been binding on 196 countries under the aegis of the World Health Organization (WHO). The IHRs require countries to report certain disease outbreaks and other public health events to WHO (WHO, 2015). However, 80% of the countries have failed to meet the requirements of the IHRs, according to the Office of Global Affairs of the U.S. Department of Health and Human Services (DHHS). Neither the United States nor the United Nations has the authority to enforce compliance—yet, when threats to public health arise anywhere in the world, the affected nations look to the United States and other developed countries to come to their aid.

U.S. government agencies lend their assistance primarily through critically needed scientific knowledge and technical expertise to address a wide range of health issues. Many U.S.-based private philanthropic organizations send supplies and aid workers to affected areas. The irony is that when major disturbances occur, the affected areas are not safe either for the locals or for foreign aid workers.

Ongoing armed conflicts, in places such as the Middle East, affect medical care and public health services. In war zones, diseases such as diarrheal episodes and acute respiratory infections can spread rapidly. In this kind of scenario, the health care infrastructure may sustain damage; health workers may be injured, killed, or evacuated; supplies dwindle; and refugees often migrate in large numbers, putting a strain on food and water supplies and sanitation. Hence, both morbidity and mortality increase. Large-scale bioterrorism has not yet occurred, but global unrest amid the rise of extremism makes it a real possibility in the future. Conflicts occurring in other parts of the globe can be "exported" to countries such as the United States.

▶ New Frontiers in Clinical Technology

Despite its role in cost escalation, technological progress will most assuredly continue, albeit accompanied by increased efforts directed toward technology assessment. At some point, assessment and use of technology based on cost-effectiveness is likely to influence health policy.

Today, technology affects many aspects of medical practice, to the point that it currently drives much of the growth in the health services industry. Several areas of technological advance are especially noteworthy.

Genetic mapping is the first step in isolating a gene. The ability to collect and interpret human genetic information has opened the way for the field of *molecular medicine*, the branch of medicine that focuses on understanding the role that genes play in disease processes and treatment of diseases through gene therapy. In gene therapy, a functioning gene is inserted into targeted cells to correct an inborn defect or provide the cell with a new function. This technique is expected to replace treatment with medications or surgery in some areas. Cancer treatment is receiving much attention as a prime candidate for gene therapy because current treatment techniques (surgery, radiation, and chemotherapy) are effective in only half of all cases and can greatly reduce a patient's quality of life.

Personalized medicine and pharmacogenomics are relatively new fields. Pharmacogenomics is the study of how genes affect a person's response to drugs. Personal characteristics of individual patients can vary so much that not all medications work for everyone. In personalized medicine, specific gene variations among patients are matched with responses to particular medications to increase effectiveness and reduce unwanted side effects.

Rational drug design is expected to shorten the drug discovery process. The chief candidates for development through this process are drugs to treat neurologic and mental disorders and antiretroviral therapies for HIV/AIDS, encephalitis, measles, and influenza. New *drug delivery* systems will be used to target specific cells. For example, cancer tumors may be treated without incurring damage to healthy tissues through the use of nanoparticles as drug delivery vehicles.

Imaging technologies have undergone some of the most dramatic advances in health care. For example, focused energy beams can now avoid damage to adjacent tissue, 3-D technology can allow faster and more accurate analysis of images, and neuroimaging can help in early detection of strokes and Alzheimer's disease.

Minimally invasive surgery is undergoing advances that include image-guided brain surgery, minimal-access cardiac procedures, and endovascular placement of grafts for abdominal aneurysms. The use of robotic surgery is in its early stages.

Vaccines have traditionally been used prophylactically to prevent specific infectious diseases. More recently, the therapeutic use of vaccines in the treatment of noninfectious diseases, such as cancer, has opened new frontiers in medicine. At the same time, development of new vaccines for emerging infectious diseases remains a key item on the research agenda.

Blood substitutes would likely be available one day for large-scale use. Substitutes for real blood are necessary when supplies fall short, particularly in war and in natural disasters.

Xenotransplantation, in which animal tissues are used for transplants in humans, is a growing research area. It presents the promise of overcoming the critical shortages of available donor organs. Organs from genetically engineered animals may one day be available for transplantation (Schneider & Seebach, 2013).

Regenerative medicine holds the promise of regenerating damaged tissues and organs in vivo (in the living body) through reparative techniques that stimulate previously irreparable organs into healing themselves. Regenerative medicine also enables scientists to grow tissues and organs in vitro (in the laboratory) and safely implant them when the body cannot be prompted into healing itself.

▶ Conclusion

Some features of U.S. health care delivery have remained stable in recent years, but the future will be determined by how certain forces of change interact. The ACA was passed in late 2010, but has not solved all problems related to health care insurance: Serious issues remain in the areas of coverage, cost, access, and affordability. Hence, a new wave of health care reform has just begun. Serious challenges lie ahead unless the United States can control its rising consumption of health care resources, the costs associated with that use, and put the economy on a growth trajectory. Eventually, the nation will have to come to grips with what it can reasonably afford in terms of health care.

The existing model of health care delivery is also likely to undergo major changes in the future. New models of care delivery are being investigated that focus on value-based shared savings, population health, community outreach, virtual consultations, and technology-driven home care.

Another critical area that must be addressed is the shortage of health care professionals. While the U.S. population is rapidly aging, little has been done to address the need for geriatric care. Addressing workforce diversity and training are other looming challenges that could threaten the adequacy of the health care workforce in a changing demographic landscape.

To combat global health threats, international readiness to respond quickly to those challenges must be maintained. Armed conflicts in unstable areas of the world not only create new health crises, but also siphon off limited resources. Catastrophic consequences could follow if global health threats are not identified and managed in a timely fashion.

Technological innovations in the areas of advanced imaging, minimally invasive surgery, genetic mapping, and regenerative medicine, among others, will help shape the delivery of medical care in ways never before imagined. Many of these developments will likely shift the focus of medicine from the acute phase of illness to prevention and aftercare.

References

1. Alcalá HE, et al. 2018. Insurance type and access to health care providers and appointments under the Affordable Care Act. *Med Care.* 56(2):186–192.
2. Centers for Medicare and Medicaid Services (CMS). 2012. The Affordable Care Act: Lowering Medicare costs by improving care. http://www.cms.gov/apps/files/aca-savings-report-2012.pdf. Accessed June 2015.
3. Centers for Medicare and Medicaid Services (CMS). 2015, July 22. The 2015 annual report of the boards of trustees of the Federal Hospital Insurance and Federal Supplementary Medical Insurance trust funds. https://www.cms.gov/Research-Statistics-Data-and-Systems/Statistics-Trends-and-Reports/ReportsTrustFunds/Downloads/TR2015.pdf. Accessed February 19, 2018.
4. Centers for Medicare and Medicaid Services (CMS). 2016, June 22. The 2016 annual report of the boards of trustees of the Federal Hospital Insurance and Federal Supplementary Medical Insurance trust funds. https://www.cms.gov/Research-Statistics-Data-and-Systems/Statistics-Trends-and-Reports/ReportsTrustFunds/Downloads/TR2016.pdf. Accessed February 19, 2018.
5. Centers for Medicare and Medicaid Services (CMS). 2017, July 13. The 2016 annual report of the boards of trustees of the Federal Hospital Insurance and Federal Supplementary Medical Insurance trust funds. https://www.cms.gov/Research-Statistics-Data-and-Systems/Statistics-Trends-and-Reports/ReportsTrustFunds/Downloads/TR2017.pdf. Accessed February 19, 2018.
6. Claxton G, et al. 2017. *Employer health benefits: 2017 annual survey.* Chicago, IL: Henry J. Kaiser Family Foundation.
7. Cohen IIJ, et al. 2002. A controlled trial of inpatient and outpatient geriatric evaluation and management. *N Engl J Med.* 346(12):906–912.
8. Cohen JJ, et al. 2002. The case for diversity in the health care workforce. *Health Aff.* 21(5):90–102.
9. Congressional Budget Office (CBO). 2015, June 16. The 2015 long-term budget outlook. https://www.cbo.gov/publication/50250. Accessed June 2015.
10. Congressional Budget Office (CBO). 2016. Federal subsidies for health insurance coverage for people under age 65: 2016 to 2026. https://www.cbo.gov/sites/default/files/114th-congress-2015-2016/reports/51385-HealthInsuranceBaseline_OneCol.pdf. Accessed February 18, 2018.

11. Congressional Budget Office (CBO). 2017, November. Repealing the individual health insurance mandate: An updated estimate. https://www.cbo.gov/system/files/115th-congress-2017-2018/reports/53300-individualmandate.pdf. Accessed February 19, 2018.

12. Davis KL. 2017, March 20. Why the American Health Care Act fell short. https://www.forbes.com/sites/kennethdavis/2017/03/20/compassion-must-drive-health-care-policy/#2d218f4caf6e. Accessed February 19, 2018.

13. Freeman B. 2017, March 13. Rasmussen poll: Public doesn't have confidence in AHCA. https://www.newsmax.com/Politics/Rasmussen-AHCA-Obamacae-repeal-and-replace/2017/03/13/id/778462/. Accessed February 19, 2018.

14. Frist WH. 2014. Connected health and the rise of the patient-consumer. *Health Aff.* 33(2):191–193.

15. Goodman JC. 2014, November 28. Why the Democrats lost the election: Obamacare. *Forbes.* http://www.forbes.com/sites/johngoodman/2014/11/28/why-the-democrats-lost-the-election-obamacare. Accessed June 2015.

16. Herman B. 2015. Deductible debate. *Mod Healthc.* 45(24):22–24.

17. Herron, J. 2016, November 1. Here's how much Obamacare premiums are rising in all 50 states. *The Fiscal Times.* http://www.thefiscaltimes.com/2016/11/01/Here-s-How-Much-Obamacare-Premiums-Are-Rising-All-50-States. Accessed February 19, 2018.

18. Hospital executives: Continued shortage of nurses, advanced practitioners, physicians. 2014. *Am Nurse.* 46(1):10.

19. Jost T. 2017, March 14. CBO projects coverage losses, cost savings from AHCA; administration signals flexibility to governors on waivers. https://www.healthaffairs.org/do/10.1377/hblog20170314.059186/full/. Accessed February 19, 2018.

20. Jost TS, Pollack HA. 2016. Making health care truly affordable after health care reform. *J Law Med Ethics.* 44(4):546–554.

21. Kiley J. 2017, June 23. Public support for "single payer" health coverage grows, driven by Democrats. http://www.pewresearch.org/fact-tank/2017/06/23/public-support-for-single-payer-health-coverage-grows-driven-by-democrats/. Accessed February 19, 2018.

22. Kvedar J, et al. 2011. E-patient connectivity and the near term future. *J Gen Intern Med.* 26:636–638.

23. Luhby T. 2017, October 30. Premiums for popular Obamacare plans soar 37% for 2018. http://money.cnn.com/2017/10/30/news/economy/obamacare-premiums/index.html. Accessed February 19, 2018.

24. McHugh K. 2013, August 10. Reid says Obamacare will lead to a single-payer healthcare system. *The Daily Caller.* http://dailycaller.com/2013/08/10/absolutely-yes-reid-says-obamacare-will-lead-to-a-single-payer-healthcare-system. Accessed June 2015.

25. Millman J. (2014, September 19). Millions have joined Medicaid under Obamacare. Here's what they think of it. *The Washington Post.* http://www.washingtonpost.com/blogs/wonkblog/wp/2014/09/19/millions-have-joined-medicaid-under-obamacare-heres-what-they-think-of-it. Accessed June 2015.

26. Moore R. 2009. Telehealth connected care. *Health Manage Technol.* 30(3):39–40.

27. National Academy of Sciences. 2010. *The future of nursing: Leading change, advancing health.* Washington, DC: Institute of Medicine.

28. National Center for Health Statistics (NCHS). 2017. *Health, United States, 2016.* Hyattsville, MD: U.S. Department of Health and Human Services.

29. Office of Actuary, Centers for Medicare and Medicaid Services. 2018, January 8. National health expenditures by type of service and source of funds, CY 1960–2016. https://www.cms.gov/Research-Statistics-Data-and-Systems/Statistics-Trends-and-Reports/NationalHealthExpendData/NationalHealthAccountsHistorical.html. Accessed February 13, 2018

30. Okrent D. 2011. *Health care workforce: Future supply vs. demand*. Washington, DC: Alliance for Health Reform.
31. Pear R. 2015, November 15. Many say high deductibles make their health law insurance all but useless. *The New York Times*, p. 22.
32. Saltsman W, Lett J. 2017, April. You had it done where? The rise of medical tourism. http://www.caringfortheages.com/article/S1526-4114(17)30093-8/fulltext. Accessed February 18, 2018.
33. Schneider MKJ, Seebach JD. 2013. Xenotransplantation literature update, July–August 2013. *Xenotransplantation*. 20(5): 308–310.
34. Spetz J, et al. 2015. Future demand for long-term care workers will be influenced by demographic and utilization changes. *Health Aff*. 34(6):936–945.
35. U.S. Census Bureau. 2001. *Statistical abstract of the United States, 2001*. Washington, DC: U.S. Census Bureau.
36. U.S. Department of the Treasury. 2018. Monthly statement of the public debt of the United States. https://www.treasurydirect.gov/govt/reports/pd/mspd/2018/opds012018.prn. Accessed February 19, 2018.
37. Weiner J, et al. 2017, March 2. Effects of the ACA on health care cost containment. https://ldi.upenn.edu/brief/effects aca health care cost containment. Accessed February 19, 2018.
38. Willis Towers Watson. 2016, August. How an aging workforce and population will impact health care in the U.S. https://www.willis.com/documents/services/Claim%20and%20Risk%20Control/15937%20THOUGHT%20LEADERSHIP_Aging%20Workforce%20and%20HealthCare.final.pdf. Accessed February 18, 2018.
39. World Health Organization (WHO). 2015. International health regulations (IHR). http://www.who.int/topics/international_health_regulations/en. Accessed June 2015.

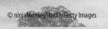
© ninjaMonkeyStudio/Getty Images

Glossary

Academic medical center: An organization in which there is active collaboration among a university, medical school, hospital/health system, and health care professionals.

Access: The ability of persons needing health services to obtain appropriate care in a timely manner.

Accountable care organization (ACO): An integrated group of providers—including hospitals, physicians, and post-discharge care delivery organizations—that work together to deliver coordinated care and take responsibility for quality and efficiency of services delivered.

Acquisition: Purchase of one organization by another.

Activities of daily living (ADLs): The most commonly used measure of disability. ADLs determine whether an individual needs assistance to perform basic activities, such as eating, bathing, dressing, toileting, and getting into or out of a bed or chair. *See* **instrumental activities of daily living (IADLs)**.

Acute condition: Short-term, intense medical care for an illness or injury usually requiring hospitalization. *See* **subacute care**.

Adaptive rehabilitation: Care that improves function despite deficits that remain.

Administrative costs: Costs associated with health insurance marketing and enrollment, contracting with providers, claims processing, utilization monitoring, and handling of denials and appeals.

Administrative information systems: Information systems that are designed to assist organizations in carrying out financial and administrative support activities such as payroll, patient accounting, materials management, and office automation.

Adult day care: A community-based, long-term care service that provides a wide range of health, social, and recreational services to elderly adults who require supervision and care while members of the family or other informal caregivers are away at work.

Adult foster care: Long-term care services provided in small, family-operated homes, located in residential communities, which provide room, board, and varying levels of supervision, oversight, and personal care to nonrelated adults.

Advance directive: A patient's wishes regarding continuation or withdrawal of treatment in the event the patient lacks decision-making capacity.

Advanced-practice nurse (APN): A general name for nurses who have education and clinical experience beyond that required of a registered nurse (RN). APNs include four areas of specialization in nursing: clinical nurse specialists (CNSs), certified registered nurse anesthetists (CRNAs), nurse practitioners (NPs), and certified nurse-midwives (CNMs).

Alliance: A joint agreement between two organizations to share their resources without joint ownership of assets.

Allied health professional: A professional who is educated and trained in a specialized field of health care and has responsibility for the delivery of services associated with medical care.

Allocative tool: A use of health policy in which there is a direct provision of income, services, or goods to groups of individuals who usually reap benefits in receiving them.

Allopathic medicine: A philosophy of medicine that views medical treatment as active intervention to counteract the effects of disease through medical and surgical procedures that produce effects opposite those of the disease. *See* **osteopathic medicine**.

Almshouse: Also called a *poorhouse*. An unspecialized institution existing during the 18th and mid-19th centuries that mainly served general welfare functions, essentially providing shelter to the homeless, the insane, the elderly, orphans, and the sick who had no family to care for them.

Alternative medicine: Also called *alternative and complementary medicine.* Nontraditional remedies—for example, acupuncture, homeopathy, naturopathy, biofeedback, yoga exercises, chiropractic, and herbal therapy.

Ambulatory: Related to walking; typically used as the opposite of inpatient.

Ambulatory care: Also referred to as *outpatient services.* Services that include (1) care rendered to patients who come to physicians' offices, outpatient departments of hospitals, and health centers; (2) outpatient services intended to serve the surrounding community (community medicine); and (3) certain services that are transported to the patient.

Asylum: Forerunner of today's inpatient psychiatric facilities. These institutions were built by state governments for patients with untreatable, chronic medical illness.

Average daily census: Average number of hospital beds occupied daily over a given period of time. This measure provides an estimate of the number of inpatients receiving care each day at a hospital.

Average length of stay (ALOS): The average number of days each patient stays in the hospital. For individual or specific categories of patients, this measure indicates severity of illness and resource use.

Balance bill: Billing of the leftover sum by the provider to the patient after insurance has partially paid the charge initially billed.

Behavioral factors: Individual lifestyles that include diet, exercise, a stress-free lifestyle, risky or unhealthy behaviors, and other individual choices that may contribute to significant health problems.

Beneficence: The ethical obligation of a health services organization to do all it can to alleviate suffering caused by ill health and injury.

Beneficiary: Anyone covered under a particular health insurance plan.

Benefit period: A period determined by a spell of illness beginning with hospitalization and ending when the beneficiary has not been an inpatient in a hospital or a skilled nursing facility for 60 consecutive days. Under Medicare rules, benefits for an inpatient stay are based on a benefit period.

Biologics: Biological products such as vaccines, blood and blood components, allergenics, somatic cells, gene therapy, tissues, and recombinant therapeutic proteins.

Biosimilar: A product that is highly similar to, or is interchangeable with, a biologic that has already been approved by the Food and Drug Administration.

Bundled payments: Payment scheme in which a number of related services are included in one price.

Capacity: The number of beds set up, staffed, and made available by a hospital for inpatient use.

Capitalism: Political and economic system that relies primarily on market forces in the production and distribution of goods and private ownership; contrasts with socialism, where collective or governmental forces prevail.

Capitation: A reimbursement mechanism under which the provider is paid a set monthly fee per enrollee (sometimes referred to as per member per month [PMPM] rate) regardless of whether the enrollee actually sees the provider and regardless of how often an enrollee sees the provider.

Carve-out: The assignment through contractual arrangements of specialized services to an outside organization because these services are not included in the contracts managed care organizations (MCOs) have with their providers or the MCO does not provide the services.

Case management: An organized approach to evaluating and coordinating care, particularly for patients who have complex, potentially costly problems that require a variety of services from multiple providers over an extended period.

Case mix: An aggregate of the severity of conditions requiring medical intervention. Case-mix categories are mutually exclusive and differentiate patients according to the extent of resource use.

Categorical programs: Public health care programs designed to benefit only a certain category of people.

Census: The number of patients in a hospital on a given day or the number of beds occupied on a given day.

Certification: Conferred by the U.S. Department of Health and Human Services, a status that entitles an organization to participate in Medicare and Medicaid. The organization must comply with the conditions of participation.

Chronic condition (chronic disease): A long-lasting medical condition that can be controlled but not cured.

Clinical decision support systems: Interactive software systems designed to help clinicians with decision-making tasks, such as determining a diagnosis or recommending a treatment for a patient.

Clinical information systems: Systems that involve the organized processing, storage, and retrieval of information to support patient care processes.

Clinical practice guidelines (medical practice guidelines): Standardized guidelines in the form of scientifically established protocols, representing preferred processes in medical practice.

Clinical trial: A research study, generally based on random assignments, designed to examine the effectiveness of a new drug, device, or treatment.

Cognitive impairment: A mental disorder that is indicated by a person having difficulty remembering, learning new things, concentrating, or making decisions that affect the individual's everyday life.

Coinsurance: Cost sharing in the form of a percent amount. A plan with an 80:20 coinsurance, for example, pays 80% of all covered medical expenses after the deductible requirement has been met until the maximum out-of-pocket liability in a given year has been met.

Community hospital: Nonfederal (i.e., Veterans Administration and military hospitals are excluded), short-term, general or specialty hospital whose services are available to the public.

Community-oriented primary care (COPC): Care that incorporates the elements of good primary care delivery as well as a population-based approach to identifying and addressing community health problems.

Comorbidity: The presence of more than one health problem in an individual.

Conditions of participation: Standards developed by the Department of Health and Human Services with which a facility must comply to participate in the Medicare and Medicaid programs.

Consumer-driven health plan: A high-deductible health plan that carries a savings option to pay for routine health care expenses.

Consumer price index: A measure of inflation in the general economy.

Copayment (coinsurance): A portion of health care charges that the insured has to pay under the terms of his or her health insurance policy. *See* **deductible**.

Corporate era: A recent period in the evolution of the U.S. medical delivery system that is characterized by the domination of corporations rather than individuals in decision making regarding care delivery and payment.

Corporatization: In this text, the ways in which health care delivery in the United States has become the domain of large organizations.

Cost-effectiveness: Evaluation of the overall usefulness of medical technology, including evaluation of the safety and efficacy of a technology in relation to its cost. *See* **cost-efficiency**.

Cost-efficiency: Delivery of services in a manner so that the benefit is greater than the cost incurred to provide the service.

Cost sharing: Sharing in the cost of health insurance premiums by those enrolled and/or payment of certain medical costs out of pocket, such as copayments and deductibles.

Cost-shifting (cross-subsidizing): In general, shifting of costs from one entity to another as a way of making up losses in one area by charging more in other areas. For example, when care is provided to the uninsured, the provider makes up the cost for those services by charging more to the insured.

Critical access hospital (CAH): Medicare designation for small rural hospitals with 25 or fewer beds that provide emergency medical services besides short-term hospitalization for patients with noncomplex health care needs. Such hospitals receive cost-plus reimbursement.

Critical pathways: Outcome-based, patient-centered case management tools that are interdisciplinary in scope, facilitating coordination of care among multiple clinical departments and caregivers. A critical pathway identifies planned medical interventions in a given case, along with expected outcomes.

Custodial care: Nonmedical care provided to support and maintain the patient's condition, generally requiring no active medical or nursing treatments.

Days of care: Cumulative number of patient days over a given period of time.

Decision support systems: Computer-based information and analytical tools to support managerial decision making in health care organizations.

Deductible: The portion of health care costs that the insured must first pay (generally up to an annual limit) before insurance payments kick in. Insurance payments may be further subject to copayment.

Deemed status: A designation used when a hospital, by virtue of its accreditation by the Joint Commission or the American Osteopathic Association, does not require separate certification from the DHHS to participate in the Medicare and Medicaid programs.

Defensive medicine: Excessive medical tests and procedures performed as a protection against malpractice lawsuits, otherwise regarded as unnecessary.

Demand-side incentive: Cost-sharing mechanism that places a larger cost burden on consumers, thereby encouraging consumers to be more cost-conscious in selecting the insurance plan that best serves their needs and more judicious in their utilization of services.

Demand-side rationing: Barriers to obtaining health care faced by individuals who do not have sufficient income to pay for services or purchase health insurance.

Dependency: (1) A person's reliance on another for assistance with common daily functions, such as bathing and grooming. *See* **activities of daily living.** (2) Children's reliance on adults, such as parents or school officials, to recognize and respond to their health needs.

Determinants of health: *See* **health determinants.**

Developmental disability: A physical incapacity that generally accompanies mental retardation and often arises at birth or in early childhood.

Developmental vulnerability: Rapid and cumulative physical and emotional changes that characterize childhood and the potential impact that illness, injury, or untoward family and social circumstances can have on a child's life-course trajectory.

Discharge: Release of a patient who has received inpatient services. The total number of discharges indicates access to hospital inpatient services as well as the extent of utilization.

Discharge planning: Part of the overall treatment plan designed to facilitate discharge from an inpatient setting. It includes, for example, an estimate of how long the patient will be in the hospital, what the expected outcome is likely to be, whether any special requirements will be needed at discharge, and what needs to be facilitated for postacute continuity of care.

Disease: Condition determined by a medical professional's evaluation; contrast with an illness, which is based on the patient's assessment. *See* **illness.**

Dispensary: A clinic during the preindustrial era that provided charity care in urban areas.

Distributive policies: Spreading of benefits throughout society. Examples are funding of medical research through the National Institutes of Health, the training of medical personnel through the National Health Services Corps, the construction of health facilities under the Hill-Burton Act program, and the initiation of new institutions (e.g., health maintenance organization).

Efficacy: The health benefit to be derived from the use of technology, or how effective a given technology is in diagnosing or treating a condition.

E-health: Health care information and services offered over the Internet by professionals and nonprofessionals alike.

Enabling characteristics: Within the access to care framework, factors that make it possible (or easier) for individuals to use available health care resources.

Enrollee: A person covered by a health plan, especially a managed care plan.

Environmental factors: Factors that encompass the physical, socioeconomic, sociopolitical, and sociocultural dimensions of life.

E-therapy: Any type of professional therapeutic interaction that makes use of the Internet to connect qualified mental health professionals and their clients.

Ethics committee: An interdisciplinary committee responsible for developing guidelines and standards for ethical decision making in the provision of health care and for resolving issues related to medical ethics.

Financing: Any mechanism that gives people the ability to pay for health care services.

Gatekeeping: The use of primary care physicians to coordinate health care services needed by an enrollee in a managed care plan.

General hospital: A hospital that provides general and specialty medical services for a variety of medical needs.

Generalist: A physician in family practice, general internal medicine, or general pediatrics. *See* **specialist.**

Genetic mapping: The first step in isolating a gene.

Globalization: Various forms of cross-border economic activities driven by global exchange of information, production of goods and services more economically in developing countries, and increased interdependence of mature and emerging world economies.

Health: A state of physical, mental, and social well-being (World Health Organization, 1948).

Health care delivery: The provision of medical care or illness care.

Health care reform: Systemic changes in how medical care is financed or delivered.

Health care system: Organizations, personnel, and activities associated with promoting, restoring, and maintaining health.

Health determinants: Factors that contribute to the general well-being of individuals and populations.

Health informatics: The application of information science to improve the efficiency, accuracy, and reliability of health care services. It requires the use of information technology (IT) but goes beyond IT by emphasizing the improvement of health care delivery.

Health plan: The contractual arrangement between the managed care organization and the enrollee, including the collective array of covered health services to which the enrollee is entitled.

Health planning: Decisions made by governments to limit health care resources, such as hospital beds and diffusion of costly technology.

Health policy: Public policy that pertains to or influences the pursuit of health.

Health technology assessment: Any process of examining and reporting properties of a medical technology used in health care, such as its safety, effectiveness, feasibility, indications for use, and cost-effectiveness.

Heredity: A key determinant of health that predisposes individuals to certain diseases.

Holistic medicine: A philosophy of health care that emphasizes the well-being of every aspect of a person, including the physical, mental, social, and spiritual aspects of health.

Horizontal integration: A growth strategy in which an organization extends its core product or service. *See* **vertical integration**.

Hospice: A cluster of special services for the dying, which blends medical, spiritual, legal, financial, and family-support services. The venue can vary from a specialized facility to a nursing home to the patient's own home.

Hospitalist: A physician who specializes in the care of hospitalized patients.

Illness: Patient condition recognized by the patient's perceptions and evaluation of how he or she feels; contrast with disease, which is determined by a medical professional. *See* **disease**.

Information technology (IT): Technology used for the transformation of data into useful information. It involves determining data needs, gathering appropriate data, storing and analyzing the data, and reporting the information generated in a user-friendly format.

Informed consent: A fundamental patient right to make an informed choice regarding medical treatment based on full disclosure of medical information by the providers.

Inpatient: Services delivered on the basis of an overnight stay in a health care institution.

Inpatient day: A night spent in the hospital by a person admitted as an inpatient; also called a patient day or a hospital day.

Instrumental activities of daily living (IADLs): A person's ability to perform household and social tasks, such as home maintenance, cooking, shopping, and managing money. *See* **activities of daily living (ADLs)**.

Insured: The individual who is covered for risk by insurance.

Integrated care: Care that embodies the concepts of comprehensive, coordinated, and continuous services that provide a seamless process of care.

Integrated delivery system (IDS): A network of organizations that provides or arranges to provide a coordinated continuum of services to a defined population and is willing to be held clinically and fiscally accountable for the outcomes and health status of the population serviced.

Interoperability: The ability to share and access patient information by various users.

Item-based pricing: The costs of ancillary services that often accompany major procedures such as surgery.

Joint venture: Creation of a new organization in which two or more institutions share resources to pursue a common purpose.

License: Permission granted by the state for an organization to legally operate.

Long-term care: A variety of individualized, well-coordinated services that are designed to promote the maximum possible independence for people with functional limitations. These services are provided over an extended period to meet the patients' physical, mental, social, and spiritual needs, while maximizing quality of life.

Maintenance rehabilitation: Care that aims to preserve the present le-vel of function and prevent further decline.

Managed care: A system of health care delivery that (1) seeks to achieve efficiencies by integrating the four functions of health care delivery, (2) employs mechanisms to control (manage) utilization of medical services, and (3) determines how much the providers get paid.

Market justice: A distributional principle according to which health care is most equitably distributed through the market forces of supply and demand rather than government interventions. *See* **social justice**.

Meaningful use: Specific criteria in quality, safety, efficiency, and other areas that providers are required to meet to comply with the Health Information Technology for Economic and Clinical Health Act (HITECH) of 2009.

Means-tested program: A program in which eligibility depends on income.

Mediating factors: Forces or conditions that moderate the effects of an intervention being studied, either positively or negatively.

Medicaid: A joint federal–state program of health insurance for the poor.

Medical center: A hospital with a high level of specialization and a wide scope of services.

Medical home: Primary care delivery based on a partnership between the patient and the provider with a focus on chronic care.

Medical loss ratio: The percentage of premium revenue spent on medical expenses.

Medical model: Delivery of health care that places its primary emphasis on the treatment of disease and relief of symptoms instead of prevention of disease and promotion of optimal health.

Medical practice guidelines: *See* **clinical practice guidelines**.

Medical system: Large organizations that may include more than one hospital to serve a large geographical area.

Medical technology: Practical application of the scientific body of knowledge for the purpose of improving health and creating efficiencies in the delivery of health care.

Medicare: A federal program of health insurance for the elderly, certain disabled individuals, and people with end-stage renal disease.

Medigap: Commercial health insurance policies purchased by individuals covered by Medicare to insure the expenses not covered by Medicare.

Member: An enrollee in a private health insurance plan.

Merger: Unification of two or more organizations into a single entity through mutual agreement.

Molecular medicine: A branch of medicine that deals with the understanding of the role that genes play in disease processes and treatment of diseases through gene therapy.

Moral hazard: Consumer behavior that leads to a higher utilization of health care services solely because people are covered by insurance.

Nanomedicine: A developing area of medicine in which materials are manipulated on the atomic and molecular level (one nanometer is one-billionth of a meter).

Need: The necessity for health services (in contrast to demand for health services), based on the individual judgment of the patient or a health care professional.

Need attributes: Within the access to care framework, factors that reflect the health status of the individual, either from a self-perceived perspective or from professional assessment.

New morbidities: Dysfunctions, such as drug and alcohol abuse, family and neighborhood violence, emotional disorders, and learning problems, from which older generations often do not suffer.

Nonmaleficence: The moral obligation of health services personnel not to harm the patients. This principle requires physicians to use their best professional judgment in choosing interventions that maximize the potential health benefits at minimum risk.

Nonphysician practitioners (NPPs): Clinical professionals, such as nurse practitioners and physician assistants, who practice in many areas similar to those in which physicians practice but who do not have an MD or a DO degree.

Occupancy rate: The percentage of a hospital's total inpatient capacity that is actually utilized.

Organized medicine: Concerted activities of physicians, mainly to protect their own interests, through such associations as the American Medical Association.

Orphan drugs: Certain new drug therapies for conditions that affect fewer than 200,000 people in the United States.

Osteopathic medicine: A medical philosophy based on the holistic approach to treatment that also emphasizes correction of the position of the joints or tissues and diet and environment as factors that might destroy natural resistance. *See* **allopathic medicine**.

Outcome: The end result of health care delivery; often viewed as the bottom-line measure of the effectiveness of the health care delivery system.

Outpatient: A person who receives health care services without being admitted to a hospital; the opposite of inpatient. *See* **ambulatory**.

Outpatient services: Any health care services that are not provided based on an overnight stay in which room and board costs are incurred. *See* **ambulatory care**.

Overutilization (overuse): Utilization of medical services, the cost of which exceeds the benefit to consumers or the risks of which outweigh the potential benefits.

Package pricing: Bundling of fees for an entire package of related services.

Palliation: Care intended to relieve or alleviate symptoms, such as pharmacologic pain management and nausea relief.

Palliative care: Pain and symptom management; it is a primary area of emphasis in hospice care.

Part A: The component of Medicare that mainly covers hospital care and limited nursing home care.

Part B: The component of Medicare in which government-subsidized voluntary insurance covers physician services and outpatient services.

Patient days: The cumulative census over a given period of time. *See* **days of care** and **inpatient day**.

Payer-driven competition: Competitive strategy used by employers that shop for the best value in terms of the cost of premiums and the benefits package (competition among insurers), and by managed care organizations that shop for the best value from providers of health services (competition among providers).

Peer review: The general process of medical review of utilization and quality when it is carried out directly or under the supervision of physicians.

Per diem: A type of reimbursement that pays a flat rate for each day of inpatient stay.

Personalized medicine: Matching of gene variations with responses to particular medications so as to increase effectiveness and reduce unwanted side effects.

Pesthouse: An institution that existed in preindustrial America to quarantine people with contagious diseases such as cholera, smallpox, or typhoid.

Pharmaceutical care: A mode of pharmacy practice in which the pharmacist not only dispenses drugs but also informs patients on the proper use of drugs and their potential misuse. When asked, the pharmacist also assists prescribers in making appropriate drug choices.

Pharmacogenomics: The study of how genes affect a person's response to drugs.

Physician–hospital organization (PHO): A legal entity formed between a hospital and a physician group to achieve shared market objectives and other mutual interests.

Planned rationing: *See* **supply-side rationing**.

Poorhouse: *See* **almshouse**.

Postindustrial era: Phase of the medical delivery system that began in the late 19th century. The medical profession grew as a result of urbanization, new scientific discoveries, and reforms in medical education.

Precertification: Requirement by some insurance plans that the enrollee or the provider call the plan administrators for approval before certain services are provided.

Preindustrial era: Phase of the medical delivery system from the middle part of the 18th century until the latter part of the 19th century. Health care was not grounded in science and was delivered in a free market.

Premium: The insurer's charge for insurance coverage; the price for an insurance plan.

Process: The specific way in which care is provided. Examples of process include correct diagnostic tests, correct prescriptions, accurate drug administration, pharmaceutical care, waiting time to see a physician, and interpersonal aspects of care delivery.

Proprietary hospital: A for-profit hospital owned by individuals, a partnership, or a corporation; also referred to as an investor-owned hospital.

Prospective reimbursement: A method of payment in which certain preestablished criteria are used to determine in advance the amount of reimbursement.

Provider-induced demand: Artificial creation of demand by providers that enables them to deliver unneeded services to boost their incomes.

Public health: A wide variety of activities undertaken by state and local governments to ensure conditions that promote optimal health for society as a whole.

Public health system: A system whose mission is to improve and protect community health.

Public hospital: A hospital owned by the federal, state, or local government.

Public policies: Authoritative decisions made in the legislative, executive, or judicial branches of government that are intended to direct or influence the actions, behaviors, or decisions of others.

Quality: The degree to which health services for individuals and populations increase the likelihood of desired health outcomes and are consistent with current professional knowledge.

Quality of life: (1) Factors considered important by patients, such as environmental comfort, security, interpersonal relations, personal preferences, and autonomy in making decisions when institutionalized. (2) Overall satisfaction with life during and following a person's encounter with the health care delivery system.

Quality-of-life indicators: Measures that demonstrate the general well-being of individuals and societies.

Redistributive policies: Policies that take money or power from one group and give it to another. An example is the Medicaid program, which takes tax revenue and spends it on the poor in the form of health insurance.

Regenerative medicine: Regeneration of damaged tissues and organs in vivo through techniques that stimulate previously irreparable organs into healing themselves. It can also be done in vitro and the tissue or organ implanted when the body cannot be prompted to heal itself.

Regulatory tools: Health policies in which the government prescribes and controls the behavior of a particular target group by monitoring the group and imposing sanctions if it fails to comply.

Reimbursement: The amount insurers pay to a provider. The payment may only be a portion of the actual charge.

Reinsurance: Stop-loss coverage that self-insured employers purchase to protect themselves against any potential risk of high losses.

Residency: Graduate medical education in a specialty that takes the form of paid on-the-job training, usually in a hospital.

Resource-based relative value scale (RBRVS): A payment method instituted by Medicare for determining physicians' fees. Each treatment or encounter by the physician is assigned a relative value based on the time, skill, and training required to treat the condition.

Respite care: A service that provides temporary relief to informal caregivers, such as family members.

Restorative care: Short-term therapy treatments to help a person regain or improve physical function.

Retail clinic: A type of proprietary, community-based, freestanding medical facility found across the country in retail establishments such as Walmart, Walgreens, and CVS pharmacies.

Retrospective reimbursement: Reimbursement rates based on costs actually incurred.

Risk: The possibility of a substantial financial loss from an event of which the probability of occurrence is relatively small.

Risk management: Limiting risks against lawsuits or unexpected events.

Rural hospital: A hospital located in a county that is not part of a metropolitan statistical area.

Safety: Protection against unnecessary harm from the use of technology.

Secondary care: Routine hospitalization, routine surgery, and specialized outpatient care, such as consultation with specialists and rehabilitation.

Self-insurance: Health insurance provided by large employers that can afford to assume the risk by budgeting funds to pay medical claims incurred by their employees.

Senior centers: Local community centers for older adults that provide opportunities to congregate and social-ize, and in some cases have a midday meal.

Single-payer system: A national health care program in which the financing and insurance functions are taken over by the federal government.

Skilled nursing care: Medically oriented long-term care provided mainly by a licensed nurse under the overall direction of a physician.

Small-area variations: Unexplained variations in the treatment patterns for similar patients and medical conditions.

Social justice: A distribution principle according to which health care is most equitably distributed by a government-run national health care program. *See* **market justice**.

Socialism: A political and economic system that advocates collective or governmental ownership and administration of the means of production and distribution of goods; contrast with capitalism, where private and market forces dominate.

Socialized medicine: Any large-scale government-sponsored expansion of health insurance or intrusion in the private practice of medicine.

Socioeconomic status: A measure of one's social position in relation to others, typically based on income, education, and occupation.

Special populations: Persons with health needs but with inadequate resources to address those needs.

Specialist: A physician who specializes in specific health care problems—for example, anesthesiologists, cardiologists, and oncologists. *See* **generalist**.

Specialty hospital: A hospital that admits only certain types of patients or those patients with specified illnesses or conditions. Examples include rehabilitation hospitals, tuberculosis hospitals, children's hospitals, cardiac hospitals, and orthopedic hospitals.

Stop-loss: An insurance provision in which an insured has a maximum out-of-pocket liability in a given year.

Structure: "The relatively stable characteristics of the providers of care, of the tools and resources they have at their disposal, and of the physical and organizational settings in which they work" (Donabedian, 1980, p. 81).

Subacute care: Clinically complex services that are beyond traditional skilled nursing care.

Subacute condition: A technically complex condition that requires services beyond traditional skilled nursing care.

Supply-side rationing: Also called planned rationing; rationing that is generally carried out by a government to limit the availability of health care services, particularly expensive technology.

Supply-side regulation: The antitrust laws passed in the United States, which prohibit business practices that stifle competition among providers, such as price fixing, price discrimination, exclusive contracting arrangements, and mergers deemed anticompetitive by the Department of Justice.

Surgicenter: A freestanding, ambulatory surgery center that performs various types of surgical procedures on an outpatient basis.

Teaching hospital: A hospital with an approved residency program for physicians.

Technological imperative: Use of technology without cost considerations, especially when the benefits to be derived from the use of technology are small compared to the costs.

Technology assessment: *See* **health technology assessment**.

Technology diffusion: The proliferation of technology once it is developed.

Telemedicine: Use of telecommunications technology that enables physicians to conduct two-way, interactive video consultations or transmit digital images, such as x-rays and magnetic resonance imaging results, to other sites.

Tertiary care: The most complex level of care, which is typically institution based, highly specialized, and highly technological. Examples include burn treatment, transplantation, and coronary artery bypass surgery.

Third-party payers: In a multipayer system, the payers for covered services—for example, insurance companies, managed care organizations, and the government. They are called third parties because they are neither the providers nor the recipients of medical services.

Title 18: The Medicare program; more precisely known as Title XVIII (18) of the Social Security Amendment of 1965.

Title 19: The Medicaid program; more precisely known as Title XIX (19) of the Social Security Amendment of 1965.

TriCare: An insurance program financed by the U.S. Department of Defense in which beneficiaries can receive care from both private and military medical care facilities.

Underutilization: Withholding of medically needed health care services, especially when potential benefits are likely to exceed the cost or risks.

Underwriting: A systematic technique used by an insurer for evaluating, selecting (or rejecting), classifying, and rating risks.

Universal access: The ability of all citizens to obtain health care when needed. It is a misnomer because timely access to certain services may still be a problem because of supply-side rationing.

Universal coverage: Health insurance coverage for all citizens.

Urgent care center: A walk-in clinic generally open to see patients after normal business hours in the evenings and weekends, which does not require patients to make an appointment.

Usual source of care: A single provider or place where patients obtain, or can obtain, the majority of their health care.

Utilization control: Limiting utilization of medical services to only those deemed appropriate and necessary.

Utilization review: A process by which an insurer reviews decisions by physicians and other providers on how much care to provide.

Value: Greater benefits or higher quality at the same or lower price levels (costs).

Vertical integration: Linking of services that are at different stages in the production process of health care—for example, a hospital system that launches hospice, long-term care, or ambulatory care services. *See* **horizontal integration**.

Veterans Integrated Service Networks (VISNs): Components of the Veterans Administration system. There are 21 geographically distributed networks that are responsible for coordinating the activities of the hospitals and other facilities located within its jurisdiction.

Virtual integration: The formation of networks based on contractual arrangements.

Virtual organization: A new organization that is formed by contractual arrangements between two or more organizations; an organization without walls.

Virtual visits: Online consultations between physicians and patients.

Voluntary health insurance: Private health insurance (in contrast to government-sponsored compulsory health insurance).

Voluntary hospital: A nonprofit hospital.

Vulnerability: Susceptibility to negative events that result in poor health or illness. Poor health can be manifested physically, psychologically, and socially.

Walk-in clinic: A freestanding, ambulatory clinic in which patients are seen without appointments on a first-come, first-served basis.

Xenotransplantation: Also called xenografting; transplanting of animal tissue into humans.

References

Donabedian A. 1980. *Explorations in quality assessment and monitoring: The definition of quality and approaches to its assessment.* Vol. 1. Ann Arbor, MI: Health Administration Press.

World Health Organization. 1948. *Preamble to the Constitution.* Geneva, Switzerland: World Health Organization.

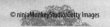© ninjaMonkeyStudio/Getty Images

Index

Note: Page numbers followed by *e*, *f*, or *t* indicate materials in exhibit, figures, or tables respectively.

A

AARP. *See* American Association of Retired Persons
ACA. *See* Affordable Care Act
academic medical center (AMC), 197
access, health care, 31
    community health centers, 176
    data on, 286–287, 289
    defining, 11–12, 286
    determinants of, 31, 287*f*
    disparities, 289–290
    elderly persons and, 321
    geographical disparities in, 119
    geographical distribution in, 259 260
    HIV/AIDS, persons with, 266
    homeless persons and, 262–263
    hospitals and, 188
    initiatives to address, 290–291
    managed care and, 219–220
    mental health and, 263–264
    primary care and, 11–12, 157*e*
    public financing and, 321
    racial/ethnic minorities and, 254–257, 254–255*e*, 290
    socioeconomic status and, 290
    surveys on, 287
    unequal in, 286–291
    uninsured persons and, 11, 16
    universal access, 23, 316
accountability
    patients and providers, 110
    primary care and, 166–167
    provider and patient, 15–16, 156
accountable care organizations (ACOs), 6, 148, 221–222, 345
ACP. *See* American College of Physicians
acquisitions and mergers, 234
Action for Mental Health, 326
Action Plan to Reduce Racial and Ethnic Health Disparities, 267

activities of daily living (ADLs), 233, 234*e*, 263
acute care
    long-term care versus, 232, 233
    Medicare benefits and, 139, 140
    technology and, 10–11
acute conditions, 29, 160, 189
ADA. *See* Americans with Disabilities Act
adaptive devices, 234
adaptive rehabilitation, 246
ADC. *See* adult day care
ADLs. *See* activities of daily living
Administration of Children and Families Head Start Program, 257*e*
administrative costs, 282
administrative information systems, 104
ADN. *See* associate's degree
adolescent females, 258
adult day care (ADC), 161, 238
adult foster care, 238
advance directives, 201
advanced medical home, 171–172
advanced-practice nurses (APNs), 89
AF4Q program. *See* Aligning Forces for Quality program
AFDC program. *See* Aid to Families with Dependent Children program
Affordable Care Act (ACA), 1, 51, 77, 115, 126, 194, 247, 261, 267, 294, 307, 312, 334, 338
    accountable care organizations and, 222
    and community health centers, 177
    expansion of Medicaid under, 135–136, 312
    health insurance exchanges and, 312
    lifetime limits and, 131
    looming shortages and, 81–83
    managed care organizations, 206
    and payment reform, 148
    political opportunism and, 50
    political will, ideologies, and legal rulings, 336

and private insurance, 135–136
quality indicators and, 208
social, demographic, and cultural trends, 334–335
uninsured under, 143, 261–262
wellness exam and, 139
age-related progression of long-term care intensity, 234e
Agency for Healthcare Research and Quality (AHRQ), 115, 256, 295, 325
AHA. *See* American Hospital Association
AHCA. *See* American Health Care Act
AHRQ. *See* Agency for Healthcare Research and Quality
Aid to Families with Dependent Children (AFDC) program, 312
AIDS. *See* HIV/AIDS
Alaska Natives, 254, 255e
Aligning Forces for Quality (AF4Q) program, 296
alliances, 12, 224–225, 315
allied health professionals, 91–93
allocative tool, health policy as, 309–310
allopathic medicine, 78–79, 198
almshouses, 55, 183–184
ALOS. *See* average length of stay
alternative medicine clinics, 162
AMA. *See* American Medical Association
ambulatory care, 155. *See also* outpatient services
clinics, 81, 81t
ambulatory payment classifications (APCs), 146–147
AMC. *See* academic medical center
American Association of Homes and Services for the Aging, 313–314
American Association of Retired Persons (AARP), 313
American Board of Examiners, 87
American Board of Opticianry, 93
American Cancer Society, 323
American College of Physicians (ACP), 171
American Dental Association, 84
American Health Care Act (AHCA), 329, 340
American Health Care Association, 313
American health care system, 308
American Heart Association, 323
American Hospital Association (AHA), 62, 182, 197, 289, 313
American Indians, 254, 255e
American Legacy Foundation, 323
American Lung Association, 323
American Medical Association (AMA), 58–59, 313
accountable care organizations and, 221–223

consolidation power of, 58
insurance industry and, 62
medical education and, 59–60, 197
opposition on national health care, 64
Physician Masterfile, 289
teaching hospitals and, 197
American Osteopathic Association (AOA), 198
American Physical Therapy Association, 93
American Speech–Language–Hearing Association, 93
Americans for Nonsmokers' Rights, 323
Americans with Disabilities Act (ADA), 327
anesthesia, discovery of, 184
Annual Survey of Hospitals (AHA), 289
antisepsis, discovery of, 184
antitrust laws, 285
anxiety disorders, 258
AOA. *See* American Osteopathic Association
APCs. *See* ambulatory payment classifications
APNs. *See* advanced-practice nurses
Area Agencies on Aging, 237
Asian Americans, 255e
assessment, technology, 120–122
assistants, medical, 92
assisted living facilities, 242
associate's degree (ADN), 88
asylums, 55
asymptomatic disease, 29
audiologists, 93
average daily census, hospital, 190, 190t
average length of stay (ALOS), 189

B

bachelor of science in nursing (BSN) degree, 88
balance bill, 143
Balanced Budget Act (1997), 140, 141, 197, 211
Baylor University Hospital, 62, 208
Beers, Clifford Whittingham, 325–326
behavioral determinants of health, 31
behavioral health carve-outs, 220
Behavioral Health IT Act, 328
behavioral health programs, 328
Behavioral Risk Factor Surveillance System (BRFSS), 270
behavioral science, 46
beneficence, 200
beneficiary, insurance, 130
benefit period, 138
Bill of the First Act to Strengthen Long-Term Care, 18
bioethics, impact on, 120

N